AIDS AND WOMEN'S REPRODUCTIVE HEALTH

REPRODUCTIVE BIOLOGY

Series Editor: Sheldon J. Segal
The Population Council
New York, New York

A Continuation Order Plan is available for this series. A continuation order will bring delivery of each new volume immediately upon publication. Volumes are billed only upon actual shipment. For further information please contact the publisher.

AIDS AND WOMEN'S REPRODUCTIVE HEALTH

Edited by
Lincoln C. Chen
Harvard School of Public Health
Boston, Massachusetts

Jaime Sepulveda Amor
Ministry of Public Health
Government of Mexico
Mexico City, Mexico

and
Sheldon J. Segal
The Population Council
New York, New York

Technical Editor:
Judith Masslo Anderson

PLENUM PRESS • NEW YORK AND LONDON

Library of Congress Cataloging-in-Publication Data

AIDS and women's reproductive health / edited by Lincoln C. Chen,
  Jaime Sepúlveda Amor, and Sheldon J. Segal ; technical editor,
  Judith Masslo Anderson.
      p.   cm. -- (Reproductive biology)
   Include bibliographical references and index.
   ISBN 0-306-44200-0
   1. AIDS (Disease) 2. Women--Diseases. 3. Women--Health and
  hygiene. 4. AIDS (Disease) in pregnancy.   I. Chen, Lincoln C.
  II. Sepúlveda Amor, Jaime. III. Segal, Sheldon J. (Sheldon Jerome)
  IV. Series.
   [DNLM: 1. Acquired Immunodeficiency Syndrome--transmission-
  -congresses. 2. Pregnancy Complications, Infectious--prevention &
  control--congresses. 3. Reproduction--congresses. 4. Risk Factors-
  -congresses. 5. Women's Health--congresses.   WD 308 A28791]
  RA644.A25A3543 1991
  616.97'92--dc20
  DNLM/DLC
  for Library of Congress   92-14052
                                                                 CIP

Proceedings of an international workshop on AIDS and Reproductive Biology,
held October 29–November 2, 1990, in Bellagio, Italy

ISBN 0-306-44200-0

© 1991 Plenum Press, New York
A Division of Plenum Publishing Corporation
233 Spring Street, New York, N.Y. 10013

PREFACE

Over the past decade, the AIDS pandemic has propagated so widely and exerted such a devastating impact that one may properly ask the question, Why not concentrate all AIDS efforts on disease control alone? Why link AIDS with women's reproductive health? What is the scientific basis for this linkage? And how might AIDS control and women's health objectives be promoted simultaneously? These questions constitute the principal themes addressed in this monograph. The 15 chapters in this volume are intended to provide state-of-the-art reviews of key interactions between AIDS and women's reproductive health for an audience of scientists and policy makers in the AIDS and population fields.

Impetus for this monograph comes in part from what we perceive to be an inadequate global response, thus far, to AIDS and women's health problems. A common platform has failed to emerge among the disparate professional communities working in the areas of AIDS, STDs, and family planning. As a result, endeavors in these fields have been isolated, and opportunities for joint action have been missed. An enormous and, as yet, unharnessed potential exists for powerful interdisciplinary collaborations that could strengthen policies and programs against these pressing health problems of humankind.

The chapters in this monograph are based on background papers contributed to an international workshop, "AIDS and Reproductive Health," held at the Bellagio Conference Center in Bellagio, Italy on October 29-November 2, 1990. The workshop was jointly organized by the AIDS and Reproductive Health Network (ARHN), the Harvard School of Public Health, and the Rockefeller Foundation. Begun in 1988, the ARHN consists of scientists and policy makers from around the world who have joined together for research, information exchange, the sharing of experiences, and the strengthening of mutual capacities. Through joint action consisting of collaborative research, problem-oriented task forces, newsletters, and semi-annual meetings, ARHN members seek to broaden the scientific basis of solutions to the interactive problems of AIDS and women's health.

This monograph begins with an introductory chapter reviewing the global scope and regional distribution of AIDS and women's health problems. This overview provides a conceptual framework for examining the linkages between AIDS and reproductive health, highlighting interactions of scientific and practical signficance. Section I, "Epidemiology and Policy," includes three chapters that bring a women's perspective to AIDS and reproductive health epidemiology and policy. Section II, " Risk Factors in Transmission," consists of six chapters that address the potential roles of sexually transmitted diseases (STDs), contraception, and sexual behavior in facilitating or interrupting HIV-1 transmission. Section III, "Perinatal Transmission," shifts the focus to the biology of mother-to-child transmission and decision-making alternatives for reducing perinatal transmission. Section IV, "Interventions," contains three chapters that explore the poorly understood domain of human sexuality and report on recent efforts to modify behavior linked to sexual transmission HIV-1 in high-risk population subgroups, expecially commercial sex workers and their clinents. The concluding chapter regarging research recommendation, organizes the recommendations of AIDS and reproductive health workshop participants, around four themes: women's empowerment and reproductive right; epidemiolol and transmission; sexual behavior; and policy and program interventions.

The 15 chapters in this volume reflect a range of perspectives on, and approaches to, research, policy, and health care issues related to AIDS and women's reproductive health. The contributors to the volume do not share identical views and positions on all issues; as such, the monograph points to the conceptual and methodological diversity that marks the AIDS and women's reproductive health fields in general. The cooperation of the contributors in preparing this monograph reflects their overarching commitment to an open, interdisciplinary exchange of views and information within the AIDs and women's reproductive health fields with the aim of shaping and supporting effective measures to combat the AIDS pandemic.

Critical to the success of this publication has been the commitment and hard work of the members of the ARHN. From its modest beginnings, the ARHN has grown and matured, due in large measure to the active participation of its members and the able leadership of the ARHN Steering Committee, which currently consists of Mukesh Kapila (United Kingdom and India), Jonathan Mann (United States), Japheth Mati (Kenya), Jaime Sepulveda (Mexico), and Debrework Zewdie (Ethiopia). The ARHN and the editors of this volume owe a special debt to Barbara de Zalduondo and David Hunter, and to Paula Johnson, Joan Kaufman, and Julie Rioux at the Harvard School of Public Health, who provided the bulk of administrative services for the ARHN.

The establishment of the ARHN and the execution of this monograph would not have been possible without the generous financial support of the ARHN's sponsors: The John Merck Fund, The Rockefeller Foundation, The Ford Foundation, and The International Development Research Centre of Canada. Special thanks are due to Frank Hatch and Ruth Hennig of The John Merck Fund. Frank Hatch had the vision to provide the flexible venture capital that launched the ARHN. Thanks also are due to Seth Berkley and Katherine LaGuardia of The Rockefeller Foundation; Richard Horowitz and Stuart Burden, formerly of the Ford Foundation; and Richard Wilson (then), Larry Gelman and Pat Trites of The International Development Research Centre of Canada; and Richard Wilson, formerly of The International Development Research Centre of Canada.

Finally, we acknowledge with deep appreciation the technical editor of this volume, Judith Masslo Anderson, as well as Jean Joseph, Colleen Murphy, Chris Cahill, and Vanessa Bingham, who provided backup support in bringing the workshop papers into publication quality and format. The shortcomings of the monograph are, of course, the sole responsibility of the editors.

Lincoln C. Chen
Jaime Supulveda Amor
Sheldon Segal

July 1, 1991

CONTENTS

PERINATAL TRANSMISSION

INTERVENTIONS

INTRODUCTION

AN OVERVIEW OF AIDS AND WOMEN'S HEALTH

Lincoln C. Chen

Harvard School of Public Health

Jaime Supulveda Amor

Ministry of Public Health, Government of Mexico

Sheldon J. Segal

The Population Council

In the brief span of a decade, the AIDS pandemic has spread to virtually all corners of the world. While data are imprecise at best, especially those related to HIV-1 prevalence, an illuminating global picture has nevertheless emerged (Table 1). Of a total world population of approximately five billion in 1990, about eight million adults are estimated to be HIV-1-infected, according to the Global Programme on AIDS of the World Health Organization (WHO) (1). Approximately 0.3% of the world's adults are HIV-1-infected. Between developing and industrialized countries, the distribution of total population and HIV-1-infected adults is approximately symmetrical. Developing countries, with about 76% of the world's population, are estimated to contain about 81% of the world's HIV-1 infections. Industrialized countries, with 24% of the world's population, contain about 19% of HIV-1-infections.

When this comparison is further disaggregated, however, marked regional imbalances become evident. Whereas Africa has only 11% of the world's population, it contains nearly two-thirds of the HIV-1 adult cases. Two other regions also contain disproportionately high shares of HIV-1 cases: North America and Latin America. In contrast, Asia, with 58% of the world's population, has only 6% of HIV-1 cases. The predominance of HIV-1 infections in Africa is dramatically confirmed by the estimated rate of 1,625 infections per 100,000 adults in Africa. This infection level is nearly three times higher than the corresponding levels in North America and Latin America. Seropositive prevalence in Africa is nearly 50 times higher than in Asia.

The potential for perinatal transmission of HIV-1 is also shown in Table 1, which demarcates the global distribution of births. Of the world's 131 million annual births, 86% occur in developing countries. African countries have 19% (25.5 million) of the world's annual births; Asian countries have 58%. Birth rates inversely reflect contraceptive use patterns, also shown in Table 1. Contraceptive use is greatest in industrialized countries; it is also increasing rapidly in Asia and Latin America. Africa, which has the lowest levels of contraceptive use, also has the highest fertility levels in the world.

Table 1. World regions according to 1990 population (millions), crude rates of births and deaths (per 1,000), contraceptive prevalence (percent), and HIV-1 infections among adults (number in thousands and rate per 100,000 population)

Continent	Popn[a]	Crude rates[b] Birth	Death	Contraceptive Prevalence[c]	HIV Infections[d] No.	Rate
World	5,272	25.7	9.3	45	8,040	152
Developed	1,210	13.8	9.6	68	1,510	125
Developing	4,062	29.2	9.2	38	6,530	161
Africa	653	42.6	12.9	3–40	5,030	770
Asia	3,085	26.0	8.7	15–65	500	16
Latin Am.	442	26.4	6.8	25–60	1,000	226
N. America	279	13.6	8.8	65	1,000	358
Europe	787	14.1	10.2	60–65	480	61
Oceania	26	19.0	8.3	–	30	115

References:

(a) and (b) Zachariah, KC and Vu, MT. World Population Projections 1987–88 Edition, Short-and Long-Term Estimates, World Bank, Washington, D.C., 1988.

(c) Mauldin, WP and SJ Segal, "Prevalence of Contraceptive Use: Trends and Issues," Studies in Family Planning 19(6):335–353, 1988.

(d) Global Program on AIDS, World Health Organization, 1990.

Note: The time period of demographics and HIV-1 data do not correspond precisely, but this mismatch does not materially affect the basic results presented.

Regional patterns of HIV-1 infection, births, and contraceptive use reflect only the current situation, of course. Furthermore, they are crude averages that undoubtedly disguise marked variability in the intensity of infection between countries and population subgroups (e.g., urban/rural, rich/poor, occupational and risk groups). No group in any region of the world is immune to the threat of AIDS nor free of reproductive health problems. Nor do current statistics forecast future trends. There is appropriate concern for the many countries with high levels of HIV-1 seropositivity and persistent, serious reproductive health problems. But in many countries with low prevalence of HIV-1 seropositivity, the potential for future transmission may be great. Of special concern are certain Latin American countries and Asian countries such as Thailand, India, and the

Philippines, all of which possess large vulnerable populations. In some of these countries, high-risk population subgroups have already been severely affected by AIDS, and transmission into the general population has recently accelerated.

AIDS AND WOMEN'S REPRODUCTIVE HEALTH

Women's reproductive health, as a field, encompasses a set of health problems associated with human reproduction. Reproductive processes are marked by major biologic events, but they involve broader social issues, including human sexuality, health behavior, the health of mothers and children, and the underlying cultural, economic, and political determinants of these process-es. Table 2 presents a framework for considering major reproductive life cycle events in relation to AIDS transmission. The reproductive life cycle is marked sequentially by key events: concep-tion, pregnancy, birth, child growth and development, adolescence, and adult sexuality. These are the fundamental landmarks of life, and their passage can entail substantial health risks. Com-monly recognized reproductive health risks are: infertility, maternal malnutrition and anemia, faulty birth practices, childhood malnutrition and infections, and the health consequences of ado-lescent and adult sexuality. HIV-1 transmission is linked to these reproductive processes because the two predominant modes of HIV-1 transmission – sexual and perinatal transmission – are inex-tricably tied to human reproduction.

The intersection between AIDS and women's reproductive health points to the potential syn-

Table 2. Estimated number of contraceptive users (million) by method, around 1985.

Method	Total	Developed Countries	Developing Countries			
			Total	Africa	Americas	Asia
Sterilization	155	19	135	1	11	123
Female	(108)	(13)	(95)	(1)	(11)	(84)
Male	(47)	(7)	(40)	(0)	(0)	(40)
Hormonal	61	20	40	5	10	26
Pill	(55)	(20)	(35)	(4)	(9)	(22)
Injectables	(6)	(0)	(6)	(1)	(1)	(4)
IUD	80	8	72	1	4	67
Condom	38	20	18	0	1	16
Vaginal	6	4	2	0	0	2
Traditional	21	15	6	0	2	4
TOTAL	398	100	297	10	32	256

Source: Mauldin, W.P. and Segal, S.J. "Prevalence of Contraceptive Use: Trends and Issues," Studies in Family Planning 19:335-353, 1988.

ergy between policy and program interventions aimed at these two health issues. As no vaccine is currently available to prevent AIDS, and as treatment to prolong the life of the infected is extraordinarily expensive, the most important currently available tool for AIDS control is the changing of reproductive behavior. Reducing the number of sexual partners, safer and less traumatic sexual practices, and the use of condoms are among the most important means of reducing HIV-1 sexual transmission. These direct approaches are complemented by other public health efforts, such as the control of sexually transmitted diseases (STDs), which may facilitate sexual transmission of HIV-1, and the promotion of birth control among seropositive mothers to prevent perinatal transmission. Other reproductive health interventions include safe obstetrical practices during delivery, abortion services, and sound counseling regarding contraception and breast-feeding.

Efforts to control AIDS can also contribute directly to reproductive health goals. In some countries, mortality from AIDS among adults and newborns has already reached significant levels. Population projections suggest that AIDS may have a powerful impact on the demographic future of severely affected societies. Beyond this, the impact of AIDS may, over time, influence reproductive decision-making, shaping future fertility performance. In many societies, it is difficult to visualize progress in reproductive health without a major concomitant effort in AIDS control.

It has been argued that the fight against AIDS and reproductive health problems would be strengthened by adopting a women's perspective, as women are the primary clients and providers of health services, and women's health is a central concern of family planning, STD, and AIDS service delivery systems. Women are not only victims with respect to AIDS and reproductive health, they also serve as advocates, caretakers, and disease preventers. Moreover, women's social status, education, and employment influence reproductive behavior. Gender relations are central to decision-making regarding human sexuality, and determine, in part, women's power to influence partner relations, sexual practices, and compliance in the practice of safe sex and condom use. The feminist focus on poor and disenfranchised women, who are often at higher risk for AIDS and reproductive health problems, is a critical perspective on effective policies and programs.

AIDS AND REPRODUCTIVE HEALTH: KEY INTERACTIONS

Harnessing the synergy between AIDS and women's reproductive health is a great challenge for the AIDS, STD, and reproductive health communities. Scientifically, the challenge involves not only the biological and epidemiological sciences, but also the social and behavioral sciences. Demography, reproductive biology, STD and family planning policy and management all have much to offer those working to advance our understanding of AIDS and AIDS control. Conversely, AIDS control programs can greatly strengthen reproductive health programs. Because AIDS and women's reproductive health intersect in so many ways, it would be useful to identify critical areas of interaction that deserve scientific priority. While the selection of these areas is to some degree arbitrary, four areas are indisputably critical: 1) STDs; 2) contraception; 3) perinatal transmission; and 4) human sexuality and health behavior.

Sexually Transmitted Diseases

From a public health perspective, STDs are the most important reportable diseases in the world. The WHO estimates that each year there are over 100 million bacterial, viral, and trichomonas infections around the world. Infertility, one of many sequelae of STDs, affects approximately 80 million couples. The regional and national prevalences of STDs are unknown, but the intensity of STDs is severe among many populations, especially in Africa. STDs deserve high priority, not only because of their own health significance, but also because of their presumed role in facilitating HIV-1 transmission.

Four of the six chapters in Section II of this book address the linkages between STDs and HIV-1 transmission. Their aim is to review the causal linkages between STDs and HIV-1 transmission. Chapters by Plummer et al. (chapter 4), Wasserheit (chapter 5), and Zewdie and Tafari (chapter 7) employ epidemiologic approaches to dissect out the complex relationships between STDs and HIV-1 transmission. Although the direction of causality can be bi-directional (i.e., AIDS may also exacerbate STDs), currently available evidence strongly supports the facilitating role of STDs in HIV-1 transmission. The data are particularly strong with regard to those STDs that disrupt the integrity of the epithelium of the reproductive track, thereby facilitating the entry of the virus into the body. Along with STDs, lack of circumcision appears to be another co-factor in HIV-1 transmission (see chapter 4).

The causal relationship between STDs and HIV-1 transmission is believed to be sufficiently powerful to rank STD control as a major instrument of AIDS control programs. Chapter 6 by Berkley examines the quantity of HIV-1 transmission attributable to STDs. The importance of STDs and other co-factors in controlling AIDS relates to their prevalence in the population. Although STD control would probably dampen HIV-1 transmission, the policy and program interventions of STD control would be essentially identical to those required for AIDS. Effective chemotherapy is available for many STDs, however, and AIDS control undoubtedly could be made more effective through drug treatment against STDs in populations with high STD prevalence.

Contraception

Contraceptive usage data by world regions are shown in Table 3. Contraceptive method usage patterns are significant not only because some methods are important tools in reducing HIV-1 transmission (e.g., condoms), but also because some methods have been reported to affect the risk of transmission (e.g., oral pills). For most contraceptive methods, however, the risks with respect to HIV-1 transmission are unknown.

Of the approximately one billion reproductive age couples in the world today, about 400 million use some form of contraception. The most commonly-used method is sterilization, accounting for 40% of contraceptive users; hormonal contraceptives are used by 15% and IUDs by 20% of contraceptive users. Fewer than 10% of contraceptive users rely on the condom, the only contraceptive method demonstrated to reduce HIV-1 transmission. Vaginal barrier methods (diaphragm, spermicides), which are of uncertain value in reducing viral transmission, have extremely low levels of use.

These data further heighten concern about Africa. Condom use is overwhelmingly concentrated in industrialized countries (53%) and Asia (43%). Contraceptive practice in Africa in general is very low, and condom use is even lower, although condom use levels may have increased in recent years. The oral pill is the most common method of contraception in Africa (40% of contraceptive users).

The promotion of contraceptive policies and programs that prevent unwanted births and protect women's and children's health is an essential public health objective. Reproductive counseling with regard to health, procreation, and human sexuality represents an important opportunity for dialogue about birth prevention and disease control. Sound contraceptive policies will depend upon knowledge of the relationships between specific methods of birth control and their roles in facilitating or inhibiting HIV-1 transmission. This is the focus of Chapter 8 by Hunter and Mati in Section II of this book, which reviews available epidemiologic evidence concerning specific contraceptive method use and HIV-1 transmission. Hunter and Mati conclude that, beyond the known protective effects of condom use, the role of other contraceptive methods in HIV-1 transmission remains uncertain.

Table 3. Major life cycle events, reproductive health and AIDS problems, and interventions.

| Life Cycle | Problems | | Reproductive/AIDS HealthIntervention |
	Reprod Health	HIV/AIDS	
Conception	Infertility	Transmission	Family planning Perinatal care
pregnancy	Malnutrition Anemia		Abortion
Birth	Birth practices Breastfeeding	Perinatal transmission	Obstetrics Breastfeeding
childhood	Infections Malnutrition	Transfusion	Child health care
adolescence			
	Sexuality STDs	Sexual transmission	Sex education STD control
adulthood			
		AIDS infection sarcoma social economic emotional	AIDS response infection control oncology counselling/care
Death			Medical care

Perinatal Transmission

With increasing HIV-1 seropositivity among adults, and an increasing number of women in the sex ratio of AIDS cases, perinatal transmission from mother-to-child is a growing problem around the world. In many countries, the number of child deaths from AIDS may soon exceed the number of child deaths from some of the major deadly childhood diseases, such as measles and diarrhea.

Chapter 10 by Meirik and Chapter 11 by Kanki et al. in Section III of this book review the biologic mechanisms postulated to be responsible for perinatal transmission of HIV-1 and HIV-2. Chapter 12 by Heymann proposes a methodology for considering alternative decision-making paths for effective counseling of HIV-1-positive mothers with the aim of reducing perinatal transmission. Heymann identifies several crucial decision-making junctures in counseling that relate to prevention of HIV-1 infection: sexual practice, birth prevention, and breast-feeding among seropositive mothers.

A special dilemma in counseling against perinatal transmission concerns the issue of breast-feeding versus alternate feeding practices (e.g., bottle-feeding, wet nursing). Some public health professionals in industrialized countries discourage seropositive mothers from breast-feeding, but in developing countries, where the health risk of breast milk substitutes may be very high, breast-feeding may be the healthiest choice. The fact that different agencies have issued different guidelines with respect to breast-feeding indicates that the issue is not yet settled.

Human Sexuality and Health Behavior

The greatest synergy between reproductive health and AIDS may be found in parallel efforts to promote healthy sexual behavior. In the past four decades, major efforts have been made in the population field to understand and change reproductive motivation. These efforts have involved knowledge, attitude, and practice (KAP) surveys as well as in-depth anthropological techniques to understand human motivation and behavior. Strong efforts have also been made in health educational interventions, involving information, education, and communication interventions. These have involved modern mass media, traditional modes of communication, and individual contact and counseling.

Despite these efforts, our understanding of human sexuality in virtually all societies is extremely modest, in part because of constraints in research methods, and in part because of sociopolitical resistance by governments to the sanction and support of research on human sexuality. New research methods and investments are desperately needed to better understand human sexuality. Studies of human sexuality can be approached from many perspectives, including identification of the actors (adolescents, men, women); type of partner arrangements (homosexuality, heterosexuality, bisexuality, celibacy); type of sexual practices (safe or hazardous vaginal, oral, anal intercourse); and the multiple purposes of sexuality (procreation, recreation, psychosocial satisfaction).

Public health information and educational efforts to change high-risk sexual behavior have expanded recently into large-scale and focused AIDS campaigns. Both the reproductive health and AIDS fields are directing substantial scientific and intervention-related resources toward changing sexual behavior. The success or failure of these efforts must be documented and evaluated, and the lessons learned disseminated. The power of the social and behavioral sciences to further our understanding of human sexual behavior should be harnessed in the effort to achieve AIDS and reproductive health programmatic goals.

Chapter 9 by Parker and Caballo in Section II of this volume examines human sexuality with particular focus on male bisexuality, which may play a role in HIV-1 transmission from high-risk groups to the general heterosexual population. Understanding human sexuality and health behavior for the purpose of designing AIDS interventions is the objective of the three chapters in Section IV of this book. Chapter 13 by Lamptey provides an overview of interventions in high-risk groups with a focus on commercial sex workers. A conceptual framework for studies of human sexuality are presented by de Zalduondo et al. in chapter 14. Chapter 15 by Hernandez et al. reports on different intervention efforts to change sexual behavior among high-risk commercial sex workers and their clients.

CONCLUSION

The proposition advanced in this book is that addressing HIV and women's reproductive health problems together may lead to mutual benefits for both fields. Indeed, the problems and solutions in these fields are inextricably linked. In this introduction, the global scale and distribution of AIDS and reproductive health problems has been examined with particular attention to the situation in African countries. A framework has been presented to specify where and how AIDS and reproductive health linkages may be approached. The scientific basis of these linkages

Table 4. Illustrative primary lines of research approaches to AIDS and women's health.

Biological
    Conception
    Contraception
    Abortion
    Maternal health and nutrition
    Child growth and development

Epidemiological
    Risk factors
    Transmission
    Behavioral epidemiology
    Intervention assessment

Behavioral
    Perceptions, attitudes, knowledge
    Sexual practices and patterns
    Human sexuality
    Gender relations
    Condom and other safe practices

Policy
    Policy technical options
    Political and economic analyses
    Ethical considerations

Program
    Design
    Mangement and implementation
    Evaluation

will be examined in the chapters of this book with an eye to determining cause-and-effect relationships, an understanding of which is necessary for the development of intervention strategies. Synergy, it has been noted, is particularly strong in four critical areas related to AIDS and reproductive health: STDs, contraception, perinatal transmission, and human sexuality and health behavior. These four areas provide the thematic structure for this volume.

Underlying these four areas of interaction between AIDS and reproductive health is the issue of women and gender relations, which lie at the heart of human sexuality. Women are both victims of disease and proactive agents for disease control. The empowerment of women, and the changing of male perceptions and actions vis-à-vis women, are required for the success of virtually all AIDS and reproductive health efforts. This issue is reflected in the process by which contraceptive decisions are made, which may directly influence contraceptive method usage patterns. It has been reported, for example, that female control could increase usage of health protecting methods, such as the condom, which is reportedly resisted by men. Decision-making regarding reproduction, human sexuality, and safe sex is a key to progress in both the AIDS and reproductive health arenas.

The future research agendas in the AIDS and reproductive health fields must incorporate a stronger social science component to complement ongoing biological research. Table 4 lists some of the research that should be considered in establishing priorities in the biological, epidemiological, behavioral, policy, and programmatic fields. These are detailed in the concluding chapter, which summarizes the research recommendations of the contributors to this monograph.

The scientific basis of interactions between AIDS and reproductive health problems is well documented and increasingly accepted. But beyond their scientific and public health dimensions, the issues of AIDS and women's reproductive health are deeply ethical and ideological. Unresolved ethical issues are confronted in addressing the issue of death control versus birth control. While death and birth prevention are not necessarily in conflict, their roots are embedded in the diverse historical roots of disparate professional communities. The potential conflict between women's and children's rights is another area that raises deep ethical and ideological issues bearing on the AIDS and reproductive health fields. Counseling potentially seropositive mothers on contraception, for example, involves information and education to inform parents of their choices and rights regarding reproduction as well as children's rights to a healthy start in life.

The future success of AIDS and reproductive health programs requires an in-depth exploration of every dimension of the problems of AIDS and reproductive health, from the biological to the political. An integrated, interdisciplinary approach to AIDS and reproductive health research, policies, and programs offers the best hope of a solution to the world's AIDS and reproductive health problems. This monograph represents a contribution to this effort.

AIDS: CHALLENGES TO EPIDEMIOLOGY IN THE 1990s

Jonathan M. Mann

Harvard School of Public Health

In the global fight against AIDS, epidemiology has played an extremely important and unusually visible role. The early history of AIDS research was dominated by the science of epidemiology, which was so rapidly and successfully applied to the AIDS problem that it became possible to develop a rational prevention strategy well before the causative agent of the disease was identified. Nevertheless, as the pandemic and efforts to understand and control it have advanced over the last decade, it may be useful to reassess the role and contribution of epidemiology to the AIDS field. Through a discussion of the epidemology of sexual transmission of HIV, this chapter will explore some of the ways in which epidemiological practice and methodology have been challenged by the HIV/AIDS pandemic.

Four interdependent approaches have characterized epidemiological studies of HIV/AIDS. Initially, in response to the discovery of AIDS, the focus in epidemiological research was on "risk groups," which included homosexual men, hemophiliacs and other recipients of blood, intravenous drug users, and Haitians. With new information on AIDS in Africa (1), widespread availability of serological tests for HIV infection, and studies among homosexual men (2), the focus shifted from "risk groups" to "risk behaviors." This led to an evolution in terminology: for example, a critical distinction was made between "homosexual" and "receptive anal intercourse," and "homosexual" was increasingly replaced by the concept of "men who have sex with men." In this phase of research, epidemiological studies began to focus on the effort to describe, measure, and link specific risk behaviors with HIV infection. The "risk behavior" approach provided the conceptual foundation for surveys of knowledge, attitudes, beliefs and practices (KABP).

The third phase emphasized the search for "biological risk factors" for HIV infection. A very productive period of epidemiological research ensued. Several factors were found to be associated with an increased risk of HIV infection: other sexually transmitted diseases (3,4); lack of male circumcision (5); stage of illness in the infected partner; and possibly cervical ectopy (6) and use of oral contraceptives (7). All of these factors share a plausible biological means of increasing the likelihood of HIV transmission during sexual exposure to an HIV-infected person.

The fourth, and most recent, stage of research reflects an evolution in epidemiological thinking — a broadening from the individual perspective to include the social, economic and political context of HIV infection. This evolution has resulted, in large part, from experience with HIV/AIDS prevention programs in different national and community settings. Increasing awareness that the "just say no" approach to prevention often reflects a cruel misunderstanding of reality has helped refocus epidemiological attention away from the isolated individual definition of

AIDS and Women's Reproductive Health
Edited by L.C. Chen *et al.*, Plenum Press, New York, 1991

risk behavior. Behaviors associated with sexual transmission of HIV are now being linked, at least conceptually, with issues of empowerment, social and economic status, education, and age and sex roles.

The combined contributions of these four epidemiological approaches have generated a complex picture of HIV transmission. Each approach has been influenced both by preceding phases in epidemiological research and by the broad, evolving social and political context of the HIV/AIDS pandemic.

Remarkable as the epidemiological contribution has been, it nevertheless remains frustratingly inadequate for the task of preventing HIV infection. From the viewpoint of those responsible for design, implementation, and evaluation of HIV/AIDS prevention programs, epidemiology has thus far not succeeded in providing a sufficiently powerful understanding of the behavioral determinants of high-risk sexual behavior. A critical gap remains between what has been measured regarding sexual behavior and what knowledge is needed to design effective behavior-based interventions to prevent sexual transmission of HIV.

For example, the attributable risk associated with identified risk factors for HIV infection are often low or relatively modest. Differences between relative risk and attributable risk are often unstated or unexamined. Available risk factor information only partly explains longitudinal observations of changing HIV incidence. The relative simplicity of the behavioral factors measured in KABP surveys seems inconsistent with the perceived, or intuitively felt, complexity and dynamic quality of sexual life. Problems in self-labelling and quantification of sexual practices lead to skepticism about the relevance of this information to understanding risk behavior.

Such problems might reasonably lead one to ask whether, to what extent, and in what manner sexual behavior is the province of epidemiology. What contributions to our understanding of human sexuality more appropriately involve anthropology, sociology, psychology, and other social sciences? While this issue merits extensive discussion, The International Epidemiological Association's "Dictionary of Epidemiology" suggests an important role for epidemiology in the study of human sexual behavior in its definition of epidemiology: "the study of the distribution and determinants of health-related states and events in populations, and the application of this study to the control of health problems" (8). Clearly, the study of the determinants (behavioral or other) of sexual exposure to HIV reflects the central concern of epidemiology as a science and as a public health discipline. At the same time, it is clear that multidisciplinary approaches uniting epidemiology with other social sciences may be the most important next phase of development in the science of AIDS research.

The present difficulties encountered in epidemiological studies of sexual behavior and HIV infection stem from problems in three areas: 1) the conceptual model of behavior underlying epidemiological studies; 2) the methodological means by which useful data is obtained; and 3) methods of data analysis.

Current epidemiological studies are based on a model of sexual behavior that is essentially deterministic and individualistic. The model works by disaggregating the presumed steps, or elements, of decision-making regarding sexual behavior. Each of these elements is presumed to be susceptible to further study, refinement, and measurement; accordingly, data are collected to fit the disaggregated schema. Surveys, case-control studies, and prospective studies seek quantitative information on elements of knowledge about AIDS, attitudes towards AIDS and sexual behavior, beliefs about AIDS and behavior, and sexual practices. Focus group approaches, while capable of generating insights into details of behavior or proximate factors influencing behavior, remain bounded by the deterministic framework within which behavior is assumed to operate.

Methods of analysis compound the determinism of the conceptual framework. Multivariate analysis, even when productive of highly significant associations and rankings, cannot begin to suggest hypotheses to address the often substantial proportion of observed effect not attributable to factors measured and incorporated into the analytic model.

The individualistic bias of current models of behavior gives rise to difficulties in conceptualizing and studying the relationship between extra-individual factors (economics, culture, politics) and individual behavior. Beyond token acknowledgement of the important role extra-individual factors may play in influencing personal behavior, available research offers little of practical utility for HIV prevention programs that must address the broader context of HIV infection in different regions.

The net result is a gap between what prevention programs need to know about sexual behavior and what they can derive from available epidemiological studies. This statement does not deny the value that descriptive information from surveys and other studies of sexual behavior has had for targeting, or otherwise improving, intervention program design, implementation, and evaluation. But an enormous gap remains between current concepts and methods of data collection and analysis on one hand, and the intuitively felt realities of sexual behavior on the other. Further progress in HIV/AIDS prevention may depend on narrowing this gap.

An example, while highly anecdotal, may help illustrate this problem. A woman meets a man at a bar and hopes to have sexual intercourse. She knows about AIDS, its modes of transmission, and the protective value of condoms. She considers her behavior "at risk" and she is concerned about AIDS, so she has made the decision to have a condom with her. All of this information is based on epidemiological studies, conveyed to her through various channels.

But now we enter a new domain of actuality in personal behavior: the realm of action. The woman is ready to suggest that she and the man leave the bar together, with the goal of having sexual intercourse. She intends to insist on condom use, counting on his eagerness to leave with her (the "good news") to gain his consent to the condom plan (the "bad news"). But just as she leans towards the man and starts to speak, a passing bartender stumbles and spills beer on the man. He leaps up and curses, angrily brushing and wiping his jacket. The intimate moment is shattered. The woman instantly reacts by changing her sexual approach: she will drop the mention of condoms, fearing that the man will react with further irritation to the condom idea, and that the whole encounter will collapse.

This small drama, involving a highly complex system with two sentient and responsive actors, may more accurately reflect real sexual behavior than do surveys of general attitudes about condom use or self-reported histories of safer sex practices. Indeed, if later questioned about her success in negotiating condom use, how would the subject of this vignette have responded? Honest answers to survey questions about her attitudes would suggest a high level of concordance with the elements of a health belief model system. Yet the realities of her sexual practices and HIV risk will have occurred at a different level. In addition, the sexual survey and its analysis would not reveal the connection between the woman's educational level, her social and economic status, and behaviors such as seeking a sexual partner in a bar; feeling uneasy about her control over condom use (and, by implication, other details of sexual practice); initiating the "towards intercourse" sequence of events; and making alcohol intake part of her sexual approach.

In conceptualizing human sexual behavior, an analogy to climate and weather might be useful. In this analogy, the general parameters of sexual behavior established under the broad influences of biology and culture represent a "climate" that generally remains relatively stable for a given individual. Elements of a "sexual climate" might include sexual preference; attitudes towards condoms; perceived relevance of AIDS; and sense of personal self-efficacy in sexual matters. Within the broad limits of that "sexual climate," the "weather" of a specific individual's sexual behavior in a particular circumstance may be unpredictable, as it is likely to be influenced by unmeasurable and unanticipated factors that cannot be included in a deterministic epidemiologic model.

New conceptualizations of risk behavior may be needed to advance our understanding of HIV-related sexual behaviors. Just as the evolution from "risk groups" to "risk behaviors" to "societal risk factors" resulted, in large part, from the influence of diverse disciplines and perspectives on epidemiology, so might advances in our ability to study human sexual behavior require new dialogue and openness to concepts and methods from other disciplines.

For example, modern theories of behavior might generate ways to approach and measure "vulnerability" to risk behavior in different scenarios. Recent theories of chaos could suggest observational studies that might reveal unanticipated patterns within apparently unpredictable behaviors. Methods of data collection might be derived from the social and physical sciences. New approaches to analysis of complex and apparently unpredictable systems may be needed.

At the same time, the strengths of epidemiology's quantitative methods must not be disregarded. The limited predictive capabilities of deterministic models may allow a better understanding of independent and intervening variables in sexual behavior. In fact, the quantitative insufficiency of existing behavioral studies may be at least as much of a problem as the conceptual over-simplicity of the deterministic model of behavior. Observational studies to suggest relevant behavioral variables, combined with appropriate quantification, may help strengthen the link between individual observations and insight and the population-level understanding that epidemiological approaches allow.

Rather than react with frustration or hopelessness to the innumerable factors that make it difficulty to describe and categorize "sexual climate," let alone predict "sexual weather," one can regard the situation as a challenge to behavioral epidemiology. Indeed, this challenge can be viewed as one that offers rich possibilities for observation from which conceptual and methodological innovations may emerge.

While the epidemiological work of the past decade has clarified important issues pertaining to sexual behavior, thereby enhancing HIV/AIDS prevention efforts, the limitations of this epidemiological work are clear. Innovative conceptual models and methodologies will be needed in epidemiology to overcome these limitations. Such innovations will not only benefit HIV/AIDS prevention programs, but will allow epidemiology to help resolve other major behavior-based public health problems.

Many challenges to epidemiology emerged during the first decade of HIV/AIDS research and response. The human rights issue is one challenge that directly relates to the preceeding discussion of sexual behavior and epidemiologic study. The use of "risk group" categories in the initial phase of epidemiologic HIV/AIDS research resulted in an inadvertant collision between epidemiology and human rights. However valuable to researchers, the "risk group" approach had significant social side effects. The most serious of these was the increased stigmatization of already marginalized people (male homosexuals, persons with hemophilia, iv drug users, and "foreigners" from developing countries). This served to fuel denial in the general population (i.e., non-"risk group" members) of the realities of heterosexual HIV transmission and the broad scope of the HIV/AIDS pandemic.

The "risk group" controversy was only part of a broader challenge to the status quo of epidemiological practice, particularly to the relationship between epidemiologic researchers and research subjects. As a result of this challenge, long-standing issues, such as informed consent, respect for privacy and confidentiality, and the longer-term responsibility of researcher for subject, are being discussed with new energy and concern. The controversy surrounding anonymous unlinked screening illustrates well the potential for conflicting values and definitions of individual autonomy and collective good in epidemiological work. Important ethical and legal issues are also being raised.

Epidemiological research on HIV/AIDS is, of necessity, international in scope; yet the occurrence of so-called "safari" or "parachute" research has been severely, and justifiably, criticized. (These terms describe the work of expatriate researchers who fail to seek genuine collaboration with local investigators and eschew efforts to strengthen the research capabilities of local institutions and investigators.) In response to these criticisms, the World Health Organization's Global Programme on AIDS initiated a process in 1989 to develop a global concensus on the ethical aspects of epidemiologic practice.

While epidemiology has contributed greatly to the understanding and prevention of HIV/AIDS, it has also been challenged by the HIV/AIDS pandemic. In epidemiology, as in many other fields, AIDS has brought to light deficiencies in existing concepts and practices. AIDS highlights the need, and provides the opportunity, to expand interactions between epidemiology and other health-related, social scientific, and biological disciplines.

These matters are vital for future studies not only of the sexual transmission of HIV, but for studies of the broad range of behavior-based health problems. The capacity of epidemiology to respond creatively to these challenges and develop improved approaches to behavior–based health problems will help shape the future of AIDS prevention, of epidemiology, and of public health in this rapidly changing world.

Acknowledgments

I would like to thank Dr. James Curran for his review of the initial draft, and the participants in the Bellagio Conference for their comments.

REFERENCES

1. Quinn TC, Mann JM, Curran JW, Piot P. AIDS in Africa: an epidemiologic paradigm. *Science* 1986; 234: 955-963.
2. Heyward WL, Curran JW. The epidemiology of AIDS in the U.S. *Scientific American*, October 1988, pp. 52-59.
3. Piot P, Laga M. Genital ulcers, other sexually transmitted diseases and the sexual transmission of HIV. *Br Med J* 1989; 298:623-4.
4. Cameron DW, Padian NS. Sexual transmission of HIV and the epidemiology of other sexually transmitted diseases. *AIDS* 1990 (suppl 1):S99-S103.
5. Simonsen JN, Cameron DW, Gakinya MN et al. Human immundeficiency virus infection among men with sexualy transmitted diseases: Experience from a centre in Africa. *N Engl J Med* 1988; 319:274-278.
6. Moss GB, D'Costa LJ, Ndinya-Achola JO et al. Cervical ectopy and lack of male circumcision as risk factors for heterosexual transmission of HIV in stable sexual partnerships in Kenya. VI International Conference on AIDS, San Francisco, California, June 1990. Final Program and Abstracts, vol. 1, pp. 267 (abstract Th.C.5770).
7. Simonsen JN, Plummer FA, Ngugi EN et al. HIV infection among lower socioeconomic strata prostitutes in Nairobi. *AIDS* 1990; 4:139-144.
8. International Epidemiological Association. *A Dictionary of Epidemiology*. Last JM, ed. New York: Oxford University Press, 1983, pp. 32-33.

Note

Responsibility for the ideas and opinions expressed in this chapter is exclusively my own.

AIDS AND REPRODUCTIVE HEALTH: WOMEN'S PERSPECTIVES

Katherine D. LaGuardia

The Rockefeller Foundation

INTRODUCTION

As a disease among women, HIV/AIDS was largely invisible until the late 1980s. During that decade, most work on the disease was done in North America, Western Europe, and Oceania, where the clinical, research, and policy focus was on the adult male whose source of infection was most likely to be homosexual contact or intravenous drug use. Only a fraction of the available research dollars was spent on investigations of heterosexual and perinatal transmission, and few women were recruited into clinical trials funded by private or public agencies (1).

Yet, tens of thousands of women are exposed to HIV/AIDS in regions where heterosexual and perinatal transmission are prominent (2), especially sub-Saharan Africa. Despite this fact, the reproductive health aspects of HIV/AIDS were not raised as a research and health policy priority (3,4) until it began to be apparent that growing numbers of women in North America were being infected sexually, that the overwhelming majority (85%) were of reproductive age, and that the majority of women with HIV infection who become pregnant were choosing to maintain their pregnancies (5). Even today, the reproductive health aspects of HIV/AIDS remain characterized by lack of research, suboptimal health care, restricted access to care, and medical and social stigmata.

The first decade of the HIV/AIDS pandemic yielded bleak, if limited, statistics about the impact of the disease on women and children. The Surveillance Unit of the Global Programme on AIDS of the World Health Organization (GPA/WHO) has estimated that, during the 1980s, there were approximately 500,000 cases globally of AIDS in women and children. Current forecasting suggests that AIDS will take an even greater toll in the 1990s: the pandemic may kill at least an additional three million women and children (6). The disparity between the two decades is due to both unrecognized cases and underreporting in the 1980s, and an overall projected increase in case mortality in women and children in the 1990s.

The concentration of HIV/AIDS in poor women of color is striking. About 80% of all women with HIV infection reside in sub-Saharan Africa, primarily in the eastern and central countries. Prevalence per 100,000 women aged 15-49 years is about 2,500, compared to fewer than 5 per 100,000 in Eastern Europe and most of Asia. Although HIV/AIDS cases among women and children have been, and will likely remain, concentrated in sub-Saharan Africa, a pattern similar to the pattern seen initially in Central Africa is now emerging in the Americas. Prevalence of HIV/AIDS is rising faster among women aged 15-49 than among men in the same age group in this hemisphere (7). The New York State AIDS Epidemiology Unit reports prevalence rates as high as 660 per 100,000 childbearing women as of March, 1990 (8). Comparable data are not available for men, but a study by Quinn et al. shows that, among men and women attending a sexually transmitted disease (STD) clinic in Baltimore, a 1:1 male to female ratio of HIV sero-prevalence is seen in the 20-25 year age group, and a roughly 6:1 ratio is seen in the 35-39 year age group (9). What is particularly striking about the epidemiology of the disease among women in the United States is its racial distribution. In the U.S., the cumulative incidence of AIDS is 13.6 times higher for African-American women and 10.2 times higher for Hispanic women than it is for white women (10).

These patterns have serious implications for the therapeutic and preventive strategies for the disease in women. Africa has very limited resources for health research and services. Even if therapeutic modalities become available to limit heterosexual and perinatal transmission, it is doubtful they could be made widely available to most of the women currently in need. In the developed world, where most of the clinical and laboratory work on the virus has been performed, resources are less of a constraint than in the developing world. However, women with HIV infection tend to be poor, of minority race, and in the drug-using culture. The relative wealth of resources in the developed world means little if these women don't have access to care. A major challenge to the international health community is to develop creative strategies to confront these issues and offer innovative solutions.

THE SIGNIFICANCE OF HETEROSEXUAL TRANSMISSION

The classic description of the global population distribution of HIV/AIDS originally postulated by GPA/WHO (11), has begun to take on a somewhat different character as the pandemic moves into the 1990s. In particular, it is becoming clear that heterosexual and perinatal transmission of HIV play an increasingly important role.

Pattern I areas are described as those in which the mode of transmission is primarily through male homosexual contact and intravenous drug use (IVDU). The regions involved in this pattern are North America, Western Europe, and Oceania. Heterosexual or perinatal transmission have not been thought to play a major role in the spread of HIV infection in these countries. Pattern II areas are those in which heterosexual and perinatal transmission do play a major role. These regions include all of sub-Saharan Africa and parts of the Caribbean. Latin America has now been entered as a Pattern II region because of the emerging evidence of heterosexual transmission in the spread of the disease. Pattern III countries have been described as those in which the virus was introduced rather late in the epidemic, and include primarily Asia, Eastern Europe, North Africa, and the Middle East. Pattern III countries have been characterized by no clear predominant mode of transmission. However, as evidence of the disease has emerged in countries such as Thailand, the Philippines, and Romania, the predominant mode of transmission in these countries appears to be heterosexual and perinatal. Thus, a re-classification of these regions may become necessary. As we move into the 1990s, the global patterns of the mode of HIV transmission will become increasingly blurred as HIV/AIDS affects more women and children.

Male-to-female seroprevalence ratios also reflect the importance of heterosexual transmission within geographic regions. In Europe, the ratio is 7.7:1; in South America, 10:1; in Haiti and parts of Africa, 1:1 (12). Further evidence of changes in transmission patterns in the United States is revealed by seroprevalence studies done on civilian applicants for military service. The male-to-female ratio reported over a three-year period was 3:1 with an incidence ratio of 1.77:1 (13). In a seroprevalence study of 26 sentinel hospitals in the United States, a strong correlation was found between high HIV seroprevalence and low male-female ratios of seroprevalence. This indicates that HIV infection is even more concentrated among women in high prevalence areas than among men, predicting a similar future for AIDS cases among women and children in these areas, and an additional burden on already financially strained hospitals (14). It also indicates a relationship between low male-female ratios of seroprevalence and potentials for heterosexual transmission. Uninfected persons of either sex have an increased likelihood of coming into contact with an HIV-infected person through unprotected intercourse in low ratio areas.

THE SIGNIFICANCE OF HIV/AIDS FOR REPRODUCTIVE HEALTH PROGRAMS AND POLICIES

The impact of HIV/AIDS on reproductive health takes many forms, not limited to the projected increased mortality among women aged 15-49 and children under five years. HIV/AIDS has created a new generation of orphans (15); has dramatically affected the child survival movement (16); has contributed to maternal morbidity (17) and probably mortality; has become a major disease of minority women in North America; and is the leading cause of death of women aged 25-34 in New York City (18,19). While reproductive health issues have always been fraught with ethical conflict and stigmatization, HIV/AIDS adds a complicated dimension to this aspect of health care for women. Clinicians and policy makers are uncertain as to whether infected women should become pregnant or whether infected mothers should breast-feed their infants. Breast-feeding is recommended by the WHO for HIV-infected mothers in developing countries; the CDC, on the other hand, does not recommend breast-feeding for HIV-infected mothers in the United States, and a similar guideline exists in England and Australia (20,21). There are conflicting data about whether certain contraceptive methods enhance or inhibit viral transmission through sexual contact. The clear association between STDs, particularly genital ulcer disease (GUD), and HIV transmission has transformed the field of venereology, but there is little concensus on whether and how to integrate STD diagnosis and treatment into women's health care.

It has only been since the recent epidemiologic trends of the disease in women in North America became apparent that the reproductive aspects of HIV/AIDS have been raised as a research and health policy priority. The AIDS and Reproductive Health Network (ARHN), founded in 1988, has played a pivotal role in focusing research work on women and children at risk for HIV infection in the developing world. The ARHN has identified and linked a wide range of reproductive health issues to HIV/AIDS. It has correctly and wisely conveyed the notion that HIV/AIDS in women and children cannot be separated from policies on contraception, STDs, breast-feeding, pregnancy management, and sexual behavior. Every aspect of reproductive behavior must now be viewed with an eye towards its interface with the HIV/AIDS pandemic. Regretfully, this association has not been widely acknowledged in reproductive health policies. It is hoped that the research generated from the ARHN and its policy implications will integrate HIV/AIDS programs more fully into reproductive health.

It is important to remember that the majority of women with HIV infection are poor. The epidemiology of the disease among women and men is quite different, particularly in the Pattern I regions. HIV/AIDS in Europe and North America began as a disease of generally well-educated, white, gay men. The fast-moving pace of AIDS research and therapeutic development has often been attributed to the financial resources and political base that exist within the gay community. The progressive, at times radical, approaches to patient advocacy and education about AIDS prevention by such groups as the Gay Men's Health Crisis (GMHC), and the AIDS Coalition to Unleash Power (ACT-UP), have had a direct impact on the conduct of clinical trials and the introduction of the concept of safe sex into sexual behavior. The downward trend seen in the U.S. in new AIDS cases among homosexuals can be largely attributed to the unity of action within the gay community.

Women with HIV infection face an entirely different set of circumstances. They are generally without financial resources, education, community, or political base. In the developed world, the majority of women with HIV infection are either drug users themselves or partners of IVDUs.

Perhaps most importantly, women have an added disadvantage in negotiating the sexual encounter. The most effective method for preventing sexual transmission of HIV, the condom, is controlled by the male. Women in high-risk groups, such as commercial sex workers, are dependent on their clients' willingness to use a condom. Additionally, there are documented cultural issues that result in some men refusing to use condoms because it is not seen as "masculine" (22). In approaching HIV/AIDS from a reproductive health perspective, a woman's status in her culture takes on increased importance as preventive strategies are constructed.

WOMEN'S REPRODUCTIVE HEALTH: WHAT IS IT AND WHERE DOES HIV/AIDS FIT INTO IT?

In the context of the definition of "health" put forth in the Constitution of the WHO, "reproductive health" has a four-fold meaning (23): 1) that people have the ability to reproduce as well as to regulate their fertility; 2) that women are able to go through pregnancy and childbirth safely; 3) that the outcome of pregnancy is successful in terms of maternal and infant survival and well-being; and 4) that couples are able to have sexual relationships free of the fear of unwanted pregnancy and disease.

If women are to achieve reproductive health, they must not only have access to necessary health services but they must also have the knowledge, ability, and right to control when, with whom, and under what conditions they have sexual relationships. This is not always the case, and is perhaps the key limiting factor in reducing heterosexual transmission of HIV. This sociologic phenomenon is revealed most vividly in data about condom use among commercial sex workers and knowledge of partners' risk factors at time of intercourse. While the condom may be efficacious in preventing transmission, it is not effective if rarely used. A study on condom use in Zaire demonstrated that only 8 of 376 sex workers interviewed used the condom more than half the time with clients. These women remained seronegative over the 12-month study period. However, these regular users comprised only 2% of the women studied (24). A study in New York City revealed that in a group of middle-class, HIV-seropositive women, 28 of 35 were partners of IVDUs and 18 of the 28 knew of the drug use; yet only 2 used the condom regularly prior to seroconversion (25). These two studies, while in different settings and among different populations, demonstrate similar points: women, for a variety of reasons, have difficulty in negotiating condom use; there is a general lack of understanding about heterosexual transmission of HIV; and there is something basically ineffective about using condoms to control heterosexual spread of the virus.

The current public health strategies to prevent sexual transmission of HIV focus on four issues: partner selection, partner number, mode of sexual expression*, and the use of condoms. By and large, these strategies restore to men the locus of control over the consequences of sexual behavior, though women may have some control over the number of partners they choose (26). Furthermore, the direction of sexual transmission of HIV clearly favors a male-to-female passage (27,28,29). The risk factors women carry in cases of sexual transmission are the behavior patterns of their male partners, such as a current or past history of IVDU, bisexuality, or contacts with female sex workers. This behavior is often clandestine, so women cannot reliably use the concept of "careful partner selection" as a preventive strategy. Clearly, women are in many ways the unacknowledged victims of the HIV/AIDS epidemic.

Concerns about perinatal transmission have also tended to overlook the woman. Perinatal transmission has generated tremendous interest in the research community, but virtually all of the

---

* The modes of sexual expression that have been strongly linked to HIV transmission are receptive anal intercourse and frequency of intercourse with an infected partner (33). Yet, it is unclear whether modes of sexual expression can be changed to reduce transmission. This is certainly true among commercial sex workers where economics, more than any other factor, determine their susceptibility to the virus and subsequent infectivity.

work has focused on the fetus and newborn. We now know that the HIV virus crosses the maternal-fetal unit very early in pregnancy (30). There are multiple research protocols within The National Institutes of Health (NIH) for early therapeutic interventions in infected newborns (31). A singular protocol for treatment with zidovudine during pregnancy is in its third year of planning and has yet to be implemented. Its objective is to reduce vertical transmission of HIV during pregnancy; it does not address the issue of reducing maternal morbidity. The slow development of this potentially beneficial intervention in pregnancy is related to concerns over possible fetal toxicity and teratogenicity.

Who is expressing concern about maternal morbidity in the presence of HIV infection? Where are the protocols to study therapeutic modalities to reduce some of the known complications of HIV infection in pregnancy? Why has the zidovudine protocol been in development for over three years? And why is there such a dearth of research protocols and clinical interventions that specifically address the impact of HIV/AIDS on women?

The advocacy groups that so effectively mobilized the research and pharmaceutical industry to make zidovudine and pentamadine available quickly and at reduced cost to the adult, primarily male population have only recently begun to speak out on behalf of women. Women themselves lack a voice in this epidemic and are victimized by their silence in many ways. Should an infected woman wish to terminate her pregnancy, she may have difficulty finding a provider willing to perform the procedure (32). Because so much of the epidemiological research on the disease in women has focused on commercial sex workersand populations attending STD clinics, there is a stigma attached to HIV/AIDS that portrays infected women as anti-social at best. And because minority women (African-American and Hispanic) in the United States carry a disproportionate share of infection, morbidity, and mortality due to HIV, there are racial implications to the disease that raise significant ethical issues in research and policy work.

KEY ISSUES AND GAPS IN RESEARCH, POLICY, AND HEALTH CARE

Given the preceding discussion of the epidemiologic trends of HIV/AIDS and its relationship to reproductive health, what are the missing links in research, policy, and health care?

Little is known about HIV/AIDS in women of reproductive age in the general population. The concept of "high risk" is inappropriate, particularly in areas of high seroprevalence where heterosexual transmission is the predominant mode of transmission. Given prevailing sexual norms and gender power relations, girls and women in the general population are often at risk of rape or incest. We must confront the reality that the possibility of exposure exists in all heterosexual encounters outside of long-term mutually monogamous relationships. There is a growing tendency, because of the demographics of the disease in the United States, to focus on minorities as a risk group. The epidemic among women must not be relegated to the ghettos and overly identified with race.

Much AIDS research and policy work has been developed in the North where, until recently, women have been largely excluded because transmission was not primarily heterosexual. This research and policy work is not widely applicable to developing countries, where resources are scarce and access to basic health services is extremely limited. There is a need for the research community to focus on heterosexual transmission and on the development of low-cost diagnostics and therapeutic modalities.

To the extent that they have been considered, women have been seen primarily as carriers ("vectors") of HIV, even though the passage of the virus favors a male-to-female direction. For both sex workers and pregnant women, the primary focus of research has been on transmission to the male partner or the fetus. These women are not representative of the general population of girls and women who are unknowingly at risk from promiscuous, drug-using, or bisexual partners, and the research and clinical work has reflected this bias. The "vector" concept underscores this skewed viewpoint. The research literature increasingly identifies women in vector terminology ("high-frequency transmitter" and "core groups" are particularly offensive new phrases) because most of the epidemiological data have been collected among high seroprevalence groups (prostitutes, women attending STD clinics, IVDUs). We must begin to shift our focus from this concept and view all women as "at risk."

Enrolling women in AIDS research and services has been difficult, and the reasons are not well understood. There is an element of exclusion by the research community in the very design of the projects and recruitment strategies used. There is also an excessive hesitancy to focus research work on reproductive issues because of fear of the effects such research may have on the fetus and on reproductive potential. As Jonathan Mann points out, there has been a "failure to articulate a commonality" in this area. The various health strategies that address reproductive health (i.e., STDs, AIDS, maternal-child health [MCH], family planning) have not been combined to create a cohesive strategy to engage women in research and services.

Too little is known about sexual behavior in general and the influence of gender power relations in particular. There is little concrete understanding of how and why women become vulnerable to infection and how they might be able to protect themselves when gender power relations are heavily weighted in favor of men. The condom is clearly not the answer. Because of the Western orientation of AIDS research, there has been a skewed assessment of sexual behavior in different cultural settings. There has not been enough work done on the diversity of sexual norms and how that behavior could be modified through preventive strategies.

The very high value many women place on fertility is poorly understood in terms of how this determines their sexual behavior and, thus, their exposure to infection and their role in transmission. Too much emphasis is placed on preventing pregnancy in preventing AIDS. There has been little discussion of fertility concerns in formulating preventive strategies (34). Many women who learn they are HIV-seropositive are psychologically devastated largely because of the impact of their HIV status on childbearing potential. The medical community has been too quick in its judgment on the reproductive rights of HIV-infected women. When we discuss HIV prevention in the sexual arena, pregnancy prevention is always a component of the technology; not enough effort has been put into the development of viral-specific technologies for use in sexual encounters by HIV-infected women who may wish to become pregnant.

RESEARCH, POLICY, AND SERVICE NEEDS

If over 80% of HIV-infected women live in Africa, and there is growing concern at the government level about women and AIDS, how will this concern be translated into effective health strategies for the women most affected? This is a question that can be asked about other reproductive health issues as well. Maternal mortality, affecting more than twice as many women of reproductive age per year as AIDS, is the focus of significant international commitment. The Safe Motherhood movement poses a question similar to one raised here: How can we use available resources to reduce preventable mortality in pregnancy? The technology exists, but the solutions require much more than technology can offer. The importance of fertility regulation in maintaining the health of women is well recognized. Yet, contraceptive prevalence remains exceedingly low in much of the developing world (35). The existence of programs, services, and methods does not necessarily translate into improved health status; family planning programs and a variety of reproductive health technologies exist worldwide. A key challenge to the public health community is how to deliver these services effectively and reach as many women as possible.

When a vaccine becomes available to prevent HIV infection, who will have access to it? When a method for preventing sexual transmission of the virus is developed that can be controlled by the woman, how will it be promoted and distributed, and to whom? When therapies become available to reduce perinatal transmission of the virus, how will they be offered to the women in need? In much of sub-Saharan Africa, HIV testing is not even possible; therefore, therapeutic strategies to reduce progression to clinical AIDS are also not possible. We continue to apply Western concepts and technologies to settings where their translation is neither possible nor understood.

There is a need to focus on the reproductive health issues in HIV/AIDS in much the same way that other successful health initiatives have been conceived. The Safe Motherhood movement has brought a wide and diverse international community together to focus on the problems of maternal mortality in the developing world. The Child Survival movement, considered highly successful until perinatal AIDS and orphanhood secondary to AIDS introduced a new agenda of needs, mobilized an academic and donor community to address illness and death among children with very creative strategies. The family planning movement has had the same kind of impact. There is a need to address HIV/AIDS and reproductive health in an equally diverse and innovative manner.

HIV/AIDS is exerting its influence on all the major maternal-child health initiatives of the past 20 years. Perhaps the donor, research, and service programs that focus on the reproductive aspects of HIV/AIDS should be more fully integrated into other maternal-child health initiatives. Clearly, a broad and powerful voice in the international health arena is needed to have an impact on the epidemic. The feminist voice, so clearly heard in the areas of maternal health, family planning, and abortion rights is sorely missing in HIV/AIDS.

HIV/AIDS stands increasingly alone as a discipline when, in fact, it needs integration with other major health initiatives. In some way, HIV/AIDS has significantly altered the agenda of each of these health initiatives, yet each continues to function independently. At the policy level, there is minimal interaction between these highly structured disciplines. In order to begin the process of integration, the following priorities should be addressed:

1) Women need information about HIV/AIDS and reproduction. This cannot be disseminated in a vacuum. Existing reproductive health programs need to learn how to integrate this information into their health education agendas. This must include information about HIV and pregnancy, sexual transmission, breast-feeding, perinatal transmission, and contraception.

2) STD programs need to become more fully integrated with reproductive health. The well-known association of HIV/AIDS with STDs, especially GUD, requires that STD programs address this connection. In addition, the long-term sequelae of reproductive tract infections secondary to STDs often result in infertility. The inability to bear a child carries heavy social stigma in many cultures. STD diagnosis and treatment needs to be made less costly, more accessible, acceptable, and associated with the health of women. Through this type of approach, HIV/AIDS preventive strategies could be introduced.

3) The development of protective technology that can be controlled by the woman, such as vaginal virucidal creams, should be given priority in research. In the development of these creams, consideration should be given to spermicidal effects as well. Ideally, two types of cream should be available, one that is virucidal only, for women who wish to conceive, and one that is both spermicidal and virucidal. The development of protective technologies that are under the woman's control and preserve fertility are essential.

4) Women need stronger advocacy in the battle against HIV/AIDS. The platforms that have been established to speak out on other aspects of women's health need to adopt HIV/AIDS as a priority. Women have been neglected in the epidemic and have been subject to unfair bias in studies. The complex ethical issues involved in HIV/AIDS and reproductive health demand serious thought and sensitivity regarding such matters as women's status; women's right to privacy; cultural differences in sexual behavior; and the high value placed on fertility by virtually every woman in the world.

5) Research priorities in HIV/AIDS need to focus more specifically on the impact of the infection on women. These priorities should include: mechanisms of heterosexual transmission;

relationship between HIV infection and reproductive tract morbidity (including STDs, cervical neoplasias, PID); impact of the infection on pregnancy, both in terms of the mother and the fetus; and development of therapeutic modalities to address aspects of the disease specific to women.

In summary, we need to begin to redefine how we approach women and women's health in the international arena in order to have an effective impact on the HIV/AIDS pandemic. The second decade of the HIV/AIDS work must shift the focus of preventive and therapeutic strategies toward the heterosexual population and strengthen its emphasis on women. In this context, all women and girls need to be addressed, not just those studied in high seroprevalence populations. This creates an opportunity to reduce the racial and social stigmata associated with the disease. Opportunity also exists to broaden the horizons of the HIV/AIDS field by integrating its research, service, and policy agenda with other major initiatives in reproductive health. Through these efforts, we may see important breakthroughs in treatment and prevention. We may also witness a revolution in our thinking about women and their reproductive health.

REFERENCES

1. National Commission on AIDS. Report No. 3: Research, the workforce and the HIV epidemic in rural America. August 1990.
2. Piot P, Taelman H, Minlangu KB et al. AIDS in a heterosexual population in Zaire. *Lancet* July 14, 1984; 1984:65-69.
3. The Centers for Disease Control. Revisions of guidelines for the prevention and management of HIV infection in women and their children. Working group meeting, Atlanta, George, August 1-2, 1990 (final draft in preparation).
4. The National Institutes of Health. Research and health care role for Obstetrician-Gynecologists involved in prevention and treatment of HIV infection in women and their children. Meeting of the Pediatric, Adolescent, and Maternal AIDS Branch (PAMA), Bethesda, Maryland, December 12-13, 1989.
5. Selwyn PA, Carter R, Schoenbaum EE et al. Knowledge of HIV antibody status and decisions to continue or terminate pregnancy among intravenous drug users. *JAMA* 1989; 261:3567-3571.
6. Chin J. Current and future dimensions of the HIV/AIDS pandemic in women and children. *Lancet* 1990; 336:221-224.
7. Gwinn M, George JR, Hannon WH, Hoff R et al. Estimates of HIV seroprevalence in child bearing women and incidence of HIV infection in infants, United States. VI International Conference on AIDS, San Francisco, CA, June 1990; Abstract F.C.43.
8. Novick LF, Glabatis DM, Stricof RL, MacCubbin PA, Lessner L, Berns DS. Newborn Seroprevalence Study: Methods and Results. *Am J Pub Health* 1991; 81(supp):15-21.
9. Quinn JC, Cannon RD, Glasser D et al. The association of syphilis with HIV infection in patients attending STD clinics. *Arch Int Med* 1990; 150:1297-1302.
10. Centers for Disease Control. Update: AIDS-United States 1981-1988. *MMWR* 1989; 38:229-326.
11. Piot P, Plummer FA, Mhalu FS et al. AIDS: An international perspective. *Science* 1988; 239:573-579.
12. Hankins CA. Issues involving women, children, and AIDS primarily in the developed world. *J AIDS* 1990; 3:443-448.
13. McNeil JG, Brundage JF, Wann F et al. The Walter Reed Retrovirus Research Group. Direct measurement of HIV seroconversions in a serially tested population of young adults in the United States Army, October '85 to October '87. *New Eng J Med* 1989; 320:1581-5.
14. St. Louis ME, Rauch KJ, Peterson LR et al. Seroprevalence rates of HIV infection at sentinel hospitals in the United States. *New Eng J Med* 1990; 323:213-218.

15. Preble EA. Impact of HIV/AIDS on African children. *Soc Sci Med* 1990; 31(6):671-680.
16. Konde-Lule JK, Serwadda D et al. The effect of HIV infection on infant and early childhood mortality in rural Rakai district, Uganda: Preliminary results. VI Internation Conference on AIDS, San Francisco, June 1990; Abstract Th.C.748.
17. Minkoff HL, Willoughby A, Mendez H et al. Serious infections during pregnancy among women with advanced HIV infection. *Am J Obstet Gynecol* 1990; 162:30-34.
18. Weinberg DS, Murray HW. Coping with AIDS — the special problems of New York City. *New Eng J Med* 1987; 317:1469-73.
19. Chu SY, Buehler JW, Berkelman RL. Impact of the HIV epidemic on mortality in women of reproductive age, United States. *JAMA* 1990; 264(2):225-29.
20. World Health Organization. Breast-feeding/breast milk and human immunodeficiency virus (HIV). *Wkly Epidem Rec* 14 August 1987; 33:245-246.
21. Oxtoby MJ. Human immunodeficiency virus and other viruses in human milk: placing the issues in broader perspective. *Pediatr Infect Dis J* 1988; 7(12):825-835.
22. Worth D. Sexual decision-making and AIDS: Why condom promotion among vulnerable women is likely to fail. *Stud Fam Plann* 1989; 20:297-307.
23. Fathalla MF. Research Needs in Human Reproduction. In: *Research in Human Reproduction: Biennial Report, 1986-1987*. Diczfalusy E, Griffin PD, Khanna J, eds. Geneva: World Health Organization, 1988; p. 341.
24. Mann J, Quinn TC, Piot P et al. Condom Use and HIV infection among prostitutes in Zaire (letter). *New Eng J Med* 1987; 316:345.
25. Glaser JB, Strange JJ, Rosati D. Heterosexual HIV transmission among the middle class. *Arch Intern Med* 1989; 149:645-649.
26. Stein ZA. HIV Prevention: The need for methods women can use. *Am J Pub Health* 1990; 80:460-462.
27. Clumeck N, Taelman H, Hermans P et al. A cluster of HIV infection among heterosexual people without apparent risk factors. *New Eng J Med* 1990; 321:1460-1462.
28. Hamberg CD, Hozburgh Jr. CR, Ward JW, Jaffe HW. Biologic factors in the sexual transmission of HIV. *J Infect Dis* 1989; 160:116-25.
29. Laga M, Taelman H, Van der Stuyft P et al. Advanced immunodeficiency as a risk factor for heterosexual transmission of HIV. *AIDS* 1989; 3:361-6.
30. Lewis SH, Reynolds-Kohler C, Fox H, Nelson JA. HIV-1 in trophoblastic and billous Hofbauer cells, and hematological precursors in eight-week fetuses. *Lancet* 1990; 335:565-8.
31. Division of AIDS, National Institute of Allergy and Infectious Diseases. Ninth AIDS Clinical Trials Group Meeting. Bethesda, Maryland, July 10-13, 1990.
32. Franke KM. Discrimination against HIV positive women by abortion clinics in New York City. V International Conference on AIDS, Montreal, Canada, June 1989.
33. Padian N, Marquis L, Francis DP et al. Male-to-female transmission of HIV. *JAMA* 1987; 258:788-90.
34. Caldwell JC, Caldwell P, Quiggin P. The social context of AIDS in sub-Saharan Africa. *Popul Dev Rev* 1989; 15(2):185-234.
35. Mauldin WP, Segal SJ. Prevalence of Contraceptive Use: Trends and Issues. *Stud Fam Plann* 1988; 19(6):335-353.

POLICY AND LEGAL ASPECTS OF AIDS INTERVENTIONS: INDIVIDUAL RIGHTS AND SOCIAL RESPONSIBILITIES

Harvey V. Fineberg

Harvard School of Public Health

INTRODUCTION

AIDS is a disease without a cure. It is spread primarily as a result of personal behaviors, some of which are regarded by some people as immoral and some of which are, in fact, illegal. Preventive measures can involve the dissemination of controversial information and other potentially provocative activities. Although the epidemic proportions of AIDS demand a response by lawmakers and policy setters, the intensity of feeling about the disease makes it difficult for decision makers to take action that ensures the protection of both the uninfected and the infected and that most effectively slows, if not stops, the spread of the disease.

The HIV epidemic intersects many concerns that bear on the health of women: human sexual behavior, reproductive health, sexually transmitted diseases, and larger social issues such as intravenous drug use and safe blood supplies. The AIDS epidemic reflects and amplifies each of these issues, focusing our attention on various aspects of the disease, including its effects on women.

In the United States, every state has enacted legislation covering some aspect of the AIDS epidemic. The best of this legislation provides guidelines for professional standards, mandates appropriate health care services and education, funds research and policy development, safeguards confidentiality, and protects against discrimination. The worst dictates the content of educational programs based on issues of morality, limits assurances of confidentiality, institutes compulsory screening of particular groups, and needlessly restricts the liberty of carriers of the AIDS virus (1).

Three areas particularly susceptible to the human rights ramifications of legislation are screening for AIDS, programs intended to effect behavior change, and discrimination against those who have AIDS or who are considered likely to have AIDS. Laws in these areas — some enlightened, some repressive — illustrate the delicacy of the balance of rights and responsibilities and the complexity of protecting society from errant individuals while protecting individuals from the undue constraints of society.

This chapter deals with policy and legal aspects of HIV screening and interventions to promote behavior change, and discusses the problem of discrimination against HIV-infected individuals. While these topics will undoubtedly suggest questions with particular significance for women (Should women in high-risk groups who are of childbearing age be required to be tested for HIV? How can women who wish to change their sexual behavior ensure the cooperation of their partners?), the principles involved pertain, in one way or another, to everyone who has AIDS/HIV infection or is at risk of contracting the virus. Those who are concerned with AIDS policies in general cannot afford to overlook their specific impact on women. At the same time, studies of AIDS and women can yield lessons for science and policy that will advance understanding of how AIDS affects everyone.

SCREENING

As a public health measure, screening for disease often has a kind of superficial appeal because it is an action that can be definitively taken. It is something a legislator or policy maker can point to as having been done. With this temptation in mind, one has to be careful in scrutinizing the purpose and reasons for advocating screening or testing.

Testing can achieve three different goals (2). One purpose of testing is surveillance, tracking the spread of an epidemic, for example, by using sentinel population groups such as newborns, hospital patients, military recruits, or college students. This is a critically important part of the overall strategy to understand and cope with an epidemic. The second goal of screening might be characterized as the medical purpose, namely to benefit the individual being tested, and at the minimum, to provide reassurance, as in a case of possible exposure to infected blood. In the event of a positive test, an individual who is infected can make a more realistic life plan and can be offered better treatment. The third goal of testing is the public health or preventive purpose. Focusing on high-risk activities, this approach aims to reduce the likelihood of spread of infection to others. This is the rationale for screening donated blood or periodically examining prostitutes in places where their activity is legal.

The first purpose described above, surveillance, is grounded in anonymity; the information sought is in the form of numbers and patterns. The second purpose is a personal one; results are (in principle) confidential, and the individual decides what if any action to take. The third purpose, prevention, raises the question of potential trade-offs between what might be best for the individual and what might represent the collective good in health terms for the community. When testing is carried out for this purpose, anonymity and confidentiality cannot be guaranteed; physicians may be required to inform specific individuals or groups of a person's HIV status or even to trace contacts. Isolation is an inappropriate measure in the case of HIV infection since the virus cannot be spread through routine social contact. However, circumstances of intentional spread — for example, by professional sex workers or intravenous drug users who know they are infected and who nevertheless persist in putting others at risk — can warrant restrictive measures, including the possibility of incarceration as punishment for past behavior and to protect others in the future. This is very different from the application of quarantine as a routine response to the HIV epidemic.

Premarital testing, which had been required by the state of Illinois, is an example of testing for the purpose of prevention. Such a policy is easy to implement because the individuals involved are often already required to have their blood tested for evidence of other diseases. However, this is a low-risk group, and the cost of administering the policy and the possibility of erroneously identifying a person as carrying the virus outweighs the advantage of detecting the relatively small number of individuals infected (3). During the first six months of testing in Illinois, only eight of the nearly 71,000 applicants for marriage licenses tested positive for the AIDS virus, at a cost of approximately $312,000 per seropositive individual tested. Because the 22.5% decline in the number of marriage licenses issued during that period was offset by a corresponding increase in the surrounding states, it is possible that individuals truly at risk for AIDS chose simply to avoid the test. The policy was eventually rescinded (4). At any rate, the condition of marriage is not required for transmission of the disease; a law such as that of the state of Utah, which prohibits marriage with a person who has AIDS, may prevent a few marriages but will do little to limit the spread of AIDS. As a restriction on the right to marriage, the law is also subject to judicial challenge.

The most widely used clinical test for HIV infection detects antibodies, the proteins created by the body in response to the infection (2). Typically, antibody tests are carried out by an initial enzyme immunoassay followed by a confirmatory test (Western blot) if the first test turns out to be positive. The accuracy of the test depends on a variety of factors, including the individual's background risk factors, the length of time since exposure to the virus, and the quality of the laboratory performing the test. Because of this possibility of error, a policy that requires all members of a group to be tested — in order, for example, to segregate those with the antibody from those without — cannot be completely effective. Individuals with false negative test results could continue to spread the disease, while those with false positives would be unjustly stigmatized. For this reason, it is significant that the principal grounds on which HIV antibody tests are now being advocated have shifted from the public health purpose of preventing spread, toward the medical purpose of benefiting the individual who is to be tested.

Many benefits may be attained by a patient who is known to be infected by HIV. For one thing, the physician is able to monitor the patient more closely, particularly in terms of the counts of the important immune defense cells called CD4 cells. The physician can initiate preventive therapy with Zidovudine (AZT) if the protective level of those cells drops too low. Complications common to HIV-infected patients, such as pneumonia, influenza A, syphilis, and tuberculosis, can be prevented or treated, and precautions can be taken to avoid certain immunizations or infections. Other advantages include the opportunity to participate in clinical trials of new agents and the ability to prevent transmission of the virus to others.

These advantages represent a compelling argument for a large-scale program of voluntary testing. A widespread program, and the treatment that would be required for those found to carry the virus, could cost billions of dollars. However, the institution of a voluntary, rather than required, testing program moves the testing question to grounds in which individual good (net benefit of medical care for the individual) is weighed against the social cost of investment and resources used to carry out a program. This puts the debate about AIDS and individual rights versus social rights and responsibilities on ground similar to that on which discussion of other expensive health conditions takes place.

Any policy about screening must therefore consider the potential conflict between individual and societal interests (2). The pertinent principles begin with the right to bodily integrity, as expressed in English common law. The idea of protecting the autonomy of the individual leads to an emphasis on informed consent and maintaining the confidentiality of medical information gathered about a patient. A second ethical principle involves balancing the good and harm to an individual that may follow so that there is a net effect of good. A third principle is to prevent harm to others in all that we do, and a fourth is to try to strive toward justice, or a fair distribution across individuals, of the burdens as well as the benefits associated with social interventions. Such ethical considerations underlie, or should underlie, the adoption of policy about screening.

Regardless of whether we base further argument about screening on individual benefit or on collective benefit, legal protection against discrimination and breach of confidentiality is the most important step to enable safe, increased use of HIV testing either for medical or public health purposes. This kind of effort must take place at legislative levels and is matched by the need to educate individuals to promote sympathetic understanding and compassion. The rights of individuals infected with HIV should include, in each jurisdiction, guaranteed access to the care that is required.

POLICIES TO PROMOTE BEHAVIOR CHANGE

Testing in and of itself is not a means of prevention. While researchers seek more effective therapies and biological preventives, education and behavior change have been repeatedly and correctly cited as the only available means of curtailing the spread of the AIDS virus. Individuals cannot take steps to avoid infecting others or becoming infected themselves unless they understand the ways in which the virus is spread and have access to the tools of prevention, such as condoms and clean needles, and are motivated to use them.

Unfortunately, this route to prevention is not as straightforward as it might seem (5). Because the disease touches upon deep-seated fears and inhibitions in American society, there is fundamental disagreement about the propriety of educational messages to prevent AIDS. For some, the only socially acceptable change is to have people abandon certain behaviors altogether. In this moralist view, it is wrong to have sexual relations outside of marriage and it is wrong to use drugs, hence it is wrong to advocate or even discuss anything that would appear to condone these activities, such as use of condoms or sterile needles. This attitude underlies the reticence of many national leaders on the subject of AIDS education, controversies over the propriety of specific educational materials, and debates among Catholic prelates over teaching about condoms. Confronting these views is a difficult political prospect, and censorship of educational materials on the grounds that they are offensive or that they encourage homosexual activities or drug use is not unusual. Nevertheless, AIDS education in some form has been mandated by federal or state governments for the general public, for high-risk groups, for health care professionals, and for schools (6).

Sustained change in behavior requires not only the personal desire to change but also a reinforcing social environment that supports the new pattern of behavior. It is not enough to know that one should practice safer sex and to want to do so; it is not even enough that one's partner secretly feels the same way. Both must feel confident that this is an important and correct decision that is supported and promoted by the society in which they live. Only by keeping this message always before people in straightforward, unambiguous terms will they be able to internalize it and truly learn the new behavior. For example, books and stories in newspapers, product advertisements on radio and television, and scenes and dialogue in television programs and films can all help engender behavior change by showing that the intended behavior is the accepted behavior. Ads for condoms, if accepted by the television networks, could promote wider use of condoms. Yet, even in 1990, no American network is willing to broadcast paid advertisements for condoms, arguing that such decisions should be left up to local affiliates more closely in touch with standards in their communities.

Homosexual communities in cities such as San Francisco and New York, hardest hit by AIDS, were earliest to organize patient support services and an extensive array of educational interventions aimed at preventing spread of infection. These have included community outreach to encourage wide participation, distribution of educational literature, broadcast media campaigns, individual counseling and testing, telephone hotlines, and peer discussion and support groups to reinforce change. These efforts proved successful in altering sexual behavior. For example, 90% of a cohort of 125 homosexual men followed at the San Francisco City Clinic between 1978 and 1985 had reduced the reported number of nonsteady partners from a median of 16 to a median of one (7).

Keeping the message before people means more than brochures and advertising campaigns. It is also necessary to see that the tools associated with the desired behavior change are readily and openly available. During World War II, the Army aggressively warned troops about the dangers of venereal disease and actively promoted condoms with the slogan, "If you can't say no, take a pro [a prophylactic or condom]." The military sold or distributed freely as many as 50 million condoms each month during the war, and between 1940 and 1943 (prior to the introduction of penicillin), the venereal disease rate in the Army fell from 42.5 to 25 per 1,000 (8). One strategy of particular controversy is that of making condoms available to high school students. As offensive as this may be to the moral beliefs of some, it must be acknowledged that those teenagers who are sexually active should be encouraged to protect themselves and others against AIDS.

AIDS is not mentioned in the President's National Drug Control Strategy, even though needle-fsharing is one of the chief modes of transmission (6). Nevertheless, a number of cities in the United States have introduced educational and behavior change programs intended to reduce dependence on intravenous drugs and to reduce the risk of HIV transmission among intravenous drug abusers. These programs have included expanded methadone and residential treatment programs (9), vouchers for entry into detoxification programs (10), and various outreach efforts to addicts (11). More controversial are proposals to decriminalize the possession of needles and syringes, to authorize the sale of needles and syringes by pharmacists to drug users undergoing treatment, to distribute bleach for the cleaning of needles, and to institute needle exchange programs (6). United States officials are particularly uncomfortable with the idea of making needles available to addicts, although needle exchange programs have been conducted in the Netherlands apparently without increasing the number of addicts or reducing entry into treatment programs (12).

Of the more than 1.2 million intravenous drug users in the United States, fewer than 250,000 are estimated to be in treatment at any one time. In some parts of the country, those who seek treatment encounter a waiting period of more than six months. In an effort to reduce the spread of AIDS by reducing the number of drug users, the President's Commission on the Human Immunodeficiency Virus Epidemic called for 2,500 new treatment sites and an additional annual investment of $1.5 billion in drug-control programs.

Such new treatment efforts could contribute simultaneously to the solution to two daunting health and social problems: illicit drug use and HIV infection. The two are interrelated and flourish in the same populations. Any intervention that reduces intravenous drug use will help deter the spread of HIV. The tension between those concerned with drugs and those concerned with AIDS arises because some interventions that diminish the risk of HIV transmission (such as needle exchange or use of bleach to clean needles and syringes) lend the appearance of condoning, or at least acknowledging, the continued use of intravenous drugs. The most sensible and effective programs will establish and maintain contact with intravenous-drug-using populations, offer means to maintain life free of HIV infection through such measures as bleach and needle exchange, and continually promote opportunities to become and to stay drug-free.

DISCRIMINATION

Through association with sex, blood, drugs, and death, AIDS provokes intense emotional responses. There is a compelling moral controversy for many people about the lifestyles and behaviors that are most closely associated with AIDS in industrialized countries. At the same time, there is still a widespread lack of understanding, or a mistrust of the facts presented, about the ways the virus can be transmitted, which can result in irrational fears and strong aversions. These factors combine to produce the risk of stigmatization, ostracism, isolation, and discrimination for the AIDS patient.

One reason for confusion about AIDS is that the public receives mixed messages, both reassuring and alarming, from responsible officials (5). Public health authorities insist that HIV is not transmitted through the air, by mosquito bites, or through everyday interaction. At the same time, the public is told that AIDS is everyone's problem, that women as well as men are at risk, and that taking protective action is wise. The public is told that HIV has been isolated from saliva and tears, but is also told that kissing on the cheek or even the lips will not transmit AIDS. To the physician or epidemiologist schooled in the transmission of viral disease, the dual message is eminently sensible. The layperson runs an understandable risk of confusion, which can easily lead to the belief that the best way to keep from becoming infected with AIDS is to avoid all contact with known carriers of the virus.

Surveys in the U.S. and other countries conducted between 1983 and 1988 point to increasing prejudice against homosexuals, to the belief that testing for AIDS will result in discrimination against those carrying the virus, and to the conviction that measures to control the spread of AIDS are more important than the privacy of those who have AIDS. The majority of respondents favored the criminalization of blood donation by a person with AIDS (84%) and believed it should be a crime for a person who knows that he or she has AIDS to have sex with another person (68%). Twice the percentage of people in 1988 (30%) as in 1985 favored tatooing those infected with the AIDS virus. Between one in five and one in four Americans — one in three in the southern states — believe that they should not be required to work with, send their children to school with, or live near someone with AIDS. In fact, a sizable minority of those questioned thought that those with AIDS should be completely isolated from the rest of society (13). Such prejudices lead to widespread discrimination against people who have AIDS or who belong to groups at risk for AIDS.

Most of the U.S. states (as well as the federal government) have declared that their handicap antidiscrimination laws apply to AIDS, and many have enacted AIDS-specific legislation. The application of handicap laws to persons with AIDS brings with it the requirement of "reasonable accommodation" to enable an otherwise qualified individual to fulfill performance criteria. Lawsuits pertaining to discrimination focus on the key areas of education, employment, housing, insurance, and access to health care and reflect a wide range of practices, from isolating a schoolchild in a glass cubicle, to evicting family members of a person with AIDS, to denying medical coverage for possibly effective drugs. Although litigation pertaining to the workplace, school attendance, housing, and provision of personal services is declining, it is anticipated that complaints will continue to increase in the areas of health care, nursing, and social services (14).

Health care professionals are not exempt from the fears and prejudices that others feel about people with AIDS. Although the risk of infection is low, precautions taken to prevent exposure to infected blood and body fluids present a constant reminder of the occupational hazard these substances pose. This fear of infection can affect the quality of treatment patients with AIDS receive. Treatment may even be denied altogether, as in the case of at least one hospital whose policy is to transfer to other institutions those patients found to carry the AIDS virus. Discrimination in this context is just as unnecessary, and just as illegal, as discrimination in other areas, while carrying the added insult of violating the medical community's moral obligation to provide care.

On an international level, the World Health Organization's Global Programme on AIDS sponsored a World Summit of Ministers of Health in 1988, which concluded with a declaration that emphasized broadening the scope of AIDS education, promoting worldwide exchange of information, and reinforcing the importance of nondiscriminatory policies. The 41st World Health Assembly in Geneva the same year adopted a formal resolution endorsing confidentiality of HIV testing and urging member states to avoid discrimination against AIDS patients in the provision of services, in employment, and in travel. A similar call for antidiscrimination laws was the first recommendation of the June 1988 report of the U.S. Presidential Commission on the HIV Epidemic.

Despite the Presidential Commission's recommendation of antidiscrimination, the U.S. Immigration and Naturalization Service still requires that prospective immigrants be tested. Visitors may be tested or may simply be excluded if evidence of HIV infection is found (14). Although there is no sound public health justification for restricting travel and immigration on the basis of HIV status, three-quarters of Americans polled on this question favored barring foreign visitors with AIDS from the United States (13). As the public becomes better educated about the disease, lawmakers will perhaps take more positive steps to recognize that AIDS can only be contained by a coordinated, international public health effort.

CONCLUSION

Civil rights legislation, such as that which protects women, minorities, and the handicapped, normally precedes general public acceptance of the rights of the protected group. The AIDS epidemic has created a new and growing minority group that requires similar protection against discrimination. Predictably, such protection is opposed by an outspoken segment of the population. Lawmakers honor their highest obligations to the public good when they resist the pressures of constituents who are not well-informed and institute policies that will ensure compassionate and dignified treatment for those affected by AIDS.

Laws regarding privacy and discrimination must be accompanied by measures to promote prevention, that is, to protect the uninfected. The best hope for prevention is education, and the most effective education is explicit, pervasive, and tailored to each group at risk. Appropriate, mandated education may offend some people. However, this is a small price to pay to control the spread of a devastating disease.

REFERENCES

1. Gostin LO. Public health strategies for confronting AIDS: legislative and regulatory policy in the United States. *JAMA* 1989; 261:1621-1630.
2. Fineberg HV. Screening for HIV infection and public health policy. *Law, Medicine & Health Care* 1990; 18:29-32.
3. Cleary PD, Barry MJ, Mayer KH, Brandt AM, Gostin LO, Fineberg HV. Compulsory premarital screening for the human immunodeficiency virus: technical and public health considerations. *JAMA* 1987; 258:1757-1762.
4. Turnock BJ and Kelly CJ. Mandatory premarital testing for human immunodeficiency virus: the Illinois experience. *JAMA* 1989; 261:3415-3418.
5. Fineberg HV. Education to prevent AIDS: prospects and obstacles. *Science* 1988; 239:592-596.
6. Gostin LO. A decade of a maturing epidemic: an assessment and directions for future public policy. *American Journal of Law & Medicine* 1990; 16:1-32.
7. Doll LS, Darrow W, O'Malley P, Bodecker T, Jaffe H. Self-reported behavioral change in homosexual men in the San Francisco City Clinic cohort. Third International Conference on AIDS, Washington DC, 1-5 June 1987. Abstracts Volume, p. 213.
8. Brandt AM. No Magic Bullet. New York: Oxford University Press, 1985.
9. Jackson J, Rodriguez G, Baxter R, Neshin S. AIDS/ARC patients in residential drug treatment therapeutic communities: a special program. Third International Conference on AIDS, Washington DC, 1-5 June 1987. Abstracts Volume, p. 45.
10. McCauliffe WE, Doering S, Breer P, Silverman H, Branson B, Williams K. An evaluation of using ex-addict outreach workers to educate intravenous drug users about AIDS prevention. Third International Conference on AIDS, Washington DC, 1-5 June 1987. Abstracts Volume, p. 40.
11. Watters JK. Preventing human immunodeficiency virus contagion among intravenous drug users: the impact of street-based education on risk-behavior. Third International Conference on AIDS, Washington DC, 1- 5 June 1987. Abstracts Volume, p. 60.
12. Buning EC. Prevention policy on AIDS among drug addicts in Amsterdam. Third International Conference on AIDS, Washington DC, 1-5 June 1987. Abstracts Volume, p. 40.
13. Blendon RJ and Donelan K. Discrimination against people with AIDS: the public's perspective. *New Engl J Med* 1988; 319:1022-1026.
14. Gostin LO. The AIDS litigation project: a national review of court and human rights commission decisions, part II: discrimination. *JAMA* 1990; 263:2086-2093.

FACTORS AFFECTING FEMALE-TO-MALE TRANSMISSION OF HIV-1: IMPLICATIONS OF TRANSMISSION DYNAMICS FOR PREVENTION

Francis A. Plummer

University of Manitoba

Stephen Moses

University of Nairobi

Jackoniah O. Ndinya–Achola

University of Nairobi

Over the past decade, HIV-1 infection has spread throughout the world, infecting millions of individuals. The problem is most severe in Africa, where the World Health Organization's Global Programme on AIDS estimated that approximately 2.5 million individuals were infected in 1988 (1). The primary route of transmission of HIV-1 is heterosexual intercourse (2).

At present, in the absence of specific biologic means of interrupting the transmission of the virus, we must rely on less direct strategies for control. To succeed, these strategies must be based on an understanding of the biologic and behavioral factors that created and have sustained the epidemic. In this chapter we review what is understood about factors affecting transmissibility of HIV-1. The main focus will be on factors known or thought to alter female-to-male heterosexual transmission. We will review data from recent studies conducted by our group in Nairobi that identify behavioral and biologic risk factors for HIV-1 infection in Africa. We will try to synthesize what we know into an overall model, and will propose ways in which our knowledge can be used for the design of interventions.

EVOLUTION OF OUR UNDERSTANDING OF FEMALE-TO-MALE TRANSMISSION OF HIV-1

In early studies from North America among hemophiliacs and their spouses (3,4), the apparent frequency of heterosexual transmission was low, leading to estimates of male-to-female transmission of 0.1-1% per sexual encounter (5,6). There were relatively few female index cases to permit estimation of the female-to-male transmission rate. By extrapolation from other sexually transmitted diseases (STDs), it was assumed that transmission from an infected woman to her male sex partners would be even less efficient. This was supported by data on behavioral risk factors for HIV-1 among gay men that showed that anal receptive intercourse was the main risk factor and that there was a much lower risk of HIV-1 acquisition associated with anal insertive intercourse (7). Apparently, the male genitalia were difficult to infect with HIV. Padian et al. have estimated the female-to-male transmission rate to be one in 1000 sexual encounters between an infected woman and a susceptible man (6).

These emerging data and estimates were hard to reconcile with the situation described in central Africa in 1984-85. In the first studies involving Africans (conducted in Europe), Clumeck et al. observed both men and women with AIDS (8). The first reports of studies in Africa showed similar results (9,10), with AIDS occurring with roughly equal frequency in men and women. Later it was shown that roughly equal numbers of men and women were infected with what later became known as HIV-1.

When HIV antibody testing became widely available, there was an explosion of information about HIV-1 prevalence in African countries with seemingly cataclysmic significance. The prevalence of HIV-1 was extremely high in samples that were probably representative of the general population of several countries, e.g., 6% in Kinshasa hospital workers (11) and 12% in pregnant women in Kampala (12). These numbers were scarcely to be believed. How could such a high prevalence of HIV-1 have occurred in such a short period of time if female-to-male and male-to-female transmission of the virus was rare? As men must be infected for women to become infected, how could female-to-male transmission be particularly rare? To achieve these prevalence levels with low female-to-male transmission rates, a long period of time, extremely high numbers of sexual partners, or another route of transmission was required.

In considering how female-to-male transmission of HIV-1 might be enhanced in some circumstances, one can conceive of two categories of risk factors: factors that alter the susceptibility of exposed men, and factors that increase the infectivity of HIV-1-infected women for their sex partners. Sexual practices or behaviors that increase the sexual exposure of susceptible men to infected women are, of course, also important as risk factors, but do not directly affect transmissibility.

In their first report, Piot et al. found that heterosexual promiscuity was an important risk factor for AIDS (9). They speculated that the uncontrolled epidemics of STDs in Africa were in part responsible for the seeming facility of heterosexual transmission of HIV-1.

In attempting to study this problem, our first work on HIV-1 in men was a retrospective study of HIV-1 seroprevalence in men with genital ulcers attending an STD clinic in Nairobi (13,14). The prevalence in these men rose from "undetectable" in 1980 to 18% in 1985. Although we did not have comparable historic sera, we found much lower rates of HIV-1 infection in men with gonococcal urethritis attending the same clinic. We hypothesized, therefore, that genital ulcers led in some way to greater female-to-male transmission of HIV-1. As a result of these initial studies, we developed a series of studies specifically designed to assess the role of genital ulcers in promoting HIV-1 transmission. (A second risk factor for HIV-1 in these early studies was place of birth. Men born in western Kenya, bordering Uganda, were at higher risk. We initially interpreted these results as indicating geographic spread from the epicenter of the epidemic in central Africa to Kenya.)

The potential relationships between STDs and HIV-1 are complex, since the primary risk factor for all STDs, including HIV-1 infection, is sexual behavior. It is difficult to separate a direct causal association from a spurious one; inevitable bias is introduced by the fact that all STDs are transmitted by sex, and the fact that the more sexual partners an individual has, the greater are the individual's chances of acquiring one or more STD. A further complication is that, through production of immune deficiency, HIV-1 could — and probably does — increase susceptibility to other STDs. In conducting epidemiologic studies, these complex relationships need to be taken into account.

Another early study of ours was a cross-sectional analysis of risk factors for HIV-1 infection in men who reported contact with a group of women working as prostitutes, whom we were following concurrently (15). These women had an extremely high seroprevalence of HIV-1 infec-

Table 1. Genital ulcers and lack of circumcision as risk factors for prevalent HIV-1 infection in men attending an STD clinic in Nairobi (adapted from reference 18).

	Odds Ratio	95% confidence intervals	p
Travel to neighbouring countries	9.0	2.3–35.2	<.002
Frequent prostitute contact	3.1	1.0–10.0	=.07
Circumcised			
no past genital ulcers	0	–	–
past genital ulcers	18.2	6.4–61.7	<.001
Uncircumcised			
no past genital ulcers	5.2	1.6–18.8	<.01
past genital ulcers	8.2	2.2–30.0	<.001

tion, with over 85% HIV-1 seropositive at the time we began the study of the men (16,17). Among men attending the Nairobi STD clinic who had an STD and reported one of these women as a source contact, 11% were HIV-1 seropositive (18).

Five factors were found to be associated with increased risk of HIV-1: a past history of genital ulcers, a current diagnosis of genital ulcers, frequent prostitute contact, lack of circumcision, and travel outside Kenya. On multivariate analysis by logistic regression, travel outside Kenya, past genital ulcers, and being uncircumcised were independently associated with an increased risk of HIV-1. (These results are summarized in Table 1). Because HIV-1 might cause increased susceptibility to genital ulcers, and because uncircumcised men are well known to have more frequent genital ulcers, particularly chancroid, this study was inconclusive as to the direction of cause and effect between these risk factors and HIV-1 infection.

The objectives of our next study were to determine if these risk factors were associated with incident HIV-1 infection and to estimate the frequency of female-to-male HIV-1 transmission (19). The study design involved following a cohort of men who reported sexual intercourse with the group of prostitutes described above. With the 85% prevalence rate of HIV-1 infection among these women, the probability of a man having sex with an HIV-1-infected woman approached one. As the risk of men acquiring another STD from these women is also high, and the incubation times of conventional STDs are much shorter than the time required to develop HIV-1 antibody, men would generally present for STD treatment before seroconversion occurred.

We recruited a cohort of 293 HIV-1 seronegative men who presented with an STD to the Nairobi STD clinic and followed them for the occurrence of seroconversion. The crude rate of seroconversion we observed was 8.2%. The probability of seroconversion, determined by survivorship analysis, was 13%. If one estimates that only 85% of men were actually exposed to HIV-1, then the overall transmission rate is 15.3% by survivorship analysis.

Three factors were associated with seroconversion: frequent prostitute contact, a presenting diagnosis of genital ulcers (primarily chancroid), and being uncircumcised. The seroconversion rate for circumcised men with ulcers was 13.4%; the rate for uncircumcised men with no genital ulcers was 29.0%. Among men with both factors, the rate of HIV-1 seroconversion was 52.6%. Seroconversion generally occurred within six weeks of exposure. Analysis of these factors by logistic regression showed that they were independently associated with seroconversion with odds ratios of 4.7 (95% CI 1.3–17.0) for genital ulcers and 8.2 (95% CI 3.0–23.0) for lack of circumcision. The same was true when we separately analyzed men who reported that their recent

Table 2. Genital ulcers and lack of circumcision increase risk of incident HIV-1 infection after prostitute contact (adapted from reference 19).

	Incidence of HIV-1 Seroconversion
Circumcised, no genital ulcers	2.5%
Circumcised, genital ulcers	13.4%
Uncircumcised, no genital ulcers	29.0%
Uncircumcised, genital ulcers	52.6%

contact with a prostitute was their first ever prostitute experience. (These results are summarized in Table 2).

GENITAL ULCERS INCREASE INFECTIVITY OF WOMEN FOR MALE SEX PARTNERS

In the male STD cohort study described above, the exposure to the STD that resulted in clinic attendance and the exposure to HIV-1 were likely to have been concomitant, i.e., both infections were probably acquired at the same time. Thus, the excess risk associated with genital ulcers in men was probably indicative of the presence of genital ulcers in the female contact. Using this logic, we observed an increased infectivity of women with both genital ulcers and HIV-1 compared to women with only HIV-1 or women with HIV-1 and another STD. We cannot absolutely rule out the possibility that pre-contact genital ulcers in exposed males increased susceptibility to HIV-1, as occurs in women. We have found, however, that, because ulcers are extremely painful, men generally cannot or do not continue to have sex after they recognize that they have a genital ulcer.

In studies conducted among the women in our prostitute population, we obtained direct evidence that genital ulcers increase HIV-1 shedding in the female genital tract (20). In HIV-1-infected women with genital ulcers, HIV-1 was isolated from 4 of 36 ulcers (11%) cultured. HIV-1 was also isolated from the cervical secretions of 2 of 4 women with positive ulcer cultures.

LACK OF CIRCUMCISION AS A FACTOR INCREASING SUSCEPTIBILITY OF MEN TO HIV-1

The presence of a foreskin appears to be a factor influencing susceptibility of men to HIV-1. The exact mechanism by which this occurs is uncertain, but several potential mechanisms can be proposed: 1) the area underneath the foreskin provides a warm, moist environment, which enhances virus survival; 2) minor inflammatory conditions are common in uncircumcised men, and these could permit virus penetration by producing mucosal breaks; and 3) the foreskin could be more susceptible to trauma and microscopic bleeding during intercourse, producing portals of entry for the virus.

There is great potential for confounding in the observed association between being uncircumcised and HIV-1 infection because circumcision is a religious and ethnic practice, which may, in turn, influence sexual behavior, and because circumcision is sometimes used as a therapy for genital ulcers. However, several other studies have since found similar associations between HIV-1 and lack of circumcision in males. Studies from Miami (21), Atlanta (22), Ivory Coast (23), and among East African truck drivers (24) have all found a higher risk of HIV-1 infection in uncircumcised men.

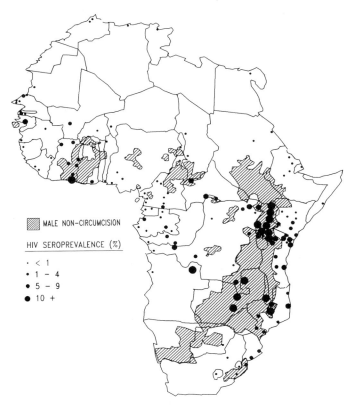

Figure 1. Seroprevalence of HIV-1 in Africa and male circumcision practices (from reference 26, used with permission).

Table 3. HIV prevalence in the general adult population and male circumcision practice in 140 geographically distinct locations in Africa (adapted from reference 26).

	General Adult Population HIV Seroprevalence (%)			
	<1	1-4	5-9	10+
male circumcision practiced	66	21	8	1
male circumcision not practiced	2	18	8	16

p<.001, Chi-square

Another approach that has been taken to study the association between male circumcision practices and the HIV-1 epidemic in Africa is comparison of the geographic patterns of HIV-1 seroprevalence with the ethnic patterns of male circumcision. Two such studies have been performed. The first, by Bongaarts et al. (25), compared the reported HIV seroprevalence in African capital cities with national male circumcision practices. They found a very strong correlation. Our group performed a similar study (26), in which the reported HIV-1 seroprevalence in general population samples from 140 locations in Africa was related to ethnic male circumcision practices gleaned from the anthropologic literature. There was a striking association. As shown in the map in Figure 1, male circumcision is not practiced in areas of highest HIV-1 prevalence. A comparison of high and low HIV prevalence areas with circumcision practice is shown in Table 3. Although these ecologic studies cannot prove that the intact foreskin renders men more susceptible to HIV-1, they are certainly very consistent with that hypothesis. Such a relationship would do much to explain some of the puzzling geographic variations in HIV prevalence, such as the fact that Nigeria and Cameroon have apparently little HIV while neighbouring Ghana and Ivory Coast have much more severe problems. It might also explain our earlier observation of increased frequency of HIV-1 in men originating in western Kenya.

The relationship between the male foreskin and HIV-1 is complicated by the fact that, as noted above, uncircumcised men are more susceptible to chancroid, and probably to other STDs as well (27). In populations in which men are uncircumcised, the overall burden of STDs that could potentially facilitate HIV-1 transmission is possibly much greater. In our assessment, both mechanisms are probably operative in communities where circumcision is not practiced. The foreskin directly increases the susceptibility of men to HIV-1 and indirectly affects the prevalence of STDs in the population. This promotes transmission of HIV-1 by rendering women more susceptible to HIV-1, and subsequently results in increased infectivity of HIV-1-infected women for their male sex partners.

An additional twist in these relationships is that chancroid, the main cause of genital ulcers in much of Africa, is more frequent, more severe, and more refractory to treatment in individuals with HIV-1 infection (28). Thus, a complex cycle of amplification or mutual facilitation between lack of circumcision, genital ulcers, and HIV-1 is involved in promoting heterosexual transmission of HIV-1: the penile foreskin increases the susceptibility of men to HIV-1 and chancroid; HIV-1 increases the susceptibility of men and women to chancroid and other genital ulcers; and genital ulcers render women more infectious for male sex partners.

FACTORS INCREASING EXPOSURE

Behavioral factors are, of course, also important for HIV-1 infection in males. In order for men to be infected with HIV-1, appropriate exposure must occur. One of the major behavioral factors that has been identified to date is the practice of sex for money. In our studies among men with STDs (18,19) and long-distance truck drivers (24), it was shown that men who have sex with women who sell sex are at higher risk of HIV-1 infection. Conveniently for the virus, women who sell sex also have a high prevalence of genital ulcers, which, if they are also infected with HIV-1, increases their HIV-1 infectivity.

There have been few studies among men who do not belong to groups at high risk of HIV-1 exposure, so information about the overall prevalence of sex-for-money activities and their contribution to the epidemic is limited. What we do know suggests that these activities occur very frequently in sub-Saharan Africa. In our study of long-distance truck drivers, who were recruited solely on the basis of their occupation, sex with prostitutes was reported by 61% of participants, with a quarter of the men visiting prostitutes at least once a week (24). This is probably one extreme of sexual behavior, but given the migrant nature of many work forces in Africa, it may not be an uncommon extreme. In a study of the work forces of two businesses in Kinshasa, Ryder et al. found that a quarter of men reported having had sex with a prostitute in the previous two years (25).

If sex-for-money is one factor affecting the transmission of HIV-1, then the socio-economic conditions that lead to women selling sex and men buying sex might be seen as another set of factors facilitating female-to-male transmission of HIV-1. These conditions are primarily the economic and social forces that deny some African women other means of livelihood and result in large pools of migrant male labour. The absence of effective health services and control programs for STDs in most African countries may also be considered factors that affect the transmission of HIV-1.

Other behavioral factors, such as sex during menses, have not been shown, in our work or in studies of couples, to be associated with HIV-1 infection in men (29,30,31,32). The reason for this is possibly that few couples have sex during menses. It would seem reasonable to assume that menstrual flow would increase viral shedding in the female genital tract. Sexual practices that result in an increased frequency of genital mucosal disruption during intercourse could possibly increase transmission as well. However, there are no data to substantiate these hypotheses.

A MODEL OF FEMALE-TO-MALE TRANSMISSION OF HIV-1

With the results of the epidemiologic studies described above, a partial model of female-to-male transmission of HIV-1 in Africa can be constructed. Socio-economic conditions (principally poverty and migrant work forces) have resulted in the frequent selling and buying of sex in many African societies. Genital ulcers, which have a high incidence in women working as prostitutes, increase the susceptibility of women to HIV-1 so the women rapidly become infected with HIV-1. Genital ulcers increase the infectivity of HIV-1-infected women by increasing viral shedding, resulting in relatively frequent transmission of the infection to men. HIV-1-induced immune deficiency results in an increased prevalence of genital ulcers in the population. Uncircumcised men are more susceptible to HIV-1 given appropriate exposure; so, in societies where male circumcision is not practiced, the foreskin serves to increase both the prevalence of genital ulcers and the prevalence of HIV-1, amplifying the entire process.

RESEARCH NEEDS

Do we completely understand female-to-male transmission of HIV-1? What factors other than those discussed might influence female-to-male transmission? Approaching these questions systematically, we need to consider factors that increase exposure, increase genital shedding of HIV-1 in infected women, and alter the susceptibility of men to HIV-1.

Many social and cultural beliefs can influence the degree of sexual exposure in a population. Why do men seek sex from prostitutes despite knowledge of the risks? Who are these men and how do we identify them so that they can be reached by targeted interventions? What are the dynamics of male populations that constitute the clients of prostitutes? There are no ready answers to these questions, but it seems safe to predict that factors influencing sexual behavior will be complex, to some extent culture- or circumstance-specific, and tied to socio-economic conditions. We must understand these factors if we hope to be able to change them.

What additional factors influence viral shedding in the female genital tract? Non-ulcerative STDs could increase HIV-1 shedding in the female genital tract in much the same way that genital ulcers appear to. Age, the presence of cervical ectopy, type of contraceptive use, and pregnancy could all conceivably alter viral shedding in women. Quantitative studies of viral shedding in both sexes are urgently needed to address these issues.

What other factors might alter the susceptibility of men to HIV-1? As discussed above, genital ulcers probably do increase men's susceptibility to HIV-1 simply by providing a portal of entry. But do men with ulcers continue to have sex? Other STDs or genital conditions, such as balanitis, could alter susceptibility in the same way. If this were so, then the teaching of improved hygienic practices could reduce the susceptibility of men to HIV-1.

POTENTIAL APPLICATION TO HIV-1 CONTROL

How does our knowledge of female-to-male transmission of HIV-1 become incorporated into control programs? Over the past two to three years, control of STDs has been adopted as a strategy for control of HIV-1. There are several reasons why this is an attractive approach in both theory and practice. The evidence that STDs increase the rate of transmission of HIV-1 is strong and makes good biologic sense. Furthermore, conventional STDs and HIV-1 affect the same population subgroups; thus, even in the absence of evidence that STDs facilitate HIV-1 transmission, it would seem logical to develop programs targeted at people with STDs. In addition, STDs are important health problems in their own right and need to be controlled.

Still, many important questions remain. Will STD control really alter HIV-1 transmission? What is STD control? Which STDs are most important to the spread of HIV-1? Our answer to the first question is an unequivocal yes. The ultimate success of an STD control approach is dependent upon the answers to the latter questions.

What is STD control? The available strategies to control STDs overlap with strategies employed to date for HIV-1 control. These strategies consist of modifying sexual behavior; encouraging use of barrier contraceptives; treating symptomatic cases; detecting asymptomatic infections; and tracing the sex contacts of infected individuals. The latter three strategies, which are specific to STD control, rely heavily on laboratory diagnosis and require substantial personnel resources for diagnosis, treatment, and contact tracing. They have had a limited impact on the incidence and complications of some STDs, even in industrialized nations.

The type of activities being proposed as STD control in many HIV-control programs consist primarily of strengthening STD diagnosis and management. This does not represent STD control so much as STD treatment. Our belief (although there is little evidence to substantiate it) is that these activities will have a relatively limited impact on STD incidence and prevalence for the following reasons. Most STD transmitters are asymptomatic, presymptomatic, or ignore symptoms, as occurs commonly among female prostitutes. Most individuals who have symptomatic STDs seek treatment rapidly and do not transmit the infection while they are symptomatic; even in the most resource poor settings, such individuals obtain some type of effective treatment. Thus, better treatment, while in itself an important goal, might do relatively little to reduce transmission of STDs. Similarly, partner referral or contact tracing will be of limited effectiveness in controlling STDs because of the sheer magnitude of the problem, the anonymity of many STD-transmitting sexual encounters, and the implications that notifying a partner may have for a relationship. Even if successful, contact tracing might be of limited benefit. Contact tracing or partner referral is much better at identifying "downstream" contacts, such as steady sexual partners, than "upstream" contacts, who are more important in the transmission dynamics of STDs. Yorke and Hethcote, who coined the term "high frequency transmission core groups" to describe those individuals in a population who are responsible for STD transmission, estimate that the maximum reduction in STD morbidity achievable through partner referral and case detection is 20% (33). Reducing HIV transmission by 20% obviously would be unsatisfactory.

With the possible exception of syphilis, and now HIV, STD control programs have not been implemented to any appreciable extent in the developing countries of Africa. It seems improbable that the industrialized-country model of STD control could be effectively implemented in African countries because of the limitations of resources and expertise, reluctance to use barrier contraceptives, and logistical difficulties. However, in the midst of the HIV epidemic, the need for tools to control the spread of STDs and HIV is urgent.

A more effective approach to STD and HIV control might be to incorporate intensive programs focusing on high frequency STD transmitters (HFTs) into current control efforts. The result would be a four-tiered, comprehensive program consisting of: 1) general educational or behavioral programs aimed at reducing the highest-risk behaviors; 2) targeted programs for HFTs aimed at changing behavior; 3) programs for the promotion of condom use among HFT groups; and 4) development and improvement of diagnostic and treatment services for HFTs. Such an approach would have the result of reducing the size of HFT populations, promoting condom use among HFT groups, reducing contact between HFT groups and the population at large, and reducing the prevalence of certain STDs within HFT groups and, ultimately, the whole population.

While these efforts must begin now, optimal implementation requires additional knowledge. What are the relative contributions of social, behavioral, and biological factors to the HIV epidemic? What is the quantitative contribution of HFTs to the burden of HIV infection in the population? How can we identify HFTs for targeting? What fraction of HIV infection in the population is attributable to the interaction of STDs and HIV?

Which STDs are most important to control? Genital ulcers, gonococcal infections, chlamydial infection, and agents causing vaginitis have all been associated with increased risk of HIV-1 transmission. Do we need to control them all to reduce HIV-1 transmission? If we must control trichomonas, which can affect up to 40% of women in African societies, the task is, indeed, formidable. Genital ulcers have been associated with increased risk of female-to-male and male-to-female HIV-1 transmission; the increase in risk observed for transmission from female to male may be as great as 100 fold, and the increase in risk for male-to-female transmission is probably greater. The increased transmissibility resulting from non-ulcerative STDs has not been quantified, but from the odds ratios and relative risks reported, it is likely to be less than that resulting from genital ulcers. On the other hand, genital ulcers are less frequent than other STDs, and despite a greater effect on transmissibility, the population attributable risk of non-ulcerative STDs could be higher. Current data do not permit a conclusion, but it is our contention that, because genital ulcers influence heterosexual transmission bi-directionally, and because they have a very clear role in altering HIV-1 transmissibility in populations of HFTs, genital ulcer control alone may be effective in significantly reducing HIV-1 transmission.

Finally, is promotion of male circumcision a viable strategy for HIV-1 and STD control? There are certain attractions to such a strategy. Circumcision is done once and is permanent and irreversible. If the data are correct, it would simultaneously reduce men's susceptibility to HIV-1 and genital ulcers, reducing the overall population prevalence of both. There is considerable indigenous expertise in circumcision in many African societies. Promoting male circumcision may be a more achievable goal than continuously providing condoms to all who need them. But there are many obstacles in the way of such an approach, particularly the strongly held cultural beliefs that would make acceptance of it difficult in some countries, and the fact that circumcision in adult men is not a trivial operation. Nevertheless, the strategy merits serious consideration. At a minimum, the introduction or re-introduction of newborn circumcision, as is increasingly ocurring in the United States, should be considered. Further study of this issue is certainly warranted.

Acknowledgments

This work was supported in part by grants from the Medical Research Council of Canada (Ottawa), the International Development Research Centre (Ottawa), the National Health Research Development Program (Ottawa), and the American Foundation for AIDS Research. Dr. Plummer is the recipient of a Scientist award from the Medical Research Council of Canada.

REFERENCES

1. Chin J, Sato PA, Mann JM. Projections of HIV infections and AIDS to the year 2000. *Bull WHO* 1990; 68:1–11.
2. Piot P, Plummer FA, Mhalu FS et al. AIDS: An international perspective. *Science* 1988; 239:573–9.
3. Kreiss JK, Kitchen LW, Prince HE et al. Antibody to human T–lymphotropic virus III in wives of hemophiliacs: Evidence of heterosexual transmission. *Ann Intern Med* 1985; 102:623–6.
4. Jason JM, McDougal JS, Dixon G et al. HTLV–III/LAV antibody and immune status of household contacts and sexual partners of persons with hemophilia. *J Amer Med Assoc* 1986; 255:212–5.
5. Peterman TA, Stoneburner RL, Allen JR, Jaffe HW, Curran JW. Risk of human immun-

odeficiency virus transmission from heterosexual adults with transfusion associated infections. *J Amer Med Assoc* 1988; 259:55–8.

6.   Padian N, Marquis L, Francis DP et al. Male to female transmission of human immunodeficiency virus. *J Amer Med Assoc* 1987; 258:788–90.

7.   Jaffe HW, Darrow WW, Echenburg DF et al. The acquired immunodeficiency syndrome in a cohort of homosexual men. A six–year follow–up study. *Ann Intern Med* 1985; 103:210–4.

8.   Clumeck N, Sonnet J, Taelman H et al. Acquired immunodeficiency syndrome in Africans. *N Engl J Med* 1984; 310:492–7.

9.   Piot P, Quinn TC, Taelman H et al. Acquired immunodeficiency syndrome in a heterosexual population in Zaire. *Lancet* 1984; ii:65–9.

10. Van de Perre P, Rouvroy D, Lepage P et al. Acquired immunodeficiency syndrome in Rwanda. *Lancet* 1984; ii:62–5.

11. Ngaly B, Ryder RW, Bila K et al. Human immundeficiency virus infection among employees in an African hospital. *N Engl J Med* 1988; 319:1123–7.

12. Carswell JW. HIV infection in healthy persons in Uganda. *AIDS* 1987; 1:223–7.

13. Piot P, Plummer FA, Rey M–A et al. Retrospective seroepidemiology of AIDS virus infection in Nairobi populations. *J Infect Dis* 1987; 155:1108–12.

14. Greenblatt R, Lukehart S, Plummer FA et al. Genital ulceration as a risk factor for human-immunodeficiency virus infection. *AIDS* 1988; 2:47–50.

15. Kreiss JK, Koech D, Plummer FA et al. AIDS virus infection in Nairobi Prostitutes: Extension of the epidemic to East Africa. *N Engl J Med* 1986; 314:414–8.

16. Simonsen JN, Plummer FA, Ngugi EN et al. HIV infection among lower socioeconomic strata prostitutes in Nairobi. *AIDS* 1990; 4:139-144.

17. Plummer FA, Simonsen JN, Cameron DW et al. Co–factors in male to female transmission of HIV–1. *J Infect Dis* (in press)

18. Simonsen JN, Cameron DW, Gakinya MN et al. Human immunodeficiency virus infection in men with sexually transmitted diseases: Experience from a center in Africa. *N Engl J Med* 1988; 319:274–8.

19. Cameron DW, Simonsen JN, D'Costa LJ et al. Female to male transmission of HIV–1: Risk factors for seroconversion in men. *Lancet* 1989; ii:403–8.

20. Kreiss JK, Coombs R, Plummer FA et al. Isolation of HIV–1 from genital ulcers in prostitutes. *J Infect Dis* 1989; 160:380–4.

21. Fischl M, Fayne T, Flanagan S et al. Seroprevalence and risks of HIV infections in spouses of persons infected with HIV. IV International Conference on AIDS, Stockholm, Sweden, June 1988.

22. Whittington WL, Jacobs B, Lewis J et al. HIV–1 in patients with genital lesions attending a North American STD clinic: Assessment of risk factors. V International on AIDS, Montreal, Canada, June 1989; Abstract T.A.P. 118.

23. Diallo MO, Alkah AN, Porter A et al. HIV–1 and HIV–2 infections in Abidjan STD clinics. V International Conference on AIDS in Africa, Kinshasa, October 1990.

24. Bwayo JJ, Omare M, Mutere A et al. HIV–1 infection in East African long distance truck drivers. *East Afr Med J* (submitted).

25. Bongaarts J, Reining P, Way P, Conant F. The relationship between male circumcision and HIV infection in African populations. *AIDS* 1989; 6:373–8.

26. Moses S, Bradley J, Nagelkerke NJD et al. Geographical patterns of male circumcision in Africa: Association with HIV seroprevalence. *Int J Epidemiol* 1990; 19:1–5.

27. Parker SW, Stewart AJ, Wren MN, Gollow MN, Straton JA. Circumcision and sexually transmissible disease. *Med J Aus* 1983; 2:288–290.

28. Tyndall M, Plourde P, D'Costa et al. Treatment ofgenital ulcer disease in HIV c o n t r o l programs. V International Conference on AIDS in Africa, Kinshasa, October 1990.

29. Cameron DW, Kosseim ML, Odour D et al. Serologic concordance and incidence of HIV in regular sexual partners in Nairobi, Kenya. V International Conference on AIDS, Montreal, Canada, June 1989.

30. Moss GM, D'Costa LJ, Plummer FA et al. Cervical ectopy and male circumcision as risk factors for heterosexual transmission of HIV in stable sexual partnerships in Kenya. VI International Conference on AIDS, San Francisco, CA, June 1990.

31. Laga M, Taelman H, Van der Stuyft P et al. Advanced immunodeficiency as a risk factor for heterosexual transmission of HIV. *AIDS* 1989; 6:361–6.

32. Johnson AM, Petherick A, Davidson A et al. Transmission of HIV to heterosexual partners of men and women. *AIDS* 1989; 6:367–73.

33. Yorke JA, Hethcote HW, Nold A. Dynamics and control of the transmission of gonorrhea. *Sex Transm Dis* 1978; 5:51–6.

EPIDEMIOLOGICAL SYNERGY: INTERRELATIONSHIPS BETWEEN HIV INFECTION AND OTHER STDs

Judith N. Wasserheit

National Institutes of Health

INTRODUCTION

The interrelationships between HIV infection and other sexually transmitted diseases (STDs)* are complex and intriguing. They may explain, in part, the heterogeneous face of the HIV/AIDS pandemic around the world (1-3), and may well provide insights into the pathogenesis of all STDs, including HIV infection. Furthermore, these interrelationships have compelling implications for HIV control efforts.

Three relationships between HIV infection and other STDs have been postulated: 1) increased transmission of HIV in the presence of other STDs; 2) accelerated progression of HIV disease in the presence of other STDs; and 3) alteration in the natural history, diagnosis, or response to therapy of other STDs in the presence of HIV infection.

What has a decade of research on HIV infection taught us about these interrelationships? This chapter examines available data on the impact of STDs on HIV transmission and progression, and the reciprocal impact of HIV infection on other STDs. It also summarizes possible mechanisms for the relationships. It considers the program and policy implications of these relationships as we currently understand them, and emphasizes that for some STDs, the "epidemiological synergy" between the relationships may be as important as the individual relationships themselves. Finally, the chapter highlights high priority research needs.

---

*Over 20 syndromes are now recognized as sexually transmitted diseases. These include infections caused by hepatitis B virus, several ectoparasites, and a number of enteric pathogens. However, as a reflection of available data and in an attempt to limit the length of the chapter, this review will focus exclusively on the classical STDs that result in primary manifestations in the genital tract.

AIDS and Women's Reproductive Health
Edited by L.C. Chen *et al.*, Plenum Press, New York, 1991

THE IMPACT OF STDs ON HIV TRANSMISSION

Methodological Considerations

Several methodological problems must be considered in a critical analysis of studies of the impact of STDs on HIV transmission. First, such studies are complicated by the fact that HIV infection is, itself, an STD. Because HIV infection and other STDs share a common dominant mode of transmission, common human reservoirs, and common behavioral risk factors, STDs could be merely surrogates for factors such as multiple partners or other multiply-infected persons, rather than causal links in HIV transmission. Analyses that control for sexual behavior are, therefore, essential to establishing whether STDs are independent, biological risk factors for HIV transmission.

Unfortunately, even when such analyses are performed, measures of sexual behavior are often imperfect for the index subject, unobtainable for partners, and difficult to validate for both. Additional complexity arises because of the frequency of multiple co-infection among individuals infected with STDs. Comprehensive STD testing and analyses that adjust for the presence of multiple STDs are necessary to ensure that spurious associations between an STD and HIV infection do not result from underlying associations between another STD and both HIV and the STD in question.

A third problem springs from the potential impact of HIV infection on other STDs. Without prospective studies documenting temporal sequence, it is impossible to determine whether STDs facilitate HIV transmission or whether they are markers for HIV-related immunosuppression. Furthermore, in case-control studies, detection bias may occur if, due to HIV infection, STDs are more prominent, more persistent, or more readily identifiable in laboratory testing.

Finally, both STDs and the populations that acquire them are heterogeneous. Relationships between specific STDs and HIV infection may not be uniform. In addition, the importance of STDs in HIV transmission may be influenced by other competing risk factors (e.g., receptive anal intercourse or circumcision), the prevalence of which differs by gender and sexual preference. Therefore, studies that use aggregate variables such as "any STD," or that provide risk estimates that are not stratified by gender and sexual preference, are difficult to interpret.

Studies of Genital Ulcer Disease and HIV Transmission

Including conference abstracts, there are over 70 publications in the international literature linking STDs with an increased risk of HIV infection (4-78). Data from at least one study support associations between HIV infection and every STD that has been examined (i.e., chancroid, syphilis, genital herpes, gonorrhea, chlamydia, trichomoniasis, genital warts, and donovanosis). Only 25 reports, however, present multivariate analyses that incorporate at least some measure of sexual behavior. These include eight analyses of prospective or nested case-control studies (7, 18, 33, 39-40, 44, 58, 76) and 17 analyses of cross-sectional case-control studies (8-10, 13, 21-22, 26, 29, 35, 41-42, 54, 60, 62, 66-68) representing 15 study populations or datasets. For the methodological reasons discussed earlier, I will focus on these studies in weighing the evidence that STDs are risk factors for HIV transmission.

Data supporting genital ulcer disease (GUD) as a risk factor for HIV transmission are currently most compelling (Table 1). GUD, either as a clinical syndrome or as an etiologic diagnosis such as syphilis or herpes, was investigated in each of the 15 study populations. The 10 reports linking syndromic GUD with HIV infection come from studies performed in two sites — Nairobi, Kenya, and Kinshasa, Zaire — covering heterosexual populations in which the majority of ulcers are due to chancroid. Controlling for sexual behavior, two of the three prospective studies found a significantly increased risk of HIV seroconversion among subjects with GUD (OR 3.7 for women; 4.7 for men) (7, 58). The third prospective study failed to demonstrate an association, but the incidence of GUD in the cohort was only 5% (44).

Four of the seven case-control studies listed also found significant associations between GUD and HIV seropositivity (26, 42, 62, 66). Risk estimates for women were similar to those detected in the prospective studies, but estimates for men based on physical diagnosis of GUD ranged from 8.2 to 18.2. The latter value was for circumcised men, and reflects an interaction between GUD and circumcision with respect to risk of HIV infection (66). Of note, the three case-control studies in which no significant association was found (13, 29, 67) were all performed in women, and two relied upon subjects' histories of GUD without any clinical or laboratory verification. The fact that all STDs (including chancroid) are frequently asymptomatic in women, and that diagnosis of GUD may be more difficult in women than in men, may explain these divergent results. Not surprisingly, a significant association between the presence of IgG antibody to *Hemophilus ducreyi* and HIV seropositivity was found among both men and women (OR 3.0, 95% CI 1.8-5.1 for men; OR 3.3, 95% CI 2.2-4.8 for women), but these risk estimates were not controlled for sexual behavior or other STDs (56).

The relationship between syphilis and HIV infection was examined in two prospective (18, 76) and nine case-control (8-9, 13, 21, 29, 35, 42, 60, 68) studies that simultaneously considered behavioral risk factors (Table 1). Significant associations were found in nine of the 11 analyses. As was the case for studies of GUD, risk estimates based on serodiagnosis of syphilis were slightly higher for heterosexual men (median OR 6.0; range 3.3-8.7) than for women (median OR 4.0; range 2.5-5.4). This may be due to more limited misclassification bias in men than in women for the reasons mentioned above. In homosexual men, the single prospective study yielded low risk estimates ranging from 1.5 for history of syphilis to 2.2 for serodiagnosis. Case-control analyses resulted in higher values (range 2.0-9.9). Since the higher odds ratios in these reports were based on syphilis serologies rather than on historical data, it is unlikely that recall bias is responsible for these differences. One of the two studies that did not demonstrate an association relied on women's histories of syphilis (35); the other was conducted among prostitutes in whom no syphilis was detected (29).

Six studies specifically addressed the relationship between genital herpes or herpes simplex virus type 2 (HSV-2) infection and HIV infection. Three prospective studies were performed in homosexual male cohorts (33, 39, 76); one documented a stronger association between HSV-2 seroconversion and HIV seroconversion (OR 4.4) than between HSV-2 seropositivity and HIV seroconversion (OR 2.5) (33). This may reflect the more fulminant course and more persistent lesions observed in primary genital herpes compared with recurrent disease. The other two prospective studies, one of which also measured HSV-2 serologies (39) and the other of which relied upon history alone (76), failed to demonstrate a significant association. Risk estimates from a case-control study of homosexual men that included serology (68) were slightly higher than those from the prospective study described above (median OR 5.9; range 3.3-8.5). A study conducted in female prostitutes did not find an association (29).

It is noteworthy that one study of Zulu STD clinic patients has investigated the role of donovanosis in HIV infection (52). Unfortunately, the method for diagnosing donovanosis is not stated and potential confounding by behavioral risk factors was not considered. Nevertheless, the presence of donovanosis of at least six weeks duration was clearly associated with HIV seropositivity among men (p=0.001).

Studies of Non-ulcerative STDs and HIV Transmission

Data on non-ulcerative STDs and HIV infection are far more limited than those on GUD. Yet, if these syndromes do facilitate HIV transmission, the proportion of HIV infection attributable to the non-ulcerative STDs (attributable risk) will far outweigh the proportion due to GUD because, in most populations, diseases such as chlamydial infection, gonorrhea, and trichomoniasis are far more common than genital ulcers.

Four studies examined chlamydial infection (Table 1). The two prospective studies (44, 58), performed in cohorts of African prostitutes, each found a significant association between chlamy-

Table 1. Summary of studies of the relationships between STDs and HIV infection by study design, study population, and methods used to document STD.

	Prospective or Nested Case-Control Studies	Cross-Sectional Case-Control Studies
Gonorrhea		
Number of studies	4	6
Number detecting significant association	2	3
Risk estimate-median (range)		
Women	3.5 Lab	5.6 (3.8-8.9) Lab
Heterosexual men	NA	NS Hx
Homosexual men	1.5 Hx	NA
Trichomoniasis		
Number of Studies	1	1
Number detecting significant association	1	0
Risk estimate-median (range)		
Women	2.7 Lab	NS Lab
Heterosexual men	NA	NA
Homosexual men	NA	NA
Anogenital Warts		
Number of studies	0	5
Number detecting significant association	0	3
Risk estimate-median (range)		
Women	NA	3.5 (3.1-4.1) Hx
Heterosexual men	NA	NS
Homosexual men	NA	3.3 Hx; 3.7 Px

KEY

NA = Not available
NS = Not significant
Hx = By history
Px = By physical examination
Lab = By laboratory studies

dial cervicitis and HIV seroconversion (median OR 4.5, range 3.2-5.7). In contrast, neither of the case-control studies (29, 67) identified chlamydial infection as a risk factor for HIV seropositivity. The latter studies were also conducted in female prostitutes and used chlamydial culture or direct antigen detection methods. Their results are not surprising: Whereas the serologic tests employed in the case-control studies of GUD detect past infection, these methods detect current infection, which is likely to be linked to prior HIV acquisition primarily through the persistence of risky sexual behavior patterns.

Gonorrhea was significantly associated with HIV infection in two of four prospective studies (44,76) and three of six case-control (35, 42, 54) analyses that attempted to adjust for sexual behavior (Table 2). Among women, risk estimates ranged from 3.5 to 8.9, with the lower figure being generated by the single prospective study. In homosexual men, gonorrhea was associated with less than a two-fold increase in risk of HIV infection. The two prospective studies that did not detect a significant association between gonorrhea and HIV infection were performed in gay male cohorts and relied on histories of gonorrhea rather than on clinical or microbiological evidence of infection (18, 40). As with studies of chlamydial infection, the frequency with which the case-control studies failed to detect an association may be related to the temporal mismatch of using laboratory tests for current gonococcal infection to examine the role of gonorrhea in HIV acquisition that occurred in the past. In at least one of these studies (29), however, an additional

Table 1. (con't)

	Prospective or Nested Case-Control Studies	Cross-Sectional Case-Control Studies
Genital Ulcers (mainly chancroid)		
Number of studies	3	7
Number detecting significant association	2	4
Risk estimate-median (range)		
Women	3.7 Px	3.3 Px
Heterosexual men	4.7 Px	2.4 Hx; 13.2 (8.2-18.2) Px
Homosexual men	NA	NA
Syphilis		
Number of studies	2	9
Number of detecting significant association	2	7
Risk estimate-median (range)		
Women	NA	1.8 Hx; 4.0 (2.5 -5.4) Lab
Heterosexual men	NA	2.0 Hx; 6.0 (3.3-8.7) Lab
Homosexual men	1.5 Hx; 2.2 Lab	3.0 Hx; 8.4 (2.0-9.9) Lab
Genital Herpes		
Number of studies	3	3
Number detecting significant association	1	2
Risk estimate-median (range)		
Women	NA	)1.9 (women and men) Lab
Heterosexual men	NA	)
Homosexual men	3.5 (2.5-4.4) Lab	2.3 Hx; 5.9 (3.3-8.5) Lab
Chlamydial Infection		
Number of studies	2	2
Number detecting significant association	2	0
Risk estimate-median (range)		
Women	4.5 (3.2-5.7) Lab	NS Lab
Heterosexual men	NA	NA
Homosexual men	NA	NA

problem was that swabs for gonococcal cultures were obtained from the vagina, rather than from the cervix.

With respect to HIV transmission, trichomoniasis remains the least well-studied of the common STDs (Table 1). A prospective study (44) detected almost a three-fold increased risk of HIV seroconversion among female prostitutes with trichomoniasis compared to those without the infection. A case-control analysis (29) found no association.

An association between anogenital warts and HIV infection has been suggested in three of five case-control studies (13, 41, 60). Risk estimates were similar for women (median OR 3.5, range 3.1-4.1) and for homosexual men (OR: 3.3 for history of genital warts, 3.7 for examination evidence of lesions). In gay men, an even stronger association was noted between the presence of human papillomavirus (HPV) DNA in anal specimens and HIV seropositivity (OR 10.4, 95% CI 1.9-56.6) (41). Among HIV-positive men in this study, the mean number of CD4 cells was lower in the HPV-infected group than in the HPV-uninfected group (p=0.10). Although these differences were not significant, they are consistent with augmented expression of HPV infection as a result of HIV-induced immunosuppression. Unfortunately, no prospective studies that include data on both genital warts and sexual behavior are yet available to clarify this issue.

Table 2. Possible impact of HIV infection on the presentation, natural history, diagnosis, and therapy of other STDs.

	Clinical Presentation		Natural History		Performance of Standard Laboratory Tests		Response to Standard Therapy	
Chancroid	(?)	Multicentric, extragenital lesions; systemic symptoms; less lymphadenitis	(?)	Larger, more persistent lesions	(#)	Altered accuracy of culture or serology for *H. ducreyi*	(++)	Increased risk of treatment failure with single dose regimens
Syphilis	(?)	Atypical presentations	(+)	More persistent 1° lesions	(?/−)	Delayed or persistently negative serologies	(+)	Increased risk of treatment failure with single dose bicillin for 2° syphilis
			(?/−)	Accelerated progression to CNS or tertiary disease	(?)	Abnormally high titers		
					(−)	Persistent elevation of titers following therapy		
					(+)	Seroreversion in advancing HIV disease		
Herpes	(?)	Atypical sites, multicentric disease	(?)	Increased frequency of recurrences	(#)	Altered accuracy of culture or serology for HSV	(+)	Increased incidence of acyclovir resistance
			(?)	Increased size and duration of lesions				
			(#)	Increased incidence of disseminated disease				
Genital Warts/HPV Infection	(?)	Multicentric disease, larger lesions	(+)	Increased incidence recurrences	(+)	Increased HPV viral load	(++)	Decreased responsiveness to topical, laser, or surgical therapy
	(+)	Increased frequency of infection with multiple HPV types	(++)	Increase incidence progression to dysplasia or neoplasia	(++)	Increased HPV detection with advancing HIV disease		

Gonorrhea

(#) Atypical presentations	(+) Increased incidence gonococcal PID	(#) Altered accuracy of culture for *N. gonorrhoea*	(+) Increased incidence of PPNG	
	(?) Increased incidence DGI		(#) Increased incidence of treatment failure	

PID

(+) Lower prevalence of leukocytosis	(?) Increased severity or duration	(#) Altered accuracy of laparoscopic or histopathologic diagnosis	(+) Decreased responsiveness to CDC regimens
(−) Altered prevalence of fever	(#) Increased incidence of sepsis		
(#) Atypical presentations	(#) Altered incidence infertility or ectopic pregnancy		

Chlamydia and Trichomoniasis No published data currently support or refute associations in any of the four categories.

Adapted from Table 2, Report of the Research Subcommittee, AIDS/STD Task Force, World Health Organization.

Key: (++) = Likely (supported by multiple studies in humans which include a comparison group).
(+) = Probable (supported by a single study in animals or humans which includes a comparison group).
(?) = Possible (supported by anecdotal information or case reports).
(#) = Unknown (supported by no published data).
(−) = Unlikely (refuted by at least one study in humans which includes a comparison group).
CDC = Centers for Disease Control.
CNS = Central nervous system.

DGI = Disseminated gonococcal infection.
HIV = Human immunodeficiency virus.
HPV = Human papillomavirus.
HSV = Herpes simplex virus.
PID = Pelvic inflammatory disease.
PPNG = Penicillinase-producing Neisseria gonorrhoeae.

THE IMPACT OF STDs ON HIV PROGRESSION

Methodological Considerations

One of the most challenging problems in studying the impact of STDs on progression of HIV disease is the need to control for duration of HIV infection. In cross-sectional case-control studies, the period between diagnosis of HIV infection and onset of AIDS or AIDS-related complex (ARC) may correlate poorly with true duration of infection. Even in prospective studies, the timing of HIV seroconversion can be established only to the level of precision permitted by the interval at which HIV testing is performed.

Adjustments for baseline immunological function and age are also important. More marked immunosuppression at enrollment, for example, may be associated with both accelerated progression of HIV disease and increased frequency or severity of recurrences of viral STDs. Age-related cohort effects in STD incidence may give rise to spurious associations between STDs and rapid progression to advanced stages of HIV infection.

Number of exposures to an STD pathogen, rather than categorical presence or absence of any exposure, may be a risk factor for accelerated HIV progression. If this is the case, the frequency of asymptomatic infection plus financial and compliance constraints on repeated STD testing may make demonstrating an association exceedingly difficult.

Studies of STDs and Progression of HIV Disease

Only a handful of studies have addressed the role of STDs in HIV progression (79-83). Most are univariate analyses that do not control for baseline immunological status or for age. Roughly half of the studies examined cohorts in which the approximate date of HIV seroconversion could be determined. Overall, the results are inconclusive.

Of three studies focusing on herpes virus infections, two (79-80) evaluated HIV seroconverters and adjusted for age. Subjects were homosexual males in one study, and persons with hemophilia in the other. Neither analysis controlled for baseline immunological function. The third study (81) analyzed seroprevalent cases of HIV infection in homosexual males and stratified by initial CD4 level, but did not consider age. No significant associations between genital herpes and rate of progression of HIV disease were noted in any of these studies, regardless of whether HSV infection was documented serologically or by clinical history, and regardless of whether HIV progression was measured by p24 antigen level, by CD4 deficit, or by clinical outcomes such as development of AIDS, ARC, or persistent generalized lymphadenopathy (PGL). Interestingly, in these studies, companion analyses of infection due to other herpes viruses such as varicella zoster (VZV), cytomegalovirus (CMV), and Epstein-Barr virus (EBV) also did not support an increased risk of progression of HIV disease.

The impact of bacterial STDs on HIV progression has received little attention. In asymptomatic HIV-positive patients enrolled in a study of neurological complications of HIV infection (82), a significant association was noted between the presence of p24 antigen and historical or serological evidence of syphilis ($p = 0.03$). These data were not controlled, however, for duration of HIV infection, immunological status, or age. Data from homosexual men in the Multicenter AIDS Cohort Study (MACS) are also equivocal. In univariate analysis, subjects who developed AIDS within 30 months of HIV seroconversion were 3.4 times as likely to report a history of syphilis at some time prior to HIV infection as were controls matched for duration of HIV infection who did not develop AIDS within 30 months (personal communication, John Phair for the MACS). This difference was borderline significant. Parallel univariate analyses of gonococcal infection also suggest a link with progression. Progression to AIDS within 30 months of seroconversion was associated with a history of rectal gonorrhea both prior to (OR 3.3, $p < 0.05$) and after (OR 9.2, $p < 0.05$) seroconversion. No significant association was found between a history of urethritis before or after seroconversion and development of AIDS within 30 months.

One study (83) of steady male partners of male AIDS patients reported that PGL was significantly more common among HIV-positive subjects with a history of an STD since last intercourse with the AIDS patient than among HIV-positive subjects without such a history (univariate OR 30, p < 0.001). Similar tantalizing data are provided by the MACS. In univariate analysis, subjects reporting any STD in the six months prior to HIV seroconversion were over six times as likely to develop AIDS within 30 months as were subjects who denied any STDs during this period (p < 0.05) (personal communication, John Phair for the MACS).

THE IMPACT OF HIV INFECTION ON OTHER STDS

Methodological Considerations

Because of its impact on other pathogens or on the host response, HIV infection could, theoretically, affect other STDs in a number of ways. HIV infection might alter STD incidence or frequency of recurrences. It might give rise to atypical presentations, including larger, more numerous, or more persistent lesions. Alternatively, HIV infection might modify the natural history of STDs, resulting in more frequent or more rapid development of complications. Performance of laboratory tests and response to standard therapy might also be affected.

Several of the methodological considerations in studies of these issues are identical to those discussed for studies of the impact of STDs on HIV transmission. For the reasons stated above, sexual behaviors and co-infection with other STDs are potential confounders in the relationship between HIV infection and STD transmission, and prospective studies are essential to establish whether STDs facilitate HIV transmission, HIV facilitates STD transmission, or both.

Additional considerations are, however, important in studies of natural history, diagnosis, and response to therapy. Health care behaviors such as rapidity of response to STD symptoms, self-medication, or compliance with STD therapy may influence each of these, and may also be related to HIV infection status. It should also be recognized that, by increasing the duration of an STD, HIV infection could increase the incidence of the STD in a community without directly facilitating its transmission through altered susceptibility or altered infectiousness in individuals.

Perhaps the most critical (and, to date, most often ignored) factor in assessing the impact of HIV infection on other STDs is the need for an HIV-negative comparison group. Our overall understanding of the natural history of STDs such as syphilis, chancroid, or HPV infection is still relatively embryonic. Furthermore, some of these syndromes are infamous for their protean clinical manifestations. In this context, case reports and case series of purported HIV/STD interactions are uninterpretable at best, and misleading at worst.

Genital Ulcer Disease

At the current time, few definitive statements can be made about the impact of HIV infection on other STDs. Although much more has been published on this topic than on the role of STDs in progression of HIV disease, the majority of this literature consists of case reports and case series. Table 2 summarizes the strength of existing data linking HIV infection with alterations in STD clinical presentation, natural history, diagnosis, and response to therapy.

Decreased responsiveness to standard therapy is the most convincingly documented effect of HIV infection on chancroid. Two randomized clinical trials of single dose therapy with a trimethoprim-sulfonamide or quinolone antibiotic (84-85) indicate that treatment failures are at least six times as common in HIV-positive as in HIV-negative patients. In one study (84), treatment failure was a useful predictor of underlying HIV infection (positive predictive value = 71%). A case report (lacking culture confirmation of *H. ducreyi* infection) and anecdotal evidence suggest that HIV infection may also result in atypical presentations, including larger, multicentric, or extra-genital lesions that may be accompanied by systemic symptoms (86-87). Lymphadenitis may be less prominent and lesions may be more persistent than in HIV-negative cases of chancroid. No data are available with respect to the impact of HIV infection on diagnosis of *H. ducreyi* infection.

A great deal of attention has been focused on the impact of HIV infection on syphilis (88-93). Numerous case reports suggest that, in the setting of HIV infection, the clinical presentation of syphilis may be atypical (94-99); progression to neurosyphilis or other tertiary disease may be fulminant (100-106); serologic tests may be both falsely positive and falsely negative (107-111); and standard therapy for early infection may be inadequate (100, 112-114). Unfortunately, few studies provide the denominator data or comparison groups necessary to assess the importance of these reports either in terms of their absolute frequency among HIV-infected syphilis patients or in terms of their relative frequency compared to that among HIV-negative syphilis patients. The pleomorphic presentations and the well-recognized limitations in serodiagnosis of syphilis in otherwise healthy individuals compound this problem. Furthermore, in weighing these data, it is worth highlighting several points that are often forgotten: Even in the absence of HIV infection, central nervous system (CNS) involvement is not uncommon in early syphilis; neurologic symptoms may occur during secondary infection; meningovascular syphilis may follow on the heels of secondary syphilis by as little as a few months; and standard benzathine penicillin therapy of early syphilis does not reliably achieve treponemicidal levels in the CNS (115-119).

Alterations in the natural history of primary syphilis are suggested by one controlled study performed in rabbits (120). Compared with rabbits infected with *Treponema pallidum* alone, rabbits latently infected with HIV and then co-infected with *T. pallidum* exhibited more extensive and more persistent cutaneous lesions.

The issue of accelerated progression to neurosyphilis has been examined in a study that compared 15 HIV-positive and 25 HIV-negative patients with untreated primary or secondary syphilis (121). Using rabbit inoculation, *T. pallidum* was isolated from cerebrospinal fluid (CSF) in a similar proportion of HIV-positive and HIV-negative subjects (27% vs 32%, p=1.00). The prevalences of reactive CSF serologic tests for syphilis, and of elevated CSF protein were also similar in the two groups. Only CSF leukocytosis was significantly associated with HIV seropositivity (p=0.02). Although HIV infection was not associated with increased risk of progression to neurosyphilis, an increased incidence of treatment failure occurred in HIV-infected patients with infectious syphilis (121). *T. pallidum* was re-isolated from three of four patients treated with CDC-recommended single dose benzathine penicillin in whom *T. pallidum* had been recovered from CSF prior to therapy. All three treatment failures occurred in HIV-infected subjects, while the single patient in whom therapy was effective was HIV-negative. In light of the extremely small sample size, these data must, of course, await confirmation.

The few available studies of the performance of serologic tests for syphilis give the impression that accuracy is similar for active disease in HIV-positive and HIV-negative individuals, but that following syphilis therapy, reactive treponemal tests (FTA-ABS or MHA-TP) may become negative with advancing HIV disease (122-124). Investigators in Zaire, for example, found no significant differences between 40 HIV-positive and 50 HIV-negative female prostitutes with syphilis in terms of the proportion with initial RPR titers ≥ 1:16, or in terms of the change in RPR titer 9-12 months following therapy (123). However, in San Francisco, among 109 homosexual men treated two months to 26 years previously for syphilis, loss of reactivity of treponemal tests occurred in 13: 36% of those with AIDS, 43% of those with ARC, 7% of asymptomatic HIV-positive subjects, and no HIV-negatives (124). In multivariate analysis, seroreversion was independently associated both with the presence of symptomatic HIV infection (OR 7.3, 95% CI 1.4-38.2) and with T4/T8 ratio ≤ 0.6 (OR 7.4, 95% CI 1.2-46.4).

Both case reports and clinical impressions suggest that the severity of herpes simplex infections may be increased in HIV-positive patients. In these patients, herpes may present as multiple necrotic ulcers in atypical locations and appears to progress to more extensive and more persistent lesions than in HIV-negative individuals (125-129). Anecdotal information also indicates that the frequency of recurrences may increase as HIV-related immunosuppression progresses

(129-131). Unfortunately, no controlled studies to date address any of these issues. Data are also lacking on the impact of HIV infection on the incidence of visceral dissemination and on the accuracy of HSV detection by culture or serology.

Data are more convincing that the incidence of resistant HSV infection is increased among HIV-infected patients. Although with dosage adjustment acyclovir remains effective in the majority of individuals co-infected with HIV and HSV (130-132), a number of reports document evolution of acyclovir-resistant HSV isolates, most of which are susceptible to other antivirals (133-141). In addition, one study evaluated sensitivity patterns of 25 HSV isolates from 16 HIV-infected patients, 40 isolates from 38 cancer patients, and 55 isolates from 54 immunocompetent individuals (142). Acyclovir-resistance was found in five isolates from a single patient with AIDS who had been on escalating doses of acyclovir for almost a year and a half. Prior acyclovir therapy had been administered in 62% of the HIV-infected patients, compared with 8% of the cancer patients, and 7% of the immunocompetent group. These data suggest that the increased incidence of acyclovir-resistance in HIV infection is due to the super-position of immunosuppression on a population with high levels of exposure to this medication.

Non-ulcerative STDs

HIV infection appears to affect many aspects of HPV infection (Table 2). Several case reports emphasize that in HIV-positive individuals, both male and female, HPV infections are often multicentric (143-146). Anecdotal information suggests that genital lesions in these individuals are frequently large. Furthermore, the incidence of infection with multiple HPV types may be increased in HIV infection. In one series, 23% of 52 HPV-infected men with CDC Group IV HIV disease had multiple HPV types (147). A second, comparative study put these results into perspective by identifying multiple HPV types in 35% of 17 co-infected women, but in none of 8 HPV-positive, HIV-negative women (148).

Both the incidence of recurrences of genital HPV lesions and their responsiveness to standard therapy are probably altered in the setting of HIV infection. In 116 homosexual men treated with laser surgery for anal warts (149), for example, the average number of recurrences was significantly greater among HIV-positive than among HIV-negative patients ($p < 0.005$). Other investigators (150-151) have reported that the median number of treatments and the median duration of anogenital warts following therapy were greater in HIV-infected homosexual men than in HIV-negatives ($p < 0.01$ for each); but comparable analyses in heterosexual men did not yield significant differences. These findings are probably due to more advanced immunosuppression among the homosexual HIV-infected men than among the heterosexual HIV-infected men, since peripheral CD4 counts were significantly lower, and intralesional CD8 levels were significantly higher, in the former group. Recurrent disease in the face of podophyllin, cryosurgery, electrocautery, and systemic alpha-2-interferon has also been noted (146, 150).

HIV infection also appears to facilitate development of anogenital dysplasia or neoplasia. A number of case series highlight the high prevalence of premalignant or malignant anogenital lesions in HIV-positive patients (143, 147, 152-156). Studies incorporating HIV-negative comparison groups (148, 157-162) have also consistently demonstrated, in both men and women, a significant association between HIV-infection and cytological or histopathological abnormalities in cervical or anal specimens (OR 4.1-7.1 for men; 3.1-10.1 for women). Four of these investigations (148, 158, 160-161) indicate that the frequency and severity of anogenital abnormalities is directly related to level of immunosuppression. Furthermore, three of four studies that specifically examined the relationship between squamous intraepithelial lesions (SIL) and HPV infection found a stronger association in the presence of HIV infection than in its absence (148, 159, 163-164). In the one multivariate analysis that controlled for sociodemographic factors and for other STDs, odds ratios for the association between SIL and HPV infection increased from 2.3 among 60 HIV-negative women, to 8.8 among 36 asymptomatic and 29 among 36 symptomatic HIV-positive women (163).

These results must be viewed with caution. Data from more than one study suggest that detection of HPV DNA may be facilitated in HIV infection, particularly in advanced disease (41, 148). The load of HPV genomes per unit amount of cellular DNA may be increased in HIV-infected individuals, for example (148). Until the functional significance of such findings is clarified, the role of HIV infection in the relationship between HPV and anogenital neoplasia will be difficult to assess.

Few data speak to the effect of HIV infection on other STDs. There are currently no data to suggest that HIV infection alters the clinical presentation or diagnosis of lower tract gonococcal or chlamydial infections, although the incidence of gonococcal infection may be increased. A prospective study of Nairobi prostitutes found a significantly greater incidence of gonococcal cervicitis among HIV-positive than among HIV-negative women (164a). Unfortunately, these data were not controlled for factors such as condom use or other incident STDs. The data are particularly difficult to interpret because a subsequent analysis in the same population and similar analyses in Kinshasa prostitutes did not confirm this association.

The risk of complications of gonococcal disease may also be increased in the setting of HIV infection. Investigators in Nairobi (53) found that HIV-infected patients with gonorrhea were more than three and a half times as likely to harbor penicillinase-producing gonococci (PPNG) as HIV-negative patients (p < 0.002). In addition, a prospective study conducted in Nairobi prostitutes documented a four-fold greater incidence of gonococcal pelvic inflammatory disease (PID) among 151 HIV-positive subjects than among 81 HIV-negatives, but no increase in the incidence of chlamydial PID (personal communication, Robert Brunham and Frank Plummer). Disseminated gonococcal infection (DGI) may also be particularly problematic among HIV-infected individuals. In contrast to the highly penicillin-sensitive AHU strains usually associated with DGI, investigators in London (165) reported a case of DGI in an AIDS patient caused by a moderately resistant isolate (auxotype P, serovar 1B7).

Anecdotal information suggests that HIV infection may affect the clinical course and response to standard therapy of PID. Currently, only one published study has examined this issue (166). Among 110 women hospitalized in New York City for acute PID, surgical intervention due to persistent fevers despite antibiotic therapy was approximately three times as common in the 15 HIV-positive women as in the 95 HIV-negatives (p=0.058), and admission leukocytosis was substantially less common in the former group (p=0.001). These differences appeared to be unrelated to microbial etiology. Unfortunately, neither the duration of symptoms of PID prior to admission nor the findings at surgery were discussed in this report.

POTENTIAL MECHANISMS

A detailed discussion of the pathophysiologic mechanisms mediating the interrelationships between HIV infection and other STDs is beyond the scope of both this review and our current knowledge. A short summary of potential mechanisms due to either the host response or to pathogen interactions is useful, however, in emphasizing the biological plausibility of the relationships described above.

One aspect of the host response to STDs that may contribute to HIV transmission is recruitment of HIV-susceptible or HIV-infected cells such as T lymphocytes or macrophages. A number of investigators have identified HIV in genital secretions (167-176) or tissue (177-178) and several have documented localization of the virus to mononuclear cells (172, 176-178). Immunohistological studies indicate that, while lymphocytes and macrophages are normally present in the tissues and secretions of the male and female genital tract (179-181) and in the rectal mucosa of homosexual men (182), these HIV target cells increase in the setting of genital tract inflammation (183-184), such as that associated with STDs (185-187). Thus, STDs potentially could augment the susceptibility of HIV-negative partners by increasing the number of cells available for invasion by the virus, and could augment the infectiousness of HIV-positive partners by increasing the number of virus-laden cells being inoculated.

Another mechanism by which some STDs might facilitate HIV transmission is disruption of epithelial barriers in the genital tract. The integrity of the genital mucosa appears to be an important host defense against infection (188) and is clearly breached in genital ulcer disease. As with STD-related genital tract inflammation, GUD-induced breaks in the lining of the genital tract could affect both susceptibility and infectiousness. In fact, HIV has been isolated directly from genital ulcers in both men and women (189-190). The consistency with which STDs appear to promote HIV transmission suggests that disruption of epithelial barriers is not the primary mechanism involved. However, the efficiency with which GUD increases HIV transmission may be due in part to the simultaneous operation of both of these mechanisms.

Both stimulation and suppression of the systemic immune response have been invoked as mechanisms to explain various aspects of the interrelationships between HIV and other STDs. Repeated STD-related activation of T lymphocytes has been postulated to play a role in susceptibility to HIV infection (191) and in progression of HIV disease, and HIV-related polyclonal B cell activation has been raised as a possible explanation for false positivity of serological tests for STDs. On the other hand, a role for STD-induced immunosuppression has been considered in susceptibility to HIV infection or in progression of HIV disease (192), and HIV-induced immunosuppression almost certainly is a factor in alterations in the natural history and response to therapy of some STDs. With the exception of the last of these points, however, few data support these hypotheses.

Interactions between HIV and STD pathogens may be responsible for increased transmission or accelerated progression of these diseases. Viral STDs might potentiate HIV infection by stimulating expression of cell surface receptors that facilitate HIV attachment, by coding for gene products that are necessary for HIV growth, or by temporarily or permanently altering HIV expression through phenotypic mixing or genetic recombination (192-193). *In vitro* data suggest, for example, that the herpesviruses (HSV, EBV, and CMV) can transactivate HIV (193-197), although the clinical significance of these observations is yet to be determined. It is also possible that HIV gene products, such as the TAT protein, could play a role in HPV-associated neoplasia, much as it appears to promote development of Kaposi's sarcoma.

CONCLUSIONS

As we enter the second decade of the HIV/AIDS pandemic, many questions about the interrelationships between HIV infection and other STDs remain unanswered. Data on HIV-STD interactions are still limited in quantity and quality, and preliminary conclusions drawn today are likely to demand revision in the near future. Yet patterns are emerging on which to base a conceptual framework for understanding these interrelationships (Figure 1). Such a framework may be useful in generating testable hypotheses for additional research. These patterns are summarized below.

Several prospective studies that control for behavioral risk factors and for other STDs support the hypothesis that the risk of HIV transmission is increased in the presence of each of the genital ulcer diseases and in the presence of non-ulcerative STDs such as chlamydial infection, gonorrhea, and trichomoniasis. HPV infection stands out as the one STD for which no well-designed, prospective studies of HIV transmission are yet available. Further studies may well demonstrate that HPV infection and anogenital warts do not facilitate HIV transmission but, instead, are themselves promoted by HIV-related immunosuppression.

In general, the role of specific STD syndromes in HIV transmission as they relate to gender is beginning to emerge. The role of STDs may be somewhat greater in heterosexual males than females, but data are still too sparse to be conclusive. It is also noteworthy that risk estimates from studies of heterosexual populations are largely similar for ulcerative and non-ulcerative STDs, and cluster in the range of a three-to-five-fold increase. Limited data currently preclude comparisons between the role of STDs in heterosexual and homosexual populations. Although specific mechanisms must be elucidated, both biologically and epidemiologically, it is highly plausible that other STDs would facilitate transmission of HIV.

The role of STDs in progression of HIV disease, on the other hand, is still unknown. The few available data come from univariate and bivariate analyses of a limited number of STDs in homosexual or hemophiliac populations. Half of the studies focus on seroprevalent cases of HIV infection in which the duration of infection cannot be ascertained. It is, therefore, difficult to interpret the results of these studies, which suggest that HSV infection plays no role in progression, while syphilis and rectal gonorrhea may possibly accelerate the pace of HIV disease. One can only emphasize the need for additional research on this issue.

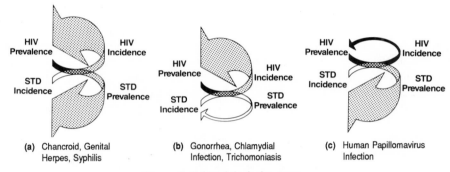

Figure 1. Epidemiological synergy.

Data on the impact of HIV infection on other STDs are also compromised by several methodological problems, the most critical of which is the dearth of studies that include comparison groups. Nevertheless, the information that is available suggests that HIV infection may have clinically significant effects on a number of STDs. It may be useful, in understanding HIV-STD interactions, to think about STDs in four categories: those in which HIV alters the course of lower tract, communicable stages of disease; those in which HIV affects the development of non-communicable sequelae of lower tract disease; those in which HIV impacts upon both aspects of disease; and those in which HIV seems to have little effect.

Genital ulcer diseases appear to fall into the first category. Available data suggest that HIV prolongs the duration of GUD through effects such as more persistent lesions, more frequent recurrences, more common treatment failures, and even through atypical presentations resulting in delayed diagnosis. At present, it is not clear whether the infectiousness as well as the prevalence of GUD is increased in the setting of HIV infection. No comparative studies currently indicate that HIV promotes the development of sequelae of GUD. Non-ulcerative STDs can be divided among the remaining categories. Gonococcal infections may represent the second category. Little evidence suggests clinically significant alterations in lower tract gonococcal infection, but the development of complications such as PID or DGI may be affected by concomitant HIV infection. In contrast, HPV infections and genital warts should be considered in the third category. HIV probably increases the prevalence (and perhaps the infectiousness) of anogenital lesions, as well as the risk of HPV-associated neoplasia. HIV seems to have little effect on chlamydial infections and on trichomoniasis, although these STDs have received minimal attention to date.

What do these patterns tell us about the HIV/AIDS pandemic and approaches to its control? The pieces of this puzzle may be most informative when the role of STDs in HIV transmission and the impact of HIV infection on other STDs are considered together. In the past, these have usually been examined as separate questions. Attention has focused primarily on the former, in the hope that identification of modifiable risk factors for transmission would lead to development of effective interventions for primary prevention (198-200). While the latter issue has concerned many involved in STD research and control efforts, it has generated little interest among HIV investigators or care providers.

Because of our compartmentalized approach, the potential significance of a bi-directional interplay between HIV infection and other STDs has not been fully appreciated. If co-infection with HIV prolongs or augments the infectiousness of individuals with specific STDs, and if the same STDs facilitate transmission of HIV, then at a community level, the two infections could greatly amplify one another (Figure 1a). Mutually reinforcing increases in HIV and STD incidence may well underpin the explosive growth of the HIV/AIDS pandemic in some heterosexual populations (1-3, 201) and may represent a uniquely effective "epidemiological synergy" between disease syndromes that are linked by common behaviors (202). The limited data available suggest that such synergy may well occur between HIV infection and genital ulcer diseases (GUD), such as chancroid, herpes, and syphilis. Other STDs, such as gonorrhea, chlamydia, and trichomoniasis appear to interact with HIV infection in a unidirectional fashion: They may promote HIV transmission, but HIV infection does not seem to result in a synergistic increase in the prevalence, and hence the incidence, of this group of STDs (Figure 1b). HPV infection may represent a different, unidirectional model closer to that of traditional opportunistic infections. HPV infection probably does not facilitate HIV transmission, but HIV may well augment expression and progression of HPV disease (Figure 1c).

Program and Policy Implications

The program and policy implications of the interrelationships between HIV and other STDs are clear and urgent. They need not and should not await additional research. As has been highlighted by others (198-199, 203-204), HIV and STD control efforts must go hand in hand in terms of clinical services, research, and training. Programmatically, this means that STD services must be strengthened or established *de novo,* and must be integrated as cornerstones of HIV prevention programs. On a policy level, countries that hope to minimize the impact of the HIV/AIDS epidemic must recognize that STDs are one of the most readily modifiable risk factors for spread of HIV within a community. They must, therefore, make STD control a major health priority.

Both individual programs and national policies should focus on the full spectrum of locally prevalent STDs, rather than exclusively on genital ulcers. The epidemiological synergy described above implies that high levels of GUD are likely to result in more rapid increase in HIV incidence than non-ulcerative STDs. However, most non-ulcerative STDs also appear to increase HIV incidence and, because of their greater prevalence in many populations, these STDs may be responsible for a larger proportion (attributable risk) of HIV transmission than genital ulcers.

Because of their complementary role both in HIV and in STD prevention, behavioral interventions, such as condom promotion, should be emphasized. Furthermore, in patients co-infected with HIV and other STDs, condoms may work where antibiotics fail. Counseling of STD patients should include information on their high risk of HIV infection.

Finally, research and training are essential components of any effective, long-term public health program. Coordination of HIV and STD activities should extend to the research and training arenas.

Research Needs and Opportunities

The complex and unique interrelationships between HIV infection and other STDs provide some of the most exciting challenges in science today. Research questions cut across a number of disciplines and demand a marriage of basic science, epidemiological, clinical, and behavioral research approaches.

Future studies of the role of STDs in HIV transmission should be prospective in design, and must control, where possible, for behavioral risk factors and for other STDs. STDs should be documented microbiologically, rather than historically. Investigators should focus on STDs and populations that have received little attention in prospective studies to date. As is apparent from Table 1, these include syphilis and herpes in heterosexuals; chlamydia, gonorrhea, and trichomoniasis in males; and HPV infections in all populations. The importance of HPV/genital warts in HIV transmission remains particularly ill-defined. As highlighted by Dr. Berkley in this volume, definition of the attributable risk of individual STDs in specific populations will be important to the rational development of program priorities.

Additional studies of the role of STDs in HIV progression are urgently needed. To minimize recall bias and permit adjustment for duration of infection, these studies should follow HIV seroconverters prospectively, controlling for factors such as age and baseline immunological status. They should be conducted in non-hemophiliac, heterosexual populations, in addition to homosexual cohorts. Investigators should consider number of episodes of STDs as well as categorical STD exposure variables.

Future studies of the impact of HIV infection on other STDs must include comparison groups. Among the highest research priorities are improved definition of HIV-induced alterations in the natural history of STDs, both as they affect the prevalence of both STDs in the community and the incidence of severe sequelae such as tertiary syphilis, anogenital malignancy, or pelvic inflammatory disease, infertility, and ectopic pregnancy. Development and testing of STD regimens that are effective in HIV-infected individuals is equally important.

Complementary research efforts should focus on the mechanisms mediating each of the HIV/STD interrelationships. In clinical studies, comparison of partners of HIV-infected individuals with and without STDs will be needed to determine whether STDs contribute to HIV transmission by increasing infectiousness as well as by increasing susceptibility to HIV. Elucidation of the molecular pathogenesis of HIV/STD interrelationships is likely to contribute substantially to our understanding of each of these diseases individually, and more broadly, to offer insights into ways in which pathogens interact to promote disease.

Ultimately, the goal of medical research is to provide the knowledge with which to control disease. Research on the interrelationships between HIV infection and other STDs must converge in the development and testing of sustainable interventions that will help contain the spread of the most devastating pandemic in the era of modern medicine. Intervention trials that conclusively demonstrate the importance of STD control in HIV prevention will be complex, expensive, and time-consuming. They may be critical, however, to informing health policy makers of the interrelationships discussed in this chapter, and to convincing them of the necessity of allocating greater resources to STD control as part of integrated HIV/STD prevention programs.

Acknowledgments

I am grateful to Willard Cates, Jr., Jeffrey Harris, and Penelope Hitchcock for their valuable input on this chapter, and to Susan Emelio, Aretha Hankinson, and Ernestine McNeill for their excellent secretarial assistance.

REFERENCES

1. Piot P, Laga M, Ryder R et al: The global epidemiology of HIV infection: continuity, heterogeneity, and change. *J Acq Imm Def Syn* 3:403-12, 1990.

2. Piot P, Plummer FA, Mhalu FS et al: AIDS: an international perspective. *Science* 239:573-79, 1988.

3. Quinn TC, Mann JN, Curran JW et al: AIDS in Africa: An epidemiologic paradigm. *Science* 234:955-63, 1986.

4. Bonneux L, Tailman H, Cornet et al: Case control study of HIV-seropositive versus HIV-seronegative European expatriates in Africa. III International AIDS Conference, Washington, D.C., 1987: abstract no. W.2.4.

5. Bulterys M, Chao A, Saah A et al: Risk factors for HIV-1 seropositivity among rural and urban pregnant women in Rwanda. VI International AIDS Conference, San Francisco, 1990: abstract no. Th.C.576.

6. Cameron DW, D'Costa LJ, Ndinya-Achola JO et al: Incidence and risk factors for female to male transmission of HIV. IV International AIDS Conference, Stockholm, 1988: abstract no. 4061.

7. Cameron DW, Lourdes JD, Gregory MM et al: Female to male transmission of human immunodeficiency virus type 1: risk factors for seroconversion in men. *Lancet* 2:403-07, 1989.

8. Cannon RO, Quinn T, Rompalo A et al: Syphilis is strongly associated with HIV infection in Baltimore STD Clinic patients independent of risk group. V International AIDS Conference, Montreal, 1989: abstract no. Th.A.O.18.

9. Cannon RO, Hook EW, Nahmias AJ et al: Association of herpes simplex virus type 2 with HIV infection in heterosexual patients attending sexually transmitted disease clinics. IV International AIDS Conference, Stockholm, 1988: abstract no. 4558.

10. Carael M, Van de Perre PH, Lepage PH et al: Human immunodeficiency virus transmission among heterosexual couples in Central Africa. *AIDS* 2:201-05, 1988.

11. Carswell JW: HIV infection in healthy persons in Uganda. *AIDS* 1:223-27, 1987.

12. Castro KG, Lieb S, Calisher C et al: AIDS and HIV infection, Belle Glade, Florida. III International AIDS Conference, Washington, D.C., 1987: abstract no. W.2.3.

13. Chiphangwi J, Dallabetta G, Saah A et al: Risk factors for HIV-1 infection in pregnant women in Malawi. VI International AIDS Conference, San Francisco, 1990: abstract no. Th.C.98.

14. Chirgwin K, Dillon S, DeHovitz J et al: Genital ulcers (GU) and HIV infection in an urban sexually transmitted disease (STD) clinic. V International AIDS Conference, Montreal, 1989: abstract no. M.B.P.57.

15. Chmiel, JS, Detels R, Kaslow RA et al: Factors associated with prevalent human immunodeficiency virus (HIV) infection in the multicenter AIDS cohort study. *Amer J Epidemiology* 128:568-575, 1987.

16. Collier A, Murphy V, Quinn T et al: Seroepidemiology of HIV infection in adults with syphilis. IV International AIDS Conference, Stockholm, 1988: abstract no. 4549.

17. Darrow WW, Cohen JB, French J et al: Multicenter study of HIV antibody in U.S. prostitutes. III International AIDS Conference, Washington, D.C., 1987: abstract no. W.2.1.

18. Darrow WW, Echenberg DF, Jaffe HW et al: Risk factors for human immunodeficiency virus (HIV) infections in homosexual men. *Am J Public Health* 77:479-483, 1987.

19. De Vindenzi I and Ancelle-Park R: Heterosexual transmission of HIV: a European study. V International AIDS Conference, Montreal, 1989: abstract no. Th.A.O.20.

20. Duerr A, Bulterys M, Dushimimana A et al: HIV-1 seropositivity and sexual history among Rwandan women. VI International AIDS Conference, San Francisco, 1990: abstract no. Th.C.575.

21. Elifson K, Soles J, Sweet H et al: Risk factors for HIV infection among male prostitutes in Atlanta. V International AIDS Conference, Montreal, 1989: abstract no. W.A.P.38.

22. European Study Group: Risk factors for male to female transmission of HIV. *Br Med J* 298:411-5, 1989.

23. Fischl MA, Dickinson GM, Flanagan S et al: Human immunodeficiency virus (HIV)

among female prostitutes in South Florida. III International AIDS Conference, Washington, D.C., 1987: abstract no. W.2.2.

24. Fischl MA, Fayne T, Flanagan S et al: Seroprevalence and risks of HIV infections in spouses of persons infected with HIV. IV International AIDS Conference, Stockholm, 1988: abstract no. 4060.

25. Freund CO, Altman R, Shahied SI et al: Prevalence of human immunodeficiency virus (HIV) infection in the sexually transmitted disease (STD) clinics of New Jersey. IV International AIDS Conference, Stockholm, 1988: abstract no. 6093.

26. Greenblatt RM, Lukehart SA, Plummer FA et al: Genital ulceration as a risk factor for human immunodeficiency virus infection. *AIDS* 2:47-50, 1988.

27. Haley CE, Anderson P, Freeman A et al: Relationship of STD history to HIV seropositivity in a cohort of homosexual men in Dallas, Texas. V International AIDS Conference, Montreal, 1989: abstract no. W.A.P.39.

28. Harrison WO, Zajdowicz T, Hendrick B et al: A comparison of history of sexually transmitted disease (STD) in HIV-positive vs HIV-negative naval personnel. IV International AIDS Conference, Stockholm, 1988: abstract no. 4636.

29. Hayes CG, Manaloto CR, Basaca-Sevilla V et al: Epidemiology of HIV infection among prostitutes in the Philippines. *J Acq Imm Def Syn* 3:913-20, 1990.

30. Hellman N, Naubuga P, Baingana B et al: HIV infection among patients in a Uganda STD clinic. VI International AIDS Conference, San Francisco, 1990: abstract no. Th.C.577.

31. Hermans P, Lee FK, Poncin M et al: Possible co-factors of human immunodeficiency virus (HIV) infection among central African patients. III International AIDS Conference, Washington, D.C., 1987: abstract no. THP.61.

32. Hira SK, Kamanga J, Macuacua R et al: Genital ulcers and male circumcision as risk factors for acquiring HIV-1 in Zambia. *J Infect Dis* 161:584-85, 1990.

33. Holmberg SD, Stewart JA, Gerber AR et al: Prior herpes simplex virus type 2 infection as a risk factor for HIV infection. *JAMA* 259:1048-50, 1988.

34. Hudson CP, Hennis AJ and Kaaha P: Risk factors for the spread of AIDS in rural Africa: evidence from a comparative seroepidemiolocal survey of AIDS, hepatitis B and syphilis in southwestern Uganda. *AIDS* 2:255-60, 1988.

35. Hunter D, Maggwa A, Mati J et al: Risk factors for HIV infection among women in a low-risk population in Nairobi, Kenya. VI International AIDS Conference, San Francisco, 1990: abstract no. Th.C.573.

36. Jaffe HW, Choi K, Thomas PA et al: National case-control study of Kaposi's sarcoma and Pneumocystis carinii pneumonia in homosexual men: part 1, epidemiologic results. *Ann Inter Med* 99:145-51, 1983.

37. Katzenstein DA, Latif A, Bassett MT et al: Risks for heterosexual transmission of HIV in Zimbabwe. III International AIDS Conference, Washington, D.C., 1987: abstract no. M.8.3.

38. Keet PM, Lee FK, Van Griansvan GJP et al: Little evidence for genital ulcerative infections as a risk factor for HIV-1 acquisition among homosexual men. VI International AIDS Conference, San Francisco, 1990: abstract no. Th.C.561.

39. Kingsley LA, Armstrong J, Rahman A et al: No association between herpes simplex virus type-2 seropositivity or anogenital lesions and HIV seroconversion among homosexual men. *J Acq Imm Def Syn* 3:773-79, 1990.

40. Kingsley LA, Kaslow R, Rinaldo CR et al: Risk factors for seroconversion to human immunodeficiency virus among male homosexuals. *The Lancet* 8529 February 14, 1987.

41. Kiviat N, Rompalo A, Bowden R et al: Anal human papillomavirus infection among human immunodeficiency virus-seropositive and -seronegative men. *J Infect Dis* 162:358-361, 1990.

42. Kreiss JK, Koech D, Plummer FA et al: AIDS virus infection in Nairobi prostitutes. *N Engl J Med* 314:414-18, 1986.

43. Laga M, Nzila N, Manoka AT et al: High prevalence and incidence of HIV and other sexually transmitted diseases (STD) among 801 Kinshasa prostitutes. V International AIDS Conference, Montreal, 1989: abstract no. Th.A.O.21.
44. Laga M, Nzila N, Manoka AT et al: Non ulcerative sexually transmitted diseases (STD) as risk factors for HIV infection. VI International AIDS Conference, San Francisco, 1990: abstract no. Th.C.97.
45. Latif AS, Katzenstein DA and Bassett MT: Genital ulcers and transmission of HIV among couples in Zimbabwe. *AIDS* 3:519-23, 1989.
46. Leonard G, Mounier M, Verdier M et al: Seroepidemiological study of sexually transmitted pathogenic agents (HIV-1, HIV-2, T. pallidum, C. trachomatis) in Ivory Coast. IV International AIDS Conference, Stockholm, 1988: abstract no. 5014.
47. Moss GB, D'Costa LJ, Ndinya-Achola JO et al: Cervical ectopy and lack of male circumcision as risk factors for heterosexual transmission of HIV in stable sexual partnerships in Kenya. VI International AIDS Conference, San Francisco, 1990: abstract no. Th.C.570.
48. Moss GB, D'Costa LJ, Plummer FA et al: HIV transmission in stable sexual partnerships in Kenya. V International AIDS Conference, Montreal, 1989: abstract no. T.A.P.88.
49. Nzila N, Ryder R, Colebunders R et al: Married couples in Zaire with discordant HIV serology. IV International AIDS Conference, Stockholm, 1988: abstract no. 4059.
50. Nzila, Kivuvu M, Manoka AT et al: HIV risk factors in steady male partners of Kinshasa prostitutes. VI International AIDS Conference, San Francisco, 1990: abstract no. Th.C.579.
51. Nzilambe N, De Cock KM, Forthal DN et al: The prevalence of infection with human immunodeficiency virus over a 10-year period in rural Zaire. *N Engl J Med* 318:276-79, 1988.
52. O'Farrell N, Windsor I and Becker P: Risk factors for HIV-1 amongst STD clinic attenders in Durban, South Africa. VI International AIDS Conference, San Francisco, 1990: abstract no. F.C.604.
53. Ombette JJ, Ndinya-Achola JO, Maitha G et al: Prevalence of HIV among men and women with H. ducreyi and Neisseria gonorrhoeae infection in Nairobi, Kenya. VI International AIDS Conference, San Francisco, 1990: abstract no. Th.C.572.
54. Piot P, Plummer FA, Rey MA et al: Retrospective seroepidemiology of AIDS virus infection in Nairobi populations. *J Infect Dis* 155:1108-12, 1987.
55. Piot P, Quinn TC, Taelman H et al: Acquired immunodeficiency syndrome in a heterosexual population in Zaire. *Lancet:*65-69, July 14, 1984.
56. Piot P, Van Dyck E, Ryder RW et al: Serum antibody to Haemophilus ducreyi as a risk factor for HIV in Africa, but not in Europe. V International AIDS Conference, Montreal, 1989: abstract no. M.A.O.32.
57. Plourde P, Plummer FA, Pepin J et al: Incidence of HIV-1 seroconversion in women with genital ulcers. VI International AIDS Conference, San Francisco, 1990: abstract no. Th.C.571.
58. Plummer FA, Cameron DW, Simonsen N et al: Co-factors in male-female transmission of HIV. IV International AIDS Conference, Stockholm, 1988: abstract no. 4554.
59. Plummer FA, Pepin J, Maitha G et al: HIV-1 infection in sexually exposed women: risk factors for prevalent and incident infections. V International AIDS Conference, Montreal, 1989: abstract no. T.A.P.87.
60. Quinn TC, Glasser D, Cannon RO et al: Human immunodeficiency virus infection among patients attending clinics for sexually transmitted diseases. *N Engl J Med* 318:197-204, 1988.
61. Rogers MF, Morens DM, Stewart JA et al: National case-control study of kaposi's sarcoma and pneumocystis carinii pneumonia in homosexual men: part 2, laboratory results. *Ann Inter Med* 99:151-58, 1983.
62. Ryder R, Hassig S, Ndilu M et al: Extramarital/prostitute sex and genital ulcer disease

(GUD) are important HIV risk factor in 7068 male Kinshasa factory workers and their 4548 wives. V International AIDS Conference, Montreal, 1989: abstract no. M.A.O.35.

63. Safrin S, Dattel BJ, Hauer L et al: Seroprevalence and epidemiologic correlates of human immunodeficiency virus infection in women with acute pelvic inflammatory disease. *Obstet & Gynecol* 75:666-70, 1990.

64. Schachter MT, Boyko WJ, Weaver MS et al: Progression to AIDS, predictions of AIDS, and seroconversion in a cohort of homosexual men: results of a four year prospective study. III International AIDS Conference, Washington, D.C., 1987: abstract no. M.3.3.

65. Shandera WX: The development of acquired immunodeficiency syndrome (AIDS) among two cohorts of sexually transmitted (STD) patients with different venereal disease histories. V International AIDS Conference, Montreal, 1989: abstract no. W.A.P.45.

66. Simonsen JN, Cameron DW, Gakinya MN et al: Human immunodeficiency virus infection among men with sexually transmitted diseases. *N Engl J Med* 319:274-78, 1988.

67. Simonsen JN, Plummer FA and Ngugi EN: HIV infection among lower socioeconomic strata prostitutes in Nairobi. *AIDS* 4:139-44, 1990.

68. Stamm WE, Handsfield HH, Rompalo AM et al: The association between genital ulcer disease and acquisition of HIV infection in homosexual men. *JAMA* 260:1429-33, 1988.

69. Stevens C, Taylor P, Holford T et al: Co-factors and cohort effects in progression to AIDS among HIV-1 infected homosexual men. V International AIDS Conference, Montreal, 1989: abstract no. M.A.P.93.

70. Telzak EE, Chiasson MA, Stoneburner RL et al: A prospective cohort study of HIV-1 seroconversion in patients with genital ulcer disease in New York City. V International AIDS Conference, Montreal, 1989: abstract no. M.A.O.34.

71. Telzak EE, Chiasson MA, Stoneburner R et al: HIV seroconversion in patients with genital ulcer disease in New York City: a prospective study. VI International AIDS Conference, San Francisco, 1990: abstract no. 3194.

72. Van de Perre P, Carael M, Nzaramba D et al. Risk factors for HIV seropositivity in selected urban-based Rwandese adults. *AIDS* 1:207-11, 1987.

73. Van de Perre P, Clumeck N, Steens M et al. Seroepidemiological study on sexually transmitted diseases and hepatitis B in African promiscuous heterosexuals in relation to HTLV-III infection. *Europ J Epid* 3:14-18, 1987.

74. Van de Perre P, Le Polain B, Carael M et al: HIV Antibodies in a remote rural area in Rwanda, Central Africa: an analysis of potential risk factors for HIV seropositivity. *AIDS* 1:213-15, 1987.

75. Van de Perre P, Rouvroy D, Lepage P et al: Acquired immunodeficiency syndrome in Rwanda. *Lancet*:62-65, July 14, 1984.

76. VanRaden M, Kaslow R, Kingsley L et al: The role of ulcerative genital diseases in promoting acquisition of HIV-1 by homosexual men. V International AIDS Conference, Montreal, 1989: abstract no. Th.A.O.17.

77. Whittington WL, Jacobs B, Lewis J et al: HIV-1 in patients with genital lesions attending a North American STD clinic: assessment of risk factors. V International AIDS Conference, Montreal, 1989: abstract no. T.A.P.118.

78. Wiznia A, Kashkin J, Caspe W et al: HIV seroprevalence in patients with syphilis. IV International AIDS Conference, Stockholm, 1988: abstract no. 4548.

79. Holmberg SD, Gerber AR, Stewart JA, et al: Herpes viruses as cofactors in AIDS. Lancet (letter) 2:746-7, 1988.

80. Webster A, Lee CA, Cook DG et al: Cytomegalovirus infection and progression towards AIDS in hemophiliacs with human immunodeficiency virus infection. *Lancet*:63-65, July 8, 1989.

81. Kaslow RA, VanRaden M, DeLoria M et al: Do clinical herpes simplex virus (HSV) and varicella-zoster (VSV) infections accelerate HIV-1-induced immunodeficiency? V International AIDS Conference, Montreal, 1989: abstract no. Th.A.P.100.

82. Berger JR, McCarthy M, Resnick L et al: History of syphilis as a cofactor for the expression of HIV infection. V International AIDS Conference, Montreal, 1989: abstract no. M.A.P.90.

83. Weber JN, McCreaner A, Berrie E et al: Factors affecting seropositivity to human T cell lymphotropic virus type III (HTLV-III) or lymphadenopathy associated virus (LAV) and progression of disease in sexual partners of patients with AIDS. *Genitourin Med* 62:177-80, 1986.

84. Cameron DW, Plummer FA, D'Costa LJ et al: Prediction of HIV infection by treatment failure for chancroid, a genital ulcer disease. IV International AIDS Conference, Stockholm, 1988: abstract no. 7637.

85. MacDonald KS, Cameron W, D'Costa LJ et al: Evaluation of fleroxacin (RO 23-6240) as single-oral-dose therapy of culture-proven chancroid in Nairobi, Kenya. *Antimicro Agents Chemo* 33:612-14, 1989.

86. Quale J, Teplitz E and Augenbraun M: Atypical presentation of chancroid in a patient infected with the human immunodeficiency virus. *Amer J Med* 88:5-43N-44N, 1990.

87. Latif AS: Epidemiology and control of chancroid. 8th ISSTDR, Copenhagen, 1989: abstract no. 66.

88. Hook EW: Syphilis and HIV infection. *J Infect Dis* 160:530-34, 1989.

89. Rufli T: Syphilis and HIV infection. *Dermatologica* 179:113-17, 1989.

90. Kinloch-de Loes S and Saurat JH: AIDS meets syphilis: Changing patterns of the syphilitic infection and its treatment. *Dermatologica* 177:261-64, 1988.

91. Matlow AG and Rachlis AR: Syphilis Serology in human immunodeficiency virus-infected patients with symptomatic neurosyphilis: case report and review. *Rev Inf Dis* 12:703-707, 1990.

92. Terry PM, Page ML and Golmeier D: Are serological tests of value in diagnosing and monitoring response to treatment of syphilis in patients infected with human immunodeficiency virus? *Genitourin Med* 64:219-22, 1988.

93. Tramont EC: Syphilis in the AIDS era. *N Engl J Med* 316:1600-01, 1987.

94. Caumes E, Janier M, Janssen F et al: Atypical secondary syphilis in HIV seropositive patients. V International AIDS Conference, Montreal, 1989: abstract no. W.B.P.49.

95. Radolf JD and Kaplan RP: Unusual manifestations of secondary syphilis and abnormal humoral immune response to Treponema pallidum antigens in a homosexual man with asymptomatic human immunodeficiency virus infection. *J Am Acad Derm* 18:423-28, 1988.

96. Cusini M, Zerboni R, Muratori S et al: Atypical early syphilis in an HIV-infected homosexual male. *Dermatologica* 177:300-04, 1988.

97. Berger JR, Hensley G, Moskowitz L et al: Syphilitic myelopathy with human immunodeficiency virus: a treatable cause of spinal cord disease. V International AIDS Conference, Montreal, 1989: abstract no. W.B.P.51.

98. Stoumbos VD and Klein ML: Syphilitic retinitis in a patient with acquired immunodeficiency syndrome-related complex. *Am J Ophthalmol* 103-4, January, 1987.

99. Carter JB, Hamill RJ and Matoba AY: Bilateral syphilitic optic neuritis in a patient with a positive test for HIV. *Arch Ophthalmol* 105:1485-1486, 1887.

100. Johns DR, Tierney M and Felsenstein D: Alteration in the natural history of neurosyphilis by concurrent infection with the human immunodeficiency virus. *N Engl J Med* 316:1569-72.

101. Reid SE: Neurosyphilis and stroke in a patient with antibodies to the human immunodeficiency virus. *Amer J Med* 87:119-21, 1989.

102. Katz DA and Berger JR: Neurosyphilis in acquired immunodeficiency syndrome. *Arch Neurol* 46:895-97, 1989.

103. Pialoux G, Jobin D, Robinet M et al: Syphilitic retinitis and uveitis in AIDS. IV International AIDS Conference, Stockholm, 1988: abstract no. 7633.

104. Armignacco O, Antonucci G, Croce GF et al: Syphilis and HIV infection. IV International AIDS Conference, Stockholm, 1988: abstract no. 7634.

105. Bari MM, Shuldin DJ and Abell E: Ulcerative syphilis in acquired immunodeficiency syndrome: a case of precocious tertiary syphilis in a patient infected with human immunodeficiency virus. *J Amer Acad Derm* 21:1310-12, 1989.

106. Dawson S, Evans BA and Lawrence AG: Short communication benign tertiary syphilis and HIV infection. *AIDS* 2:315-16, 1988.

107. Centers for Disease Control: Recommendations for diagnosing and treating syphilis in HIV-infected patients. *MMWR* 37:600-08, 1988.

108. Hicks CB, Benson PM, Lupton GP et al: Seronegative secondary syphilis in a patient infected with the human immunodeficiency virus (HIV) with kaposi sarcoma. *Ann of Int Med* 107:492-95, 1987.

109. Morgello S and Laufer H: Quaternary neurosyphilis in a Haitian man with human immunodeficiency virus infection. *Hum Path* 20:808-11, 1989.

110. Malessa R, Bahro M, Brockmeyer N et al: Neurosyphilis in HIV-infected patients: evidence of unreliable serologic responses. V International AIDS Conference, Montreal, 1989: abstract no. W.B.P.50.

111. Feraru ER, Aronow HA and Lipton RB: Neurosyphilis in AIDS patients: initial CSF VDRL may be negative. *Neurol* 40:541-43, 1990.

112. Berry CD, Hooton TM, Collier AC et al: Neurologic relapse after benzathine penicillin therapy for secondary syphilis in a patient with HIV infection. *N Engl J Med* 316:1587-89.

113. Richards BW, Hessburg TJ, Nussbaum JN et al: Recurrent syphilitic uveitis. *N Engl J Med* 320:60-61, 1989.

114. Duncan WC: Failure of erythromycin to cure secondary syphilis in a patient infected with the human immunodeficiency virus. *Arch Dermatol* 125:82-84, 1989.

115. Hook EW: Treatment of syphilis: current recommendations, alternatives, and continuing problems. *Rev Inf Dis* 11:S1511-17, 1989.

116. Beck-Sague CM, Alexander ER and Jaffe HW: Neurosyphilis and HIV infection. *N Engl J Med* (letter) 317:1473, 1987.

117. Jordan KG: Neurosyphilis and HIV infection. *N Engl J Med* (letter) 317:1473-74, 1987.

118. Fiumara N: Human immunodeficiency virus infection and syphilis. *J Amer Acad Derm* 21:141-42, 1989.

119. Fernandez-Guerrero ML, Miranda C, Cenjor C et al: The treatment of neurosyphilis in patients with HIV infection. *JAMA* (letter) 259:1495-96, 1988.

120. Tseng CK, Hughes MA and Sell S: Altered immunity to syphilis in HIV-1-infected rabbits. *Immunol* 31:234 abstract no. 1383, 1990.

121. Lukehart SA, Hook EW, Baker-Zander SA et al: Invasion of the central nervous system by Treponema pallidum: implications for diagnosis and treatment. *Ann Int Med*:588-62, 1988.

122. Schultz S, Araneta MR, Joseph S et al: Neurosyphilis and HIV infection. *N Engl J Med* (letter) 317:1474, 1987.

123. Manoka AT, Laga M, Kivuvu M et al: Syphilis among HIV and HIV prostitutes in Kinshasa: prevalence and serologic response to treatment. VI International AIDS Conference, San Francisco, 1990: abstract no. S.B.27.

124. Haas JS, Bolan G, Larsen S et al: Sensitivity of treponemal tests for detecting prior treated syphilis during human immunodeficiency virus infection. *J Infect Dis* 162:862-866, 1990.

125. Quinnan GV, Masur H, Rook AH et al: Herpesvirus infections in the acquired immune deficiency syndrome. *JAMA* 252:72-77, 1984.

126. Sooy CD and Mills J: Herpes virus infection presenting as giant herpetic nasal ulcers in AIDS. IV International AIDS Conference, Stockholm, 1988: abstract no. 7096.

127. Siegal FP, Lopez C, Hammer GS et al: Severe acquired immunodeficiency in male homosexuals, manifested by chronic perianal ulcerative herpes simplex lesions. *N Engl J Med* 305:1439-44, 1981.

128. Maier JA, Bergman A and Ross MG: Acquired immunodeficiency syndrome manifested by chronic primary genital herpes. *Am J Obstet Gyn* 155:756-58, 1986.
129. Corey, L: Genital Herpes. In: Sexually Transmitted Diseases, Holmes KK (ed). New York, McGraw Hill, Inc., 1990, p 399.
130. Gold D and Corey L: Acyclovir prophylaxis for herpes simplex virus infection. *Antimicro Agents Chemo* 31:361-67, 1987.
131. Thin RN: Management of genital herpes simplex infections. *Amer J Med* 85:3-6, 1988.
132. Conant MA: Prophylactic and suppressive treatment with acyclovir and the management of herpes in patients with acquired immunodeficiency syndrome. *J Amer Acad Derm* 18:186-88, 1988.
133. Birch CJ, Tachedjian G, Doherty RR et al: Altered sensitivity to antiviral drugs of herpes simplex virus isolates from a patient with the acquired immunodeficiency syndrome. *J Infect Dis* 162:731-34, 1990.
134. Chatis PA, Miller CH, Schrager LE et al: Successful treatment with foscarnet of an acyclovir-resistant mucocutaneous infection with herpes simplex virus in a patient with the acquired immunodeficiency syndrome. *N Engl J Med* 320:297-300, 1989.
135. Norris SA, Kessler HA, and Fife KH: Severe, progressive herpetic whitlow caused by an acyclovir-resistant virus in a patient with AIDS (letter). *J Infect Dis* 157:209-210, 1988.
136. Schinazi RF, del Bene V, Scott RT et al: Characterization of acyclovir-resistant and -sensitive herpes simplex viruses isolated from a patient with an acquired immune deficiency. *J Antimicrob Chemother* 18(suppl):127-134, 1986.
137. Youle MM, Hawkins DA, Collins P et al: Acyclovir-resistant herpes in AIDS patients treated with Foscarnet (letter). *Lancet* 2:341-342. 1988.
138. Causey DM, Rarick MU, Melancon H: Foscarnet treatment of acyclovir-resistant herpes simplex proctitis in an AIDS patients. IV International AIDS Conference, Stockholm, 1988: abstract no. 3589.
139. Erlich K, Mills J, Chatis P et al: Acyclovir-resistant herpes simplex virus infections in patients with the acquired immunodeficiency syndrome. *N Engl J Med* 320:293-296, 1989.
140. Safrin, S, Assaykeen T et al: Foscarnet therapy for acyclovir-resistant mucocutaneous herpes simplex virus infection in 26 AIDS patients: preliminary data. *J Infect Dis* 161:1078-1084, 1990.
141. Doherty R, Hayes K, Birch C et al: Evolution of foscarnet and acyclovir resistant herpes simplex infection in response to therapy. VI International AIDS Conference, San Francisco, 1990: abstract no. Th.B.446.
142. Englund JA, Zimmerman M, Erice A et al: Development of herpes simplex virus (HSV) resistance to acyclovir in HIV infected patients. IV International AIDS Conference, Stockholm, 1988: abstract no. 7095.
143. Byrne MA, Taylor-Robinson D, Munday PE et al: The common occurrence of human papillomavirus infection and intraepithelial neoplasia in women infected by HIV. *AIDS* 3:379-82, 1989.
144. Caubel P, Poulques H and Katlama C: Multifocal human papillomavirus infections of the genital tract in HIV seropositive women. *NYS J Med*:162-63, 1990.
145. Milburn PB, Brandsma JL, Goldsman CI et al: Disseminated warts and evolving squamous cell carcinoma in a patient with acquired immunodeficiency syndrome. *J Amer Acad Derm* 19:401-05, 1988.
146. Rudlinger R, Grob R, Buchmann P et al: Anogenital warts of the condyloma acuminatum type in HIV-positive patients. *Dermatologica* 176:277-88, 1988.
147. Palefsky J, Gonzales J, Greenblatt RM et al: Anal intraepithelial neoplasia and anal papillomavirus infection among homosexual males with group IV HIV disease. *JAMA* 263:2911-16, 1990.
148. Feingold AR, Vermund SH, Burk RD et al: Cervical cytologic abnormalities and papillomavirus in women infected with human immunodeficiency virus. *J Acq Imm Def Syn* 3:896-903, 1990.

149. Thomas G, Geraci A, Lavigne J et al: Recurrent anogenital warts and HIV status. VI International AIDS Conference, San Francisco, 1990: abstract no. Th.B.362.

150. McMillan A and Bishop PE: Clinical course of anogenital warts in men infected with human immunodeficiency virus. *Genitourin Med* 65:225-28, 1989.

151. Bishop PE, McMillan A and Fletcher S: Immunological study of condylomata acuminata in men infected with the human immunodeficiency virus. *Inter J STD & AIDS* 1:28-31, 1990.

152. Bradbeer C: Is infection with HIV a risk factor for cervical intraepithelial neoplasia? *Lancet*:1277-78, November 28, 1987.

153. Bradbeer CS, Heyderman E: The risk of progression of cervical dysplasia in women with HIV. V International AIDS Conference, Montreal, 1989: abstract no. M.B.P.58.

154. Henry MJ, Stanley MW, Cruikshank S et al: Association of human immunodeficiency virus-induced immunosuppression with human papillomavirus infection and cervical intraepithelial neoplasia. *Am J Obstet Gynecol* 160:352-53, 1989.

155. Hiller KF, Lutz R, Baur M et al: High rates of cervical dysplasias, cervical intra-epithelial neoplasias (CIN) and human papilloma virus infection in HIV infected female patients. V International AIDS Conference, Montreal, 1989: abstract no. M.B.P.60.

156. Pomeroy L, Boylan P, Murphy J et al: Cervical intraepithelial neoplasia in HIV seronegative drug abusers. VI International AIDS Conference, San Francisco, 1990: abstract no. S.B.518.

157. Schrager LK, Friedland GH, Maude D et al: Cervical and vaginal squamous cell abnormalities in women infected with human immunodeficiency virus. *J Acq Imm Def Syn* 2:570-75, 1989.

158. Schafer A, Wolfgang F, Mielke M et al: Increased frequency of cervical dysplasia/neoplasia in HIV-infected women is related to the extent of immunosuppression. VI International AIDS Conference, San Francisco, 1990: abstract no. S.B.519.

159. Muggiasca ML, Conti E, Ravasi L et al: Human immunodeficiency virus and human papilloma virus in the cervical intraepithelial neoplasia (CIN) in development of past intravenous drug abusers (PIVDA) women. V International AIDS Conference, Montreal, 1989: abstract no. M.B.P.56.

160. Goedert JJ, Caussey D, Palefsky J et al: Anal pap smears and human papilloma viruses (HPV) in a 7-year cohort study of homosexual men. Proc Ann Meet Am Soc Clin Oncol 9:A6, 1990.

161. Frazer IH, Medley G, Crapper RM et al: The association between anorectal dysplasia, human papillomavirus, and human immunodeficiency virus infection in homosexual men. *Lancet*:657-60, September 20, 1986.

162. LaVigne J, Thomas G, Geraci A et al: Occurrence of malignancy in the setting of anogenital warts in the gay male population. VI International AIDS Conference, San Francisco, 1990: abstract no. S.B.520.

163. Vermund SH, Kelley DF, Burk RD et al: Risk of human papillomavirus (HPV) and cervical squamous intraepithelial lesions (SIL) highest among women with advanced HIV disease. VI International AIDS Conference, San Francisco, 1990: abstract no. S.B.517.

164. Crocchiolo P, Lizioli A, Goisis F et al: Cervical dysplasia and HIV infection. *Lancet* (letter) 238-39, January 30, 1988.

164a. Plummer FA, Simonsen JN, Chubb H, et al: Epidemiological evidence for the development of serovar-specific immunity after gonococcal infection. *J Clin Invest* 83:1472-6, 1989.

165. Moyle G, Barton SE, Rowe IF et al: Gonococcal arthritis caused by auxotype P in a man with HIV infection. *Genitourin Med* 66:91-92, 1990.

166. Hoegsberg B, Abulatia O, Sedlis A et al: Sexually transmitted diseases and human immunodeficiency virus among women with pelvic inflammatory disease. *Am J Obstet Gynecol*, in press.

167. Alexander NJ: Sexual transmission of HIV: virus entry into male and female tract. *Fertility & Sterility* 54:1-18, 1990.

168. Bagasra O, Freud M, Condoluci D et al: Presence of HIV-1 in the sperms of HIV-seropositive individuals by DNA-hybridization and immunogold methods. V International AIDS Conference, Montreal, 1989: abstract no. M.C.P.86.

169. Borzy MS, Connell RS and Kiessling AA: Detection of human immunodeficiency virus in cell-free seminal fluid. *J Acq Imm Def Syn* 1:419-24, 1988.

170. Krieger JN, Coombs R, Collier A et al: HIV recovery from semen: minimal impact of clinical stage of infection and minimal effect of semen analysis parameters. VI International AIDS Conference, San Francisco, 1990: abstract no. Th.C.102.

171. Krieger JN, Coombs AC, Collier SO et al: Patterns of human immunodeficiency virus excretion in semen of seropositive men: a cross-sectional and longitudinal study. 30th ICAAC, Atlanta: abstract no. 309.

172. Van de Perre P, De Clercq A, Cogniaux-Leclerc J et al: Detection of HIV p17 antigen in lymphocytes but not epithelial cells from cervicovaginal secretions of women seropositive for HIV: implications for heterosexual transmission of the virus. *Genitourin Med* 64:30-33, 1988.

173. Vogt MW, Witt DJ, Craven DE et al: Isolation of HTLV-III/LAV from cervical secretions of women at risk for AIDS. *Lancet* 525-30, March 8, 1986.

174. Vogt MW, Witt DJ, Craven DE et al: Isolation patterns of the human immunodeficiency virus from cervical secretions during the menstrual cycle of women at risk for the acquired immunodeficiency syndrome. *Ann Inter Med* 106:380-82, 1987.

175. Wofsy CB, Cohen JB, Hauer LB et al: Isolation of AIDS-associated retrovirus from genital secretions of women with antibodies to the virus. *Lancet* 527-29, March 8, 1986.

176. Wolff H, and Anderson DJ: HIV im sperma. *Hautarzt* 40:737-40, 1989.

177. Donegan SP, de la Monte S, Steger KA at al: HIV-1 infection of the lower female genital tract. VI International AIDS Conference, San Francisco, 1990: abstract no. F.C.750.

178. Pomerantz RJ, de la Monte M, Donegan SP et al: Human immunodeficiency virus (HIV) infection of the uterine cervix. *Ann Inter Med* 108:321-27, 1988.

179. Edwards JN and Morris HB: Langerhans' cells and lymphocyte subsets in the female genital tract. *Br J Obstet Gynecol* 92:974-82, 1985.

180. Meltzer MS, Skillman DR, Gomatos PJ et al: Role of mononuclear phagocytes in the pathogenesis of human immunodeficiency virus infection. *Annu Rev Immunol* 8:169-94, 1990.

181. Wolff H, Anderson DJ: Immunohistologic characterization and quantitation of leukocyte subpopulations in human semen. *Fert & Ster* 49:497-504, 1988.

182. Bishop PE, McMillan A and Gilmour HM: Immunological study of the rectal mucosa of men with and without human immunodeficiency virus infection. *Gut* 28:1619-24, 1987.

183. Mayer KH, Zierler S, Feingold L et al: Sexually transmitted diseases and genital tract inflammation among U.S. heterosexuals at increased risk for HIV infection. 30th ICCAC, Atlanta: abstract no. 307.

184. Wolff H, and Anderson DJ: Male genital tract inflammation associated with increased number of potential human immunodeficiency virus host cells in semen. *Androl* 20:404-10, 1988.

185. Cunningham AL, Turner RR, Miller AC et al: Evolution of recurrent herpes simplex lesions. *J Clin Invest* 75:226-33, 1985.

186. Lukehart SA, Baker-Zander SA, Lloyd RM et al: Characterization of lymphocyte responsiveness in early experimental syphilis. *J Immunol* 124:461-67, 1980.

187. Schmitz L, Holmes KK, Kiviat N: Histopathology of STDs in the Female Genital Tract. Submitted.

188. Miller CJ, Alexander NJ, Sutjipto S et al: Genital mucosal transmission of simian immunodeficiency virus: animal model for heterosexual transmission of human immunodeficiency virus. *J Virol* 63:4277-84.

189. Kreiss JK, Coombs R, Plummer FA et al: Isolation of human immunodeficiency virus from genital ulcers in Nairobi prostitutes. *J Infect Dis* 160:380-84, 1989.

190. Plummer FA, Wainberg MA, Plourde P et al: Detection of human immunodeficiency virus type 1 (HIV-1) in genital ulcer exudate of HIV-1-infected men by culture and gene amplification. *J Infect Dis* 161:810-11, 1990.

191. Quinn TC, Piot P, McCormick JB, et al: Serologic and immunologic studies in patients with AIDS in North America and Africa. *JAMA* 257:2617-21, 1987.

192. Hirsch MS, Schooley RT, Ho DD et al: Possible viral interaction in the acquired immunodeficiency syndrome (AIDS). *Rev Infect Dis* 6:726-31, 1984.

193. Laurence J: Molecular interactions among herpesviruses and human immunodeficiency viruses. *J Infect Dis* 162:358-346, 1990

194. Margolis DM, Parrott C, Leonard J et al: The role of DNA binding motifs in transactivation of the HIV long terminal repeat (LTR) by herpes simplex virus type 1 (HSV-1). VI International AIDS Conference, San Francisco, 1990: abstract no. S.A.229.

195. Borkowski JA, Albin R, Schwartz J et al: The Epstein Barr virus (EBV) BZLF 1 gene product activates the HIV-1 5'LTR. VI International AIDS Conference, San Francisco, 1990: abstract no. S.A.230.

196. McCormack MH, Azad RF, Rosen JI et al: Cytomegalovirus (CMV) induces HIV transcriptional activity in human fibroblasts. VI International AIDS Conference, San Francisco, 1990: abstract no. S.A.225.

197. Skolnik PR, Kosloff BR and Hirsch MS: Bidirectional interactions between human immunodeficiency virus type 1 and cytomegalovirus. *J Infect Dis* 157:508-14, 1988.

198. Pepin J, Plummer FA, Brunham RC et al: The interaction of HIV infection and other sexually transmitted diseases: an opportunity for intervention. *AIDS* 3:3-9, 1989.

199. Piot P and Laga M: Genital ulcers, other sexually transmitted diseases, and the sexual transmission of HIV. *Br Med J* 298:623-24, 1989.

200. Kreiss JK, Carael M, Meheus A et al: Role of sexually transmitted diseases in transmitting human immunodeficiency virus. *Genitourin Med* 64:1-2, 1988.

201. Piot P, Kreiss JK, Ndinya-Achola JO et al: Editorial review: heterosexual transmission of HIV. *AIDS* 1:199-206, 1987.

202. Piot P and Carael M: Epidemiological and sociological aspects of HIV-infection in developing countries. *Brit Med Bull* 44:68-88, 1988.

203. World Health Organization: Report of the Research Sub-Committee of the AIDS/STD Task Force. July, 1990.

204. World Health Organization: Consensus statement from consultation on sexually transmitted diseases as a risk factor for HIV transmission. *J Acq Imm Def Syn* 2:248-55, 1989.

THE PUBLIC HEALTH SIGNIFICANCE OF SEXUALLY
TRANSMITTED DISEASES FOR HIV INFECTION IN AFRICA

Seth Berkley

The Rockefeller Foundation

INTRODUCTION

In sub-Saharan Africa, the primary mode of transmission of HIV is through heterosexual intercourse. Numerous studies, both retrospective (1-13) and prospective (14-16), have demonstrated a relationship between sexually transmitted diseases (STDs) and HIV infection. Initially, it was thought that STDs might just be markers of high-risk sexual behavior. It is now postulated that STDs are co-factors in facilitating the sexual transmission of HIV. As a result, scientists and public health officials have called for the urgent enhancement of existing STD programs, or implementation of new programs, as an important strategy in AIDS prevention.

STDs are an important cause of morbidity and mortality in the developing world, and for that reason alone, deserve increased attention. Furthermore, there is no question that primary prevention of STDs by safer sex practices (condom use, monogamy with an uninfected partner, or abstention) would also reduce HIV transmission. However, studies have also shown that STDs – particularly genital ulcerative diseases (GUD), and more recently, chlamydia, gonorrhea, and trichomonas – are independent risk factors for HIV transmission (16,17). If this is true, it follows that aggressive treatment of STDs could reduce transmission of HIV even if no change occurred in sexual practices. As the implementation of extensive new STD control programs would require major financial and logistical resources, it is important to assess the impact that STD control programs might have on the transmission of HIV infection. This chapter reviews some of the key concepts and assumptions that are required to make calculations concerning the potential impact of STD control on HIV infection.

MEASUREMENT OF THE ASSOCIATION BETWEEN HIV AND STDs

The measure of the relative risk, or risk ratio, is used to study the association between a disease and a certain factor (or exposure) in a group exposed to this factor as compared to an unexposed group. The relative risk (risk ratio) is defined as the incidence of disease in the exposed group divided by the incidence of disease in the unexposed group, and is a measure of how many times more likely the disease occurs in the exposed group than in the unexposed group. The relative risk (or the odds ratio, which will be used as an approximation of the relative risk) provides information beyond that conveyed by significance testing alone (i.e., reporting a p-value only), as it gives additional information about the magnitude of the association.

To understand the practical importance of an association, one needs to know not only the strength of the association, but also the prevalence of exposure to the risk factor in the general population. For example, it is known that there is a strong association between receiving an HIV-infected blood transfusion and the subsequent development of AIDS in the recipient. If, however, blood transfusions are only rarely given in a certain area, the association, although still present and of the same magnitude, is of limited public health significance. A relative risk of 2 can be generated from incidence rates of 80% in the exposed group compared to 40% in the unexposed group, or from an incidence of 2 per million in the exposed group versus 1 per million in the unexposed group – two very different scenarios.

One way to determine the public health importance of an association is to ask how many cases of disease transmission could be prevented by the removal of a certain risk factor. More specifically, in this chapter we address the question, What percentage of HIV transmission would be prevented by removing other STDs without changing any other behaviors? This measurement is called the attributable risk.*

Figure 1 demonstrates the calculation of the attributable risk of a risk factor, expressed as a percentage, based on its strength of association (relative risk) and on the proportion of the population exposed (prevalence) to the risk factor. As can be seen, a risk factor with a weak association and a high prevalence may be responsible for more transmission in the population than one that has a strong association and is rare. For example, if 1% of the population is exposed to a risk factor that increases the risk of disease tenfold, it can be estimated that 8% of all cases could be eliminated by removal of the factor. On the other hand, if an exposure to the risk factor is common, with a prevalence of 25% in the general population (like some STDs in certain areas of Africa), with a relative risk of 2 (which is one-fifth the association in the previous example), this exposure would be responsible for 20% of all cases.

PUBLIC HEALTH SIGNIFICANCE OF THE HIV-STD ASSOCIATION: ISSUES TO CONSIDER

Four issues must be considered in understanding the public health significance of the association between STDs and HIV infection: 1) Are STDs risk factors for the transmission of HIV infection?; 2) If so, what is the magnitude of the association?; 3) How common are STDs in the general population, or in relevant subgroups?; and 4) Is the control of STDs feasible and if so, what would be the effect of this control?

To simplify matters, discussion will be limited to STDs and heterosexual transmission of HIV infection in Africa.

STDs as Risk Factors

This issue has been studied by a number of authors and is reviewed by Judith Wasserheit in this volume (17,18). It is clear that further studies are necessary. Studies have varied by methodology and have found some conflicting results. Most studies are observational in nature; as such,

---

* The terms used for this concept are not yet standardized. Different authors use the terms "etiologic fraction," "attributable risk," and "risk difference" to define this concept, often calculating the ratio with different denominators. It should be noted that the concept of attributable risk does imply a causal relationship — an assumption often difficult to prove.

the association found between STDs and HIV may be confounded by other risk factors and not be causal. Despite these problems, a consensus on the issue of HIV and STD association was reached at a 1988 consultancy at the World Health Organization (WHO), and for the purposes of this chapter, it will be assumed that at least some STDs are independent risk factors for transmission of HIV infection (19). It is important to realize, however, that this issue is not yet adequately resolved.

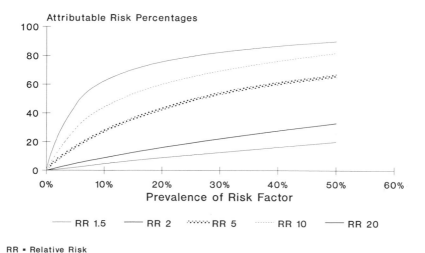

Attributable Risk Percentages

Prevalence of Risk Factor

—— RR 1.5   —— RR 2   ······ RR 5   ······ RR 10   —— RR 20

RR ▪ Relative Risk

Figure 1. Calculation of attributable risk percentage using relative risk and prevalence of risk factor.

Magnitude of the Association

The estimatation of the magnitude of the association between HIV infection and STDs suffers from the same methologic problems. As HIV in Africa is primarily transmitted sexually, it is by definition an STD. Because HIV and other STDs are so closely associated in terms of transmission, it is extremely difficult to separate all of the common factors and behaviors to show a 'clean' (i.e., non-confounded) association. For example, as thoughtfully discussed and demonstrated in a recent paper (20), this association may be artifactually high or low, as persons with multiple sexual partners who are at risk for one STD are also at risk for all other STDs, including HIV infection. The association seen may be a result of common risk behaviors rather than the result of a causal effect on transmission.

A proper study should account for all of the potential factors that may confound the relationship between general STD transmission and transmission of HIV, including number of sexual contacts and partners, contacts with prostitutes, and even specific sexual behaviors. There is evidence to suggest that persons infected with HIV are more susceptible to STDs, and more likely to have prolonged, classical STDs; this makes it important to determine the temporal sequence of infection.

Table 1. Selected retrospective and cross-sectional studies demonstrating a relationship between a specific STD and HIV infection in Africa.

Country	Group	STD Ascertainment History/Exam	Type STD	Approximate Odds Ratio
Tanzania (1)	STD clinic	E	Genital Ulcers	4.4
Kenya (2)	Prostitutes low status	E	Genital Ulcers	3.3*
Kenya (2)	Prostitutes low status	E	Syphilis	2.5*
Kenya (2)	Prostitutes low status	E	Gonorrhea	3.8*
Uganda (3)	STD Clinic	E	Genital Ulcers	1.8
Kenya (4)	Males in STD clinic	H	Genital Ulcers	7.2
Kenya (4)	Males in STD clinic	E	Genital Ulcers	2.0
Zaire (5)	Male employees	H	Genital Ulcers	2.7
Kenya (6)	STD clinic	H	Genital Ulcers	2.4
Kenya (7)	Females family planning clinic	E	Gonorrhea	5.6*
Kenya (8)	Prostitutes	E	Gonorrhea	5.6

* Adjusted odds ratio by logistic regression

Table 1 shows some of the major retrospective and cross-sectional studies done to date in Africa addressing the interaction between STDs and HIV. As can be seen, studies demonstrate a range of relative risks of HIV transmission in persons with genital ulcers (1.8 to 7.2), syphilis (2.5), and gonorrhea (3.8 to 5.6). These studies were conducted in high- and lower-risk settings among prostitutes, antenatal clinic attendees, and STD clinic patients. Data for chancroid are somewhat limited due to the difficulty of culturing the organism; but using serum antibody against *H. ducreyi*, the odds of association between *H. ducreyi* serologic markers and HIV infection varied from 1.8 to 3.3 in different groups in Africa (21).

Since these studies were done with different methodologies and different populations, they are not directly comparable. Yet, all show a consistent association between the presence of STDs and an increased risk of HIV infection.* The magnitude of association as measured by the relative risk, or odds ratio, varies from 1.8 to 7.2 based on the group studied, the particular STD, and the methodology. However, only a few of these studies are controlled for potential confounding factors, and these studies are not prospective; thus, they are not ideally suited to document the temporal association between the presence of an STD and HIV infection.

---

* There is a well-known bias that non-associations are probably less likely to be reported. We cannot use the lack of reported studies demonstrating non-associations as definitive.

Table 2. Prospective studies in Africa demonstrating a relationship between an STD and HIV infection.

Country	Group	Type STD	Odds Ratio	Adjusted OR by Logistic Regression
Kenya (14)	Male Prostitute Clients	Genital Ulcers		4.7
Kenya (15)	Female Prostitutes	Genital Ulcers	2.4	3.7
Kenya (15)	Female Prostitutes	Chlamydia trachomatis	3.3	5.7
Zaire (16)	Female Prostitutes	Gonorrhea		3.5
Zaire (16)	Female Prostitutes	Chlamydia		3.2
Zaire (16)	Female Prostitutes	Trichomonas		2.7

The few studies in Africa that are prospective, and have been carefully controlled for the influence of confounding factors, are shown in Table 2. These studies show associations similar to the retrospective studies discussed above. However, these studies have been performed in selected groups that may limit their generalizability to other members of the population. For example, despite the strong associations seen between STDs and HIV in female prostitutes in Kinshasa (16), a study done by the same group of researchers in antenatal clinic attendees failed to shown an association between these STDs and HIV infection (22). To understand the importance of these findings in terms of the general population, high quality prospective studies of this association in normal heterosexual populations are urgently needed.

Prevalence of STDs

The data to determine the prevalence of STDs in the general population in Africa are even more limited than are studies of the association between STDs and HIV. There are very few current population-based STD studies in Africa, and none that were prospectively done using physical examination and microbiological isolation for diagnosis. However, there does exist some data on STD prevalences in selected groups in Africa.

Table 3 lists studies done in high-risk groups, such as prostitutes, or in selected populations, such as attendees of STD clinics. The data show large differences in STD prevalences in different areas and groups. Although these figures have relevance for studies done in these populations, they are not representative of the prevalence in the general population, nor are they likely to be representative of the prevalence among prostitutes generally. Furthermore, cross-sectional studies only describe part of the epidemiology of these infections; persons may have multiple episodes of STDs in any study period.

Table 4 contains information on the prevalence of STDs from prenatal clinic attendees, a group that may best reflect the prevalence of STDs in the general female population. However, this data may be biased by the fact that it is derived only from sexually active, fertile women who are coming to a clinic and may have to pay for the services rendered. Studies in this population group have shown serologic evidence of syphilis in 1-15%, culture evidence of gonorrhea in 2-11%, serologic and bacteriologic evidence of chlamydia in 6-19%, and microscopic identification of trichomonas in 17-32% of attendees.

Table 3. Prevalence of STDs in selected studies conducted in prostitutes in Africa.

Country	Reference	STD	Group	Percentage Infected
Uganda	(23)	Syphilis		46%
Kenya	(24)	Syphilis		41%
Kenya	(25)	Syphilis	Low Status	31%
Zaire	(26)	Syphilis		18%
Kenya	(25)	Syphilis	High Status	14%
Kenya	(24)	Gonorrhea		47%
Zaire	(26)	Gonorrhea		35%
Somalia	(27)	Chlamydia		33%
Zaire	(26)	Chlamydia		20%
Zaire	(26)	Trichomonas		16%
Kenya	(24)	Trichomonas		28%

Data on chancroid are not available on a population basis, but there is evidence that *H. ducreyi* is the etiology in a substantial percentage of all the genital ulcer disease (GUD) in sub-Saharan Africa (>50% in studies in Kenya [37,38]). Table 5 lists some studies of GUD and chancroid. As GUD has been the STD syndrome most strongly associated with HIV, studies to clarify the epidemiology of this infection are required.

The Effect of STD Control

The attributable risk of a disease in the general population can only be generated with population-based data. However, an attempt to estimate the magnitude of the attributable risk using the data that exists as a surrogate for population-based studies is warranted and will be attempted here.

Using data available from a prospective study in Kenya, an attributable risk of 33% for genital ulcers in female prostitutes can be generated (13). This suggests that the eradication of genital ulcer disease in this group would result in a 33% reduction of HIV infection in these prostitutes.* As these high-risk persons are thought to be responsible for a large percentage of female-to-male transmission in the total Nairobi population, such eradication may have a profound impact on the propagation of HIV transmission. Difficulties in generalization, however, are shown by another prospective study in prostitutes in Zaire (16). In that study, genital ulcers were not shown to be a risk factor, probably due to the low prevalence of genital ulcers in the prostitutes (5%).

It is unknown whether these associations and prevalences are valid for the general population. It is known, however, that the dynamics of STD transmission in prostitutes are different from those in the general population, as are the prevalences of genital ulcers and other STDs. This

---

* The imprecision of the estimate can be shown by the 95% confidence interval of the attributable risk percentage of 10-56% (40). The figures generated in this chapter are for conceptual purposes only.

Table 4. Prevalences of STDs in selected studies conducted in antenatal clinic attendees in Africa.

Country	Reference	STD	Percentage Infected
Malawi	(28)	Syphilis	15%
Zambia	(29)	Syphilis	13%
Mozambique	(30)	Syphilis	6%
Gambia	(31)	Syphilis	1%
Zaire	(22)	Syphilis	1%
Zambia	(33)	Gonorrhea	11%
Gambia	(31)	Gonorrhea	7%
Tanzania	(34)	Gonorrhea	6%
Zaire	(22)	Gonorrhea	2%
Somalia	(27)	Chlamydia	19%
Gabon	(35)	Chlamydia	10%
Kenya	(36)	Chlamydia	10%
Gambia	(31)	Chlamydia	7%
Zaire	(22)	Chlamydia	6%
Gambia	(31)	Trichomonas	32%
Zaire	(22)	Trichomonas	17%

problem is demonstrated by the difference between the 0.3% point prevalence of chancroid in one study of outpatients in Nairobi (Table 5) and the prevalence of chancroid estimated to be 50 times higher in Nairobi prostitutes over a 54-month period, based on the occurrence of genital ulcers.

In a cross-sectional study of postpartum women in Nairobi, the prevalence of any STD (i.e., syphilis, gonorrhea, or chlamydia) was 9%. Using seroprevalence data from that study, an attributable risk of 8% for STDs can be estimated (personal communication, Marlene Temmerman, University of Nairobi). This sub-population is more representative of the general population of females than are prostitutes, but cannot be considered representative of the general population. The difference in attributable risk between prostitutes and members of the general population cannot be dismissed lightly. As previously mentioned, another study in Kinshasa, Zaire of 701 first attendees at antenatal clinics showed no statistical association between STDs and HIV infection (22).

Even in a small geographic area, prevalences of STDs vary dramatically depending on the group studied. This results in different attributable risks among different subgroups of the population (Table 6). Furthermore, the consensus of most researchers in Africa is that the HIV epidemic has moved from high-risk groups in the urban areas to the general population in both urban and rural areas. What would STD control do in these areas?

As mentioned above, there are no data from prospective studies of STDs in the general population. A retrospective general population-based study in Uganda showed a self-reported STD

Table 5. Genital ulcers and chancroid: selected studies in Africa.

Author	Country	Group	Percentage
Genital Ulcers			
Nzila (26)	Zaire	Prostitutes	15% [65% Chancroid]
Ndinya-Achola (15)	Kenya	Prostitutes	51% [50% Chancroid]
Chancroid			
Mbugua (39)	Kenya	Urban Outpatients	0.3% [100% Chancroid]

rate of 15%. This rate was associated with a relative risk for HIV infection of 1.5, resulting in a population attributable risk in this study of only 7% (41). However, it is known that many STDs are only mildly symptomatic or even asymptomatic, especially in women. Thus, STDs that are self-reported or reported by passive surveillance are probably grossly underestimated, yielding an underestimated population attributable risk (PAR). Population-based studies must be repeated in a prospective fashion with laboratory evaluation of STDs.

Although the case for an association between the occurrence of an STD and increased transmission of HIV infection has been most persuasively made for GUD, recent data suggest that other STDs – including gonorrhea, chlamydia, trichomonas, and candida – may also increase the efficacy of transmission. This is an enormously important issue. Genital ulcers, which have a high relative risk, are probably rare in the general population, and thus contribute to a low attributable risk. But most very sexually active persons in Africa will contract at least one of the other STDs at some point. With high lifetime probabilities of contracting an STD other than GUD, the attributable risk for those non-ulcerative STDs might be high even if, for the population, the relative risk for that STD is not as high as for GUD.

The final issue is perhaps the most crucial: Even if the attributable risk is of a high magnitude, can an STD control program successfully remove the risk factor? Can theory be translated into practice? Only experience will reveal the answer to this question. It is important to remember that the amount of infection that can be prevented by the elimination of a risk factor (as expressed by the calculation of an attributable risk) assumes complete eradication of the factor in the population. Proportionally smaller reductions in the presence of the risk factor will generate a smaller reduction in the associated transmission of infection and a correspondingly smaller public health significance for the interventions.

To gather relevant data on the feasibility and impact of such interventions, an advisory group to the WHO's Global Programme on AIDS recommended STD intervention studies as its highest priority. An essential component of these studies will be cost effectiveness comparisons of different interventions. With the per capita health expenditures of many African countries under 10 U.S. dollars per year, and with shortages of health care providers and public health officials, limited health and educational resources must be prioritized. Economic analyses should not only calculate the effect of the program on HIV transmission, but also the derivative benefits of an STD program, such as reductions in involuntary infertility, congenital STD syndromes, and STD morbidity and mortality, as well as better general health education and family planning.

Table 6. Estimated attributable risk of STD on HIV infection from selected studies in Africa.

Disease	Group	Prevalence of STD in Controls	Approximate Odds Ratio	Approximate Attributable Risk (%)
Nairobi, Kenya				
Genital Ulcers (13)	Female Prostitutes	36%	2.4	33%
C. Trachomatis (13)	Female Prostitutes	18%	2.4	20%
S.T.D. (gonorrhea, syphilis, chlamydia)	Post-partum Women	9%	2.0	8%
Chancroid	General Outpatients	0.3%		?
Kinshasa, Zaire				
Gonorrhea (16)	Female Prostitutes	19%	3.5	32%
Trichomonas (16)	Female Prostitutes	18%	2.7	23%
C. Trachomatis (16)	Female Prostitutes	6%	3.2	12%

CONCLUSION

In summary, there is some evidence to suggest a role for some STDs in increasing the risk of HIV transmission. The strength of the association and the prevalence of different STDs in the general population are still not well delineated, although in some selected high-risk populations, such as prostitutes, the attributable risk appears to be high. The evidence of strong association in these selected subgroups, along with the high prevalence of STDs in some African communities, imply a considerable attributable risk for STDs in some groups and warrant STD intervention trials. Because the relationships between HIV and other STDs are not well delineated, all control programs should be accompanied by an active evaluation and research component.

This analysis has, of course, oversimplified the relationship between HIV and STDs. The PAR may differ depending on the particular STD, its clinical stage, the sex and age of the patient, and other potential risk factors, such as male circumcision. Furthermore, since the calculation of attributable risk assumes a direct relationship between an association and a risk factor, it represents a conservative estimate of the maximum benefit of an intervention. Other factors peculiar to the HIV epidemic, such as the high numbers of sexual partners or the increase in susceptibility and expression of STDs, may act as multipliers of the association. The magnitude of the attributable risk might, in fact, be stronger than calculated. Studies in the future need to address not only the biologic interaction of STDs and HIV, but also their relative public health significance. Population-based studies in rural as well as urban communities are desperately needed.

REFERENCES

1. Dielly SA, Shao JF, Mbena E, Mhalu FS. Relationship between infection with HIV and other sexually transmitted diseases among patients attending a referral clinic for sexually transmitted diseases. III International Conference on AIDS and Associated Cancers in Africa, Arusha, Tanzania, September 1988; Abstract W.5.1.
2. Kreiss JK, Koech D, Plummer FA, Holmes KK, Lightfoote M, Piot P, Ronald AR, Ndinya-Achola, D'Costa LJ, Roberts P, Ngugi E, Quinn TC. AIDS virus infection in Nairobi prostitutes—Spread of the epidemic to East Africa. *N Engl J Med* 1986; 314:414-418.
3. Nsubuga P, Mugerwa R, Nsibambi J, Sewankambo N, Katabira E, Berkley S. The association of genital ulcer disease and HIV infection in attendees at a dermatology/STD clinic in Uganda. *J Acq Imm Def Synd* 1990; 3:1002-1005.
4. Simonsen JN, Cameron DW, Gakinya MN, Ndinya-Achola JO, D'Costa LJ, Karasira P, Cheang M, Ronald AR, Piot P, Plummer FA. Human immunodeficiency virus infection among men with sexually transmitted diseases, experience from a center in Africa. *N Engl J Med* 1988; 319:274-278.
5. Ryder RW, Ndilu M, Hassig SE, Kamenga M, Sequeira D, Kashamuka M, Francis H, Behets F, Colebunders RL, Dopagne A, Kambale R, Heyward W. Heterosexual transmission of HIV-1 among employees and their spouses at two large businesses in Zaire. *AIDS* 1990; 4:725-732.
6. Greenblatt RM, Lukehart SA, Plummer FA et al. Genital ulceration as a risk factor for human immunodeficiency virus infection. *AIDS* 1988; 2:47-50.
7. Hunter D, Maggwa A, Mati J, Tukei P, Solomon M, Mbugua S, Bhullar V, Mohammedali Y. Risk Factors for HIV infection among women in a low risk population in Nairobi, Kenya. VI International Conference on AIDS, San Francisco, California, June 1990; Abstract Th.C.573.
8. Piot P, Plummer FA, Rey MA, Ngugi EN, Rouzioux C, Ndinya–Achola JO, Veracauteren G, D'Costa LJ, Laga M, Nsanze H, Fransen L, Haase D, van der Groen G, Brunham RC, Ronald AR, Brun–Vezinet F. Retrospective seroepidemiology of AIDS virus infection in Nairobi populations. *J Infect Dis* 1987; 155:1108-1112.
9. Van de Perre P, Le Polain B, Carael M, Nzaramba D, Zissis G, Butzler JP. HIV antibodies in a remote rural area in Rwanda, Centeral Africa: An analysis of potential risk factors for human HIV seropositivity. *AIDS* 1987; 1:213-215.
10. Berkley SF, Widy-wirski R, Okware SI, Downing R, Linnan MJ, White KE, Sempala S. Risk factors associated with HIV infection in Uganda. *J Infect Dis* 1989:160;22-30.
11. Konde-Lule J, Berkley SF, Downing R. Knowledge, attitudes and practices concerning AIDS in Ugandans. *AIDS* 1989; 3:513-518.
12. Mhalu F, Bredberg-Raden U, Mbena E, Pallangyo K, Kiango J, Mbise R, Nya-muryekunge K, Biberfeld G. Prevalence of HIV infection in healthy subjects and groups of patients in Tanzania. *AIDS* 1987; 1:217-221.
13. Van de Perre P, Carael M, Nzaramba D, Zissis G, Kayihigi J, Butzler J-P. Risk factors for HIV seropositivity in selected urban based Rwandese adults. *AIDS* 1987 1:207-211.
14. Cameron DW, Simonsen JN, D'Costa LJ, Ronald AR, Maitha GM, Gakinya MN, Cheang M, Ndinya-Achola JO, Piot P, Brunham RC, Plummer FA. Female to male transmission of Human Immunodeficiency Virus type 1: Risk factors for seroconversion in men. *Lancet* 1989; ii:403-407.
15. Ndinya-achola JO, Cameron W, Simonsen N, Maitha MG, Kreiss J, Waiyaki P, Ronald A, Ngugi E. Co-factors in male-female transmission of HIV. III International Conference on AIDS and Associated Cancers in Africa, Arusha, Tanzania, September 1988; Abstract W.P.45.

16. Laga M, Nzila N, Manoka AT, Malele M, Bush TJ, Behets F, Heyward WL, Piot P, Ryder R. Non-ulcerative sexually transmitted diseases (STD) as risk factors for HIV infection. VI International Conference on AIDS, San Francisco, California, June 1990; Abstract Th.C.97.

17. Pepin J, Plummer FA, Brunham RC, Piot P, Cameron DW, Ronald AR. Editorial Review: The interaction of HIV infection and other sexually transmitted diseases: an opportunity for intervention. *AIDS* 1989; 3:3-9.

18. Wasserheit JN. Epidemiological Synergy: Interrelationships between HIV infection and other STDs. Chapter 6 in this volume.

19. Consensus statement from consultation on sexually transmitted diseases as a risk factor for HIV transmission. Global Programme on AIDS and Programme of STD, World Health Organization, 1989, Geneva, Switzerland; WHO/GPA/INF/89.1.

20. Mertens TE, Hayes RJ, Smith PG. Epidemiologic methods to study the interaction between HIV infection and other sexually transmitted diseases. *AIDS* 1990; 4:57-65.

21. Piot P, Van Dyck E, Ryder RW, Nzila N, Laga M. Serum antibody to Haemophilus Ducreyi as a risk factor for HIV infection in Africa. V International Conference on AIDS, Montreal, Quebec, Canada, 1989; Abstract M.A.O.32.

22. Luyeye M, Gerniers M, Lebughe N, Behets F, Nzila N, Edidi B, Laga M. Prevalence et facterus de risque pour les MST chez les femmes enceintes dans les soins de sante primaries a Kinshasa. VI International Conference on AIDS, San Francisco, California, June 1990; Abstract T.P.C.6.

23. Hudson CP, Hennis AJ, Kataaha P et al. Risk factors for the spread of AIDS in rural Africa: evidence from a comparative seroepidemiological survey of AIDS, hepatitis B and syphilis in southwestern Uganda. *AIDS* 1988; 2:255-60.

24. DaCosta LJ, Plummer FA, Bowmer I et al. Prostitutes are the major reservoir of sexually transmitted diseases in Nairobi, Kenya. *Sexually Transmitted Diseases* 1985; 12:64-67.

25. Mabey DC. Syphilis in sub–Saharan Africa. *Afr J Sex Transm Dis* 1986; 2:61-64.

26. Nzila N, Laga M, Bomboko B, Behets F, Hassig SE, Ryder R. STD prevention program in a cohort of prostitutes, Kinshasa, Zaire. III International Conference on AIDS and Associated Cancers in Africa, Arusha, Tanzania, September 1988; Abstract P.S.7.4.

27. Jama H, Ismail SO, Isse A, Omar K, Lidbrink P, Bygdeman S. Genital Chlamydia trachomatis infection in pregnant women and female prostitutes in Magadishu, Somalia. *The African Journal of Sexually Transmitted Diseases* 1987; 3:17-20.

28. Watson PA. The use of screening tests for sexually transmitted diseases in a Third World community–a feasibility study in Malawi. *European Journal of Sexually Transmitted Diseases* 1985; 2:63-5.

29. Hira SK. Sexually transmitted disease–a menace to mother and children. *World Health Forum* 1986; 7:243-7.

30. Liljestrand J, Bergstrom S, Nieuwenhuis F, Hederstedt B. Syphilis in pregnant women in Mozambique. *Genitourinary Medicine* 1985; 61:355-358.

31. Mabey DC, Lloyd-Evans NE, Conten S, Forsey T. Sexually transmitted diseases among randomly selected attenders at an antenatal clinic in the Gambia. *Br J Vener Dis* 1984; 60:331-6.

32. Arya OP, Nsanzumuhire H, Taber SR. Clinical, cultural and demographic aspects of gonorrhea in a rural community in Uganda. *Bull WHO* 1973; 49:587-95.

33. Ratham AV, Din SN, Chatterjee TK. Gonococcal infection in women with pelvic inflammatory disease in Lusaka, Zambia. *Am J Obster Gynecol* 1980; 138:965-8

34. Urassa EJ. Some aspects of sexually transmitted diseases in obstetrics and gynecology. Proceedings of the Symposium on Sexually Transmitted Diseases, Dar es Salaam, September 17, 1985, 23-28.

35. LeClerc A, Frost E, Collet M, Goeman J, Bedjabaga L. Urogenital chlamydia trachomatis in Gabon: an unrecognized epidemic. *Genitourin Med* 1988; 64:308-311.

36. Laga M, Plummer F, Nsanze H, Epidemiology of ophthalmia neonatorum in Kenya. *Lancet* 1986; ii:1145-1148.

37. Nsanze H, Fast MV, DaCosta LJ, Tukei P, Curran J Ronald A. Genital ulcers in Kenya. Clinical and laboratory study. *Br J Vener Dis* 1981; 57:378-381.

38. Plummer FA, D'Costa LJ, Nsanze H, Karasira P, Maclean IW, Piot P, Ronald AR. Clinical and microbiologic studies of genital ulcers in Kenyan women. *Sexually Transmitted Diseases* 1985; 42:193-197.

39. Mbuga G, Kimata J, Maina J, Khamala J, Oogo S, Mutuura C, Muthami L, Miriti S, Achola P, Waiyaki PG. Prevalence of HIV and other sexually transmitted diseases (STD) in Nairobi. III International Conference on AIDS and Associated Cancers in Africa, Arusha, Tanzania, September 14–16, 1988; Abstract W 5.2.

40. Walter SD. Calculation of attributable risks from epidemiologic data. *International Journal of Epidemiology* 1978; 7:175-182.

41. Berkley S. Population attributable risk of sexually transmitted diseases (STDs) in HIV infection. V International Conference on AIDS, Montreal, Quebec, Canada, 1989; Abstract Th.G.O.14.

HUMAN IMMUNODEFICIENCY VIRUS AND SYPHILIS INFECTION IN WOMEN OF CHILDBEARING AGE IN ADDIS ABABA, ETHIOPIA

Debrework Zewdie

National Research Institute of Health, Ethiopia

Nebiat Tafari

Addis Ababa University

INTRODUCTION

As the HIV/AIDS pandemic progresses, it is becoming apparent that heterosexual transmission represents the major mode of spread of HIV infection in most regions of the world, especially in Africa. The rapid spread of AIDS in Africa, therefore, indicates a high rate of heterosexual transmission. Possible factors contributing to the HIV epidemic in Africa include sexual behavior as influenced by pre-existing cultural attitudes and practices, ineffective disease control measures, or co-infection with other sexually transmitted diseases (STDs).

Although there are no formal studies of sexual practices in Ethiopia, most sexually active adults are presumed to be heterosexual. The extent of homosexuality or bisexuality in men is unknown. Other risk factors for HIV infection, such as intravenous drug use, are nonexistent, mainly for economic reasons. The main modes of transmission of HIV-1 infection in Ethiopia are, therefore, heterosexual contact, blood transfusion, and perinatal vertical transmission.

Heterosexual contact does not appear to be an efficient way of transmitting HIV-1 in many industrialized countries. But in African cities in which the steep rise in incidence of HIV-1 infection has been noted, heterosexual contact is thought to be the main mode of transmission. A number of investigators have identified co-infection with other STDs as a factor in HIV-1 infection (1-6) and have noted that this observation provides an opportunity for intervention.

Two hypotheses have been advanced to explain how STDs can affect the rate of transmission of HIV-1. One hypothesis states that STDs — especially those that cause disruption of epithelial integrity or those that evoke an inflammatory response — increase the number of infected lymphocytes in a seropositive person or the pool of potential target cells for HIV-1 in the seronegative individual (4-7). A second hypothesis suggests that the association between HIV-1 infection and other STDs may be spurious. Those with multiple sexual partners are at increased risk of infection with any STD. A second reason for the apparent association between HIV and other STDs may be the effect of HIV-1 infection on the clinical course of some STDs, thereby unmasking subclinical infections. In either case, if it can be shown that STDs enhance the transmission of HIV-1, and that HIV adversely affects the clinical course and outcome of treatable STDs (8), intensive campaigns to control STDs may help to slow down the spread of HIV infection (5).

HIV INFECTION IN ETHIOPIA

The first official report of HIV/AIDS in Ethiopia was made in 1986. During that year a sero-survey of 5,300 army recruits tested for HIV-1 infection yielded a prevalence of only 0.7%. Since there is no system of surveillance, the risk of HIV-1 infection in the general population in Ethiopia remains unknown. The main sources of current information on the progress of HIV infection are the occassional serological surveys conducted by the Department of AIDS Control Program of the Ministry of Health. These are done mainly in such high-risk behavior groups as female commercial sex workers and long-distance truck drivers. Other sources of information regarding the trend of HIV-1 infection are blood donors and college students seeking foreign scholarships. Some countries require information on the serological status of applicants with regard to HIV-1 before awarding scholarships. Data from all these sources suggest a rapid increase in the burden of HIV infection among all groups surveyed.

The highest HIV-1 infection rate was found in female sex workers in major towns, among whom the prevalence of HIV-1 infection increased from 6.7% in 1986, to 29% in 1989, to 50% in some cities in 1990. The second highest prevalence was in long-distance truck drivers, among whom the mean prevalence increased from 13% in 1988, to 17% in 1989, to 20% in 1990. The prevalence of HIV-1 in blood donors increased from 0.9% in 1987, to 2.4% in 1989, to 3.9% in 1990 (double ELISA only). The prevalence among scholarship students in 1990 was 3.2% (Western blot confirmed), a result comparable to the level among blood donors. The observed prevalence rate among blood donors and scholarship students best approximates the level of HIV-1 infection in the non-high-risk group of the urban population.

The results of the above surveys and screenings indicate that HIV-1 infection is well established in urban Ethiopia. HIV-1 infection appears to be associated with urban residence and is particularly high among female sex workers. Urban youth who have not completed their education and who are unemployed constitute the bulk of the reservoir of HIV-1 infections. The frequency gradient of infection observed in several risk categories in Ethiopia is reminiscent of the pattern observed in Rio de Janeiro (9).

Surveys in 1985 and 1987 involving nearly 1,000 persons in different rural areas yielded no positive cases. But in 1990 a few cases of HIV infection were reported from these rural areas.

STDs IN ETHIOPIA

Syphilis, chancroid, lymphogranuloma venereum, gonorrhea, and non-gonococcal urethritis are endemic to Ethiopia. Of these, the best documented is syphilis, which was noted in Ethiopia as far back as the eighteenth century. Numerous surveys over the past three decades indicated that the prevalence of syphilis infection was high, varying from 4% to 40% in both urban and rural populations.

The main reasons for the sustained high prevalence of syphilis in Ethiopia are lack of effective health services for case identification and treatment and the fact that syphilis infection remains asymptomatic for long periods of time. If major morbidities or deaths in adults occur as a result of syphilis, these are not generally appreciated. But a necropsy study of about 1,000 consecutive perinatal deaths in Addis Ababa during 1974-75 showed that congenital syphilis was the fourth highest cause of death, accounting for about 8% of fetal and early neonatal mortality (10).

THE PRESENT STUDY

The purpose of the present study was to examine the epidemiologic aspects of HIV infection in a population with relatively high prevalence of syphilis. The study focused on pregnant women and persons attending prenatal, family planning, general outpatient, and STD clinic services. The reasons for this focus were:

1) Syphilis is a leading cause of perinatal morbidity and mortality (10). In a country with a high total fertility rate (11), prenatal infections with syphilis and HIV should constitute a significant source of the overall national morbidity and mortality burden.

2) Pregnant women attending prenatal clinics best approximate the normal risk, general population (12).

3) The most cost-effective intervention for syphilis is, perhaps, the prevention of congenital syphilis. However, the efficacy and efficiency of current treatment of maternal syphilis can be adversely affected by co-infection with HIV (8). Thus, a measure of the frequency of HIV and syphilis co-infection is appropriate at this stage of HIV infection in the country.

Sample population and study design

We surveyed patients attending the first level of the formal health services in Addis Ababa and in two roadside towns within 100 kilometers of the capital city. The subjects of the current report are women of childbearing age attending prenatal, STD, family planning, and general outpatient clinics.

Following health education on the prevention of syphilis and HIV by the staff of the specific clinic, patients were invited to participate in the study by responding to a pretested questionnaire designed to obtain demographic, social, and economic data. The questionnaires were administered by trained female field enumerators. The identity of patients was known only to the clinic personnel. Upon enrollment, questionnaires and blood samples were identified with pre-assigned study numbers only. The questionnaires were forwarded to the Department of Pediatrics and Child Health of the Addis Ababa University for coding and data entry.

Blood was obtained by venepuncture from those patients who agreed to respond to the questionnaire. Rapid plasma reagin (RPR) tests for syphilis were done during the clinic session. Patients with positive test results were referred to the treating physician or nurse who administered therapy for syphilis according to the CDC recommendations (13). Excess serum was transferred to vials bearing the study number only, then forwarded to the AIDS Laboratory at the National Research Institute of Health for anonymous testing for HIV and confirmatory serologic testing for syphilis. Patients who wished to know the results of HIV testing were informed that test results would be made available through the treating physician or nurse, who subsequently arranged for counseling in accordance with procedures established by the National Program on AIDS. The study protocol was reviewed and approved by the National Committee on AIDS.

Laboratory methods

Syphilis serologic study was carried out using RPR testing as screening and the fluorescent treponemal-antibody absorption test (FTA) for confirmation. Cases of syphilis were those giving positive test by RPR and/or VDRL and subsequently confirmed by FTA testing. Of the 4,266 women screened, 3,599 (84%) were correctly classified by RPR test using FTA as the reference test. This corresponds to a kappa value of 0.84, which indicates excellent agreement between the two tests (14).

Table 1. Prevalence of HIV and syphilis infections by selected demographic and socio-economic characteristics.

Characteristics	Serological status			
	WB positive		FTA positive	
	% (n)	p	% (n)	p
Domicile				
Rural	0.0(112)	<0.01	12.7(112)	NS
Urban	6.1(4161)		14.9(4161)	
Clinic service				
Prenatal	4.2(3337)	<0.001	13.0(3337)	<0.001
Family planning	5.9(471)		15.1(471)	
STD	25.4(197)		35.5(197)	
General outpatients	13.9(267)		22.5(267)	
Age				
Under 25 years	8.4(1630)	<0.001	13.4(1630)	<0.001
25 and over	4.4(2638)		15.8(2638)	
Number of sexual partners				
Multiple	13.9(1210)	<0.001	21.2(1210)	<0.001
Single	2.8(3063)		12.4(3063)	
Employment status				
Irregular	15.8(859)	<0.001	21.2(859)	<0.001
Regular	3.6(3288)		13.4(3288)	
Monthly income in US $				
Under 100	7.7(2561)	<0.001	17.4(2561)	<0.001
100 and over	3.1(1475)		10.9(1475)	
Level of formal education				
Under 5 years	6.4(2176)	NS	18.2(2176)	<0.001
5 years and over	5.5(2092)		11.4(2092)	
Religious affiliation				
Christian	6.2(3783)	<0.02	15.8(3783)	<0.001
Moslem	3.5(485)		7.8(485)	

(n) = number of patients screened. FTA = fluorescent treponemal antibody.
WB = western bolt test. NS = not significant

Screening for HIV-1 antibody was carried out using the enzyme-linked immunosorbent assay (ELISA) Wellcozyme second generation (Wellcome Diagnostics, Dartford UK). All samples that were positive on the first ELISA test were repeated with the Abbot ELISA (Abbot Laboratories). The Western blot test (Bio-rad) was used as a confirmatory test. A sample was considered to be positive if there were two envelope bands +/– one pol band or +/– one gag band.

Table 2. Bivariate analysis of potential risk factors in HIV, syphilis, and HIV-syphilis infection with women without either infection serving as reference.

Risk factor	% Frequency	OR (95% CI)	p
HIV infection (N = 157)			
Age			
Under 25	6.2(1412)		
25 and over	3.1(2221)	2.1(1.5,2.8)	<0.001
Number of sex partner			
Multiple	10.0(954)		
Single	2.3(2684)	4.7(3.5,6.3)	<0.001
Employment status			
Informal and irregular	11.2(677)		
Formal and regular	2.8(2849)	4.3(3.2,5.8)	<0.001
Monthly cash income in US $			
Under 100	5.3(2116)		
100 and over	2.7(1315)	2.0(1.4,3.0)	<0.001
Years of formal education			
Under 5	4.6(1780)		
5 and over	4.1(1854)	1.1(0.8,1.5)	NS
Religious affiliation			
Non-Moslem	4.6(3186)		
Moslem	2.7(447)	1.7(1.0,3.1)	NS
Syphilis infection (N = 539)			
Age			
Under 25	11.3(1493)		
25 and over	14.7(2522)	0.7(0.6,0.9)	<0.01
Number of sex partner			
Multiple	17.6(1042)		
Single	12.0(2978)	1.6(1.3,1.9)	<0.001
Employment status			
Informal and irregular	16.7(723)		
Formal and regular	12.7(3171)	1.3(1.1,1.7)	<0.01
Monthly cash income in US $			
Under 100	15.3(2365)		
100 and over	10.4(1429)	1.5(1.3,1.9)	<0.01
Years of formal education			
Under 5	16.7(2038)		
5 and over	10.0(1977)	1.8(1.5,2.2)	<0.001
Religious affiliation			
Non-Moslem	14.3(3547)		
Moslem	7.1(468)	2.2(1.5,3.1)	<0.001
HIV-syphilis co-infection (N = 96)			
Age			
Under 25	3.6(1373)		
25 and over	2.1(2199)	1.7(1.1,2.5)	<0.02
Number of sex partner			
Multiple	7.8(932)		
Single	0.9(2645)	9.7(6.5,14.4)	<0.001
Employment status			
Informal and irregular	9.1(661)		
Formal and regular	1.3(2804)	7.7(5.3,11.0)	<0.001
Monthly cash income in US $			
Under 100	4.0(2088)		
100 and over	0.9(1291)	4.9(2.7,8.7)	<0.001
Years of formal education			
Under 5	3.2(1754)		
5 and over	2.2(1819)	1.5(1.0,2.2)	NS
Religious affiliation			
Non-Moslem	2.9(3132)		
Moslem	1.1(440)	2.6(1.1,6.2)	<0.04

Figures in parenthesis refer to number of patients screened.

Data analysis

Demographic, socio-economic, and clinical data and results of laboratory tests were entered into a microcomputer and analyzed using Statistical Analysis System (SAS) software. Variables of possible epidemiologic significance for HIV infection, syphilis infection, and HIV-syphilis co-infection were screened by analysis of two-way contingency tables using the Cochran-Mantel-Haenszel statistic in the Frequency Procedure of SAS. Variables of possible epidemiologic significance derived from analysis of contingency tables were subsequently entered into a main effects model. Multivariate logistic regression (maximum likelihood) analysis was used to identify factors that were independently associated with syphilis and HIV-1 seropositivity.

Results

In the period between May 1, 1989 and March 31, 1990, we surveyed 4,273 women in the age group of 15 to 49 years, attending government health care facilities in Addis Ababa and two roadside towns to the southeast of the city (Table 1). Of these, 112 (2.6%) were residing in rural areas and engaged in farming. There were no cases of HIV infection among the 112 rural women, though the prevalence in rural areas was only slightly less than in urban centers. The prevalence of syphilis and HIV was highest in women attending STD clinics and lowest in those seeking prenatal services. Both HIV and syphilis appear to be influenced by the following factors: age, number of sex partners, employment status and income, cultural practice, and religious affiliation.

When patients were stratified by type of infection (Table 2), there were 157 (3.9%) with HIV infection, 539 (13.4%) with syphilis infection, and 96 (2.4%) with syphilis and HIV co-infection.

Table 3. Multivariate logistic regression analysis of risk factors in HIV infection.

Risk factor	% Positive (Western blot)	OR (95% CI)	p
Syphilis infection	15.1(635)	3.1(2.5,4.4)	<0.001
Multiple sexual contact	13.9(1210)	2.8(1.9,4.2)	<0.001
Irregular or no employment	15.8(859)	1.7(1.1,2.5)	<0.01
Age under 25 years	8.4(1630)	1.5(1.1,2.0)	<0.02
Monthly income under under US $ 100	7.7(2561)	1.5(1.1,2.1)	<0.03
Non-Moslem religious affiliation	6.2(3783)	1.4(0.8,2.4)	NS
Formal education under 5 years	6.3(2176)	1.2(0.8,1.8)	NS

Figures in parenthsis number of patients screened. NS = not significant.

There were no patients with AIDS, using the modified WHO Bangui case definition (15). Most cases giving positive FTA were thought to have early latent syphilis; there were no cases with genital ulcers. Bivariate stratified analysis of risk factors indicate that syphilis is significantly more common among women who are older than 24 years, those with multiple sex partners, the poor and unemployed, those with rudimentary education, and those with non-Moslem religious affiliation. HIV infection has the same risk profile as syphilis except that the level of formal education and category of religious affiliation did not significantly affect its prevalence. HIV-syphilis co-infection shares the same risk factors as the individual infections.

Table 3 summarizes risk factors in HIV infection. The woman with HIV has significantly higher odds of co-infection with syphilis. The following additional factors are independently associated with risk of HIV infection: multiple sexual contacts, unemployment, poverty, and young age.

Discussion

Our data confirm that both syphilis and HIV are more prevalent in those attending STD and general outpatient clinics. Patients in STD and general outpatient clinics may represent a higher-risk category for the acquisition of both infections. Most women attending prenatal clinics reported stable relationships with a single partner, hence the relatively low prevalence of HIV infection among pregnant women seeking prenatal care. The prevalences of syphilis and HIV in family planning clinic attendees were intermediate; a higher proportion of these women reported previous risk behavior, such as sex with multipe partners.

The acquisition of HIV infection among urban women in central Ethiopia appears to be through multiple sexual contacts. Such behavior seems to be reinforced by unemployment and poverty. Lack of education or training and lack of employment opportunities in the face of a rapidly expanding urban youth population underlies the current epidemic in central Ethiopia. The epidemiology of HIV closely resembles that of syphilis. Syphilis is presently equally prevalent in urban and rural areas. It can be expected, therefore, that, given time, the epidemic of HIV infection will spread to rural areas. The spread of infection to rural areas may be accelerated by rapid movement of large populations to escape the ravages of war and natural disasters, which continue to happen on a large scale.

We encountered no cases of intravenous drug use. Of those who gave a positive serologic reaction for HIV-1 and syphilis, 1.7% and 1.8% respectively gave histories of blood transfusion during the past 12 years. It is not known whether the positive sero-status was related to the transfusion. The question of homosexuality is difficult to ascertain in Ethiopia, as this sexual practice is stigmatized and is likely to be under-reported in this traditional society.

CONCLUSION

Our study of the epidemiology of HIV and syphilis in women of childbearing age showed prevalences of HIV infection of 3.9%, syphilis infection of 13.4%, and HIV-syphilis co-infection of 2.4%. Thus, 38.4% of women with HIV infection have additional infection with syphilis.

The following factors were independently associated with HIV infection: syphilis infection, multiple sexual contacts, age under 25 years, unemployment, and poverty. Syphilis can serve as a marker for other STDs, such as chlamydia, which may increase the risk of HIV infection as shown elsewhere in Africa. It is, therefore, possible that HIV infection is also more common in women with other STD infections.

From the present survey it is impossible to determine if syphilis infection preceded HIV infection. If it can be shown that prior syphilis infection increases the risk of acquisition of HIV, then an intensive program of control of STDs can be expected to slow down the current HIV epidemic. But until proof of such a causal relationship is available, we will have to assume that a temporal relationship exists and aim at controlling STDs through case finding and treatment, and through sexual behavior modification. As Brown et al. advise (16), the time to act is now.

Acknowledgments

We are indebted to Mr. Solomon Zewdie, B.Sc. (Biometrics) for his valuable assistance in data analysis. We express our gratitude to clinic and hospital staff for their assistance in patient recruitment.

The study was partially supported by the Swedish Agency for Research Cooperation with Developing Countries (SAREC), the Swedish International Development Authority (SIDA), and The Rockefeller Foundation through the AIDS and Reproductive Health Network.

REFERENCES

1. Jaffe HW, Choi K, Thomas PA et al. National case–control study of Kaposi's sarcoma and Pneumocystis carinii pneumonia in homosexual men: part 1, epidemiologic results. *Ann Intern Med* 1983; 99:145-151.
2. Quinn TC, Glasser D, Cannon RO et al. Human immunodeficiency virus infection among patients attending clinics for sexually transmitted diseases. *New Engl J Med* 1988; 318:197-203.
3. Simonson JN, Cameron DW, Gakinya et al. Human immunodeficiency virus infection among patients attending clinics for sexually transmitted diseases. Experience from a center in Africa. *J Med* 1988; 319:274-8.5
4. Kreiss J, Caraee M, Meheus A. Role of sexually transmitted diseases in transmitting human immunodeficiency virus. *Genitourin Med* 1988; 64:1-2.
5. Pepin J, Plummer FA, Brunham RC et al. The interaction of HIV infection and other sexually transmitted diseases: an opportunity for intervention. *AIDS* 1989; 3:3-9.
6. Mertens TE, Hayes RJ and Smith PG. Epidemiological methods to study the interaction between HIV infection and other sexually transmitted diseases. *AIDS* 1990; 4:57-65.
7. Van De Perre P, De Clercq A, Cogniaux–Leclerc J, Nzaramba D, Butzler J, Sprecher–Goldberger S. Detection of HIV p17 antigen in lymphocytes but not epithelial cells from cervicovaginal secretions of women seropositive for HIV: implications for heterosexual transmission of the virus. *Genitourin Med* 1988; 64:30-33.
8. Lukehart SA, Hook III EW, Baker–Zander SA et al. Invasion of the central nervous system by *Treponema pallidum*: Implications for diagnosis and treatment. *Annals Internal Medicine* 1988; 109:855-62.
9. Cortes E, Detels R, Aboulafia D et al. HIV-1, HIV-2 and HTLV-1 infection in high-risk groups in Brazil. *New Engl J Med* 1989; 320:953-62.
10. Naeye RL and Tafari N. *Risk Factors in Pregnancy and Diseases of the Fetus and Newborn*. Baltimore: William and Wilkins, 1983, pp. 125-128.
11. Central Statistical Authority. Population and Housing Census of Ethiopia, 1984. Analytical Report on Results for Addis Abba, 1987.
12. Hoff R, Berardi VP, Weiblen BJ et al. Seroprevalence of human immunoeficiency virus among childbearing women. Estimates by testing samples of blood from newborns. *New Engl J Med* 1988; 318:525-30.
13. Sexually transmitted diseases treatment guidelines, 1982. *MMWR* 1982; 31(suppl):33S–62S.
14. Landis JR and Koch GG. The measurement of observers agreement for categorical data. *Biometrica* 1977; 35:159-173.
15. Widy-Wirski R, Berkley S, Downing R et al. Evaluation of the WHO case definition for AIDS in Uganda. *JAMA* 1988; 260:3286-9.
16. Brown ST, Zacarias FRK, Aral SO. STD control in less developed countries: The time is now. *Inter J Epidemiol* 1985; 14:505-509.

CONTRACEPTION, FAMILY PLANNING, AND HIV

David J. Hunter

Harvard School of Public Health

Japheth K. Mati

University of Nairobi

Throughout the world the predominant mode of HIV transmission is heterosexual intercourse. It is to be expected, therefore, that the HIV/AIDS epidemic will have an impact on reproductive behaviors and choices, including those involving contraception. The fact that individual methods of contraception may decrease or increase the risk of acquiring HIV, given exposure, broadens this impact considerably.

Modern contraceptive methods play a crucial role in efforts to reduce population growth in developing countries. Contraceptive methods (e.g., condoms) may also have a direct utility in the control of the HIV epidemic and in providing choices, such as pregnancy prevention, to HIV-infected persons. Because of their link to sexual behavior and the fact that they may be the only available infrastructure in many settings, family planning services need to reassess the advice they give to clients in light of the HIV/AIDS epidemic. It is important that the associations between HIV transmission and individual contraceptive methods are known, and that appropriate changes are made in family planning services to confront this new challenge.

We begin this chapter by briefly examining the difficulties in studying associations between contraceptive methods and HIV transmission. We then review the evidence suggesting that oral contraceptives, intrauterine devices, and spermicides may enhance HIV transmission, while barrier methods protect against it. Finally, we discuss the implications of these results for individuals making contraceptive choices and for the family planning programs that serve them.

METHODOLOGIC DIFFICULTIES IN STUDIES OF CONTRACEPTIVE USE AND HIV TRANSMISSION

While *in vitro* studies are helpful in looking at some issues (such as condom permeability to HIV), epidemiologic evidence in humans is needed to guide policy regarding contraceptive use and HIV transmission. For certain methods of contraception, particularly those expected to be

AIDS and Women's Reproductive Health
Edited by L.C. Chen *et al.*, Plenum Press, New York, 1991

protective against HIV (e.g., condoms), it may be feasible to perform intervention studies to evaluate protective efficacy. In the case of methods that may enhance transmission probability, interventions are clearly unethical. For these methods, observational study designs are the only sources of epidemiologic information. Unfortunately, it is not easy to design observational studies in this area that give unambiguous results.

Case-Control Studies

The most rapid method of evaluating associations between contraceptive use and HIV transmission is to perform a case-control study. In this design, seropositive women and otherwise comparable seronegative women are compared with respect to current and previous contraceptive use. The cases in such a study are usually prevalent cases (seropositive women detected by screening for HIV antibodies) rather than incident cases (women identified at the time of acquisition of these antibodies, i.e., shortly after infection).

The chief problem with using prevalent cases is that it is usually impossible to tell when individuals became infected with HIV. For exposures that are constant over time (such as blood type), it is reasonable to conclude that current exposure matches exposure at the time of infection. For intermittent exposures (such as ulcers), it is impossible to know exposure status at the time of infection. In addition, most contraceptive methods are used intermittently (with varying periodicity), so it is not possible to establish definitively the type of contraceptive method in use at the time of infection (and, thus, whether the method facilitated transmission). This potential misclassification decreases the ability of a case-control study to observe the underlying result (bias to the null). A null result from a case-control study of contraceptive method use and HIV infection may obscure an underlying association. The strength of any positive or negative result observed may be an underestimate of the true relationship.

Prospective studies

These problems of case-control studies can be mitigated in a prospective study, in which exposure data is obtained and updated and seroconversion is observed. The major difficulty in prospective studies is acheiving the high follow-up necessary to avoid bias. If we compare oral contraceptive users and non-users in a prospective design, for instance, then bias would result if all non-users, but only half of the users, were completely followed up, and all seroconversions occurred among the half who were lost to follow-up. This would lead to an underestimation of the effect of oral contraceptives. Another serious difficulty in designing a prospective study is forming a cohort among whom enough endpoints will occur to give the study sufficient power. In a low-risk population (say 1% seroconversion per year), a very large number of women would need to participate (at least several thousand for several years). In high-risk populations, the starting size of the cohort can be much smaller (perhaps 100 or more). Here, the principal problem is the ethical one of observing seroconversions among a group under study. It is likely, therefore, that very few prospective studies of the effect of contraceptive methods on HIV transmission probabilities will be conducted.

Couples studies

A third type of study design that may shed light on transmission co-factors is the "partners" or "couples" study, in which regular sex partners are enrolled. These may be cross-sectional in nature, looking at predictors of whether couples are concordant or discordant in sero-status, or they may be prospective, following discordant couples over time to examine factors associated with seroconversion of the negative partner. Prospective couples studies reported to date have been small.

Confounding

As if these measurement and design issues were not enough, investigations of the relationship between contraceptive methods and HIV transmission are highly susceptible to confounding. Contraceptive use and choice of methods may be associated with number and type of sexual partners. Some evidence links individual contraceptive methods with certain sexually transmitted diseases that have been independently linked to facilitation of HIV transmission. An attempt to control for these potential confounding factors, and some assessment of the probability of residual confounding, should be mandatory in the analysis of studies of contraceptives and HIV transmission.

The above considerations should be kept in mind in reviewing the evidence on contraceptives and HIV. Given the predominant role of exposure to the HIV virus as a primary risk factor for HIV infection, the relative risks associated with a contraceptive method that facilitates transmission are likely to be small, on the order of 1.5-3. The presence of misclassification and bias of the sorts mentioned above could very easily conceal this small relative risk. On the other hand, these biases could easily lead to an observed relative risk in this range when there is no true underlying elevation in risk. The situation is analogous to the oral contraceptive use and cervical cancer issue about which, after many years of investigation and many studies, little consensus has been reached. So far, few studies of contraceptives and HIV transmission have been reported. Even if available studies were highly consistent, it would be difficult to reach confident conclusions at this stage.

POSTULATED MECHANISMS FOR INCREASED OR DECREASED RISK OF HIV TRANSMISSION ASSOCIATED WITH CONTRACEPTIVE USE

A number of mechanisms have been proposed by which individual contraceptive methods alter the risk of HIV transmission (Table 1). Some of these are backed up by research data, but the evidence for most of them remains limited. For each of the main contraceptive methods, these mechanisms are discussed below, along with the epidemiologic evidence for each individual association.

Table 1. Suggested mechanisms by which individual contraception methods may influence risk of HIV infection.

METHOD	POSTULATED BASIS FOR INCREASED RISK	POSTULATED BASIS FOR DECREASED RISK

Oral Contraceptives	Increased cervical ectropion
	Increased STD's,
	  especially chlamydia
	Increased menstrual bleeding
	
	Systemic immune suppression
		
		Decreased menstrual
		  bleeding

Injectable hormones	Re-use of unsterilized needles Increased menstrual bleeding	 Decreased menstrual bleeding
IUD	Increased STD's Chronic inflammation of cervix and uterus	
Spermicides	Inflammation of vagina and cervix	Anti-virucidal action
Condoms		Prevention of exhange of HIV-infected fluids

Oral Contraceptives and HIV

The studies of Simonsen et al. and Plummmer et al., discussed in detail below, have raised the possibility that the use of oral contraceptives (OCs) may facilitate HIV transmission (39,47). Where prevalence of OC use is very low, as it is in most of sub-Saharan Africa, it is clear that OC use could account for only a small part of heterosexual transmission, even in areas where HIV prevalence is high. In some areas of sub-Saharan Africa, however, OC use is high, and efforts are being made in these areas to increase OC use for family planning purposes. Should OCs prove to be a co-factor for HIV tranmission, this would be important to know, as information on this association is needed to guide family planning policy.

Listed below (and in Table 1) are some of the biological mechanisms that may play a part in the interaction between hormonal contraceptives and HIV transmission:

1. Increased probability of cervical ectropion associated with OC use.
2. Increased risk of certain STDs, particularly chlamydia, among OC users.
3. Interruption of menstrual pattern and irregular uterine bleeding (leading to a "raw" endometrium) associated with long-acting steroidal methods.
4. Systemic immunologic changes associated with steroids.

Cervical Ectropion

Cervical ectropion (or "ectopy") refers to the outgrowth of the columnar epithelium of the cervix, replacing the squamous epithelium of the exocervix. It is normally observed in newborns, around the time of puberty, and during pregnancy. It is believed to be caused by higher levels of circulating estrogens during these periods. (Cervicitis caused by infections such as *Trichomonas vaginalis*, and chlamydia may cause punctate hemorrhages on the exocervix which, if severe, may be confused with cervical ectropion.) Columnar epithelium is more vascular than squamous epithelium, and therefore more easily traumatized. Thus, cervical ectropion may lead to bleeding during coitus, possibly increasing the probability that infection will be acquired after sexual contact with an infected partner. Cervical ectopy has been associated with HIV seropositivity among couples in Nairobi (32). The women in this study were identified after seroconversion, however; thus, it is not possible to be certain that the ectopy was not a consequence of HIV seropositivity.

It is the general impression of clinicians that cervical ectropion occurs more frequently among users of OCs. However, data to document the association are limited. Most of the data have been derived from cross-sectional studies based at STD clinics. To our knowledge, no one has studied women before the initiation of OC use to establish prospectively when the cervical ectropion develops. Another problem is the lack of a standardized classification of cervical ectropion. Some investigators have recorded presence or absence of ectropion (4); others have estimated the size and classified the ectropion according to whether the diameter was less or greater than 2 cm (12); while others used the term cervical "discontinuity" and graded the degree of discontinuity in percentages ranging from 0 to 100 (36). In addition, the possibility that chlamydial infection causes the appearance of ectropion makes the association difficult to assess in studies that have not assessed chlamydial infection.

Goldacre et al. examined 1,498 women attending family planning clinics and observed the highest prevalence of ectropion among users of OCs (51%), compared to non-contraceptors (32%), users of an intrauterine device (26%), and users of a diaphragm or condom (26%) (12). In a study by Burns et al., data on chlamydial infection are available (4). Among the OC users not infected with chlamydia, cervical ectropion was found in 12 of 33 women (36.4%), compared to 3 of 41 (7.3%) non-OC users (including users of other non-hormonal contraceptive methods). This indicates that OC use may be associated independently with cervical ectropion. Among women infected with chlamydia, the rates of ectropion were higher: 21 of 37 (56.7%) OC users and 16 of 37 (43.2%) non-OC users. These data suggest that both OCs and chlamydial infection are independently associated with cervical ectropion.

Sexually Transmitted Diseases

Any infection that leads to macro- or micro-ulceration of the genital tract epithelium may facilitate infection with HIV. An association between chancroid and increased risk of HIV infection has been established (39). The relation between chancroid (and other diseases that cause visible ulceration) and OCs is uncertain. Chlamydia can cause cervicitis with varying degrees of micro-ulceration. In addition, infection with chlamydia accompanied by an inflammatory exudate may provide target cells for viral infection. The same could be true for any lower genital tract infection, such as anaerobic vaginosis. The use of OCs and hormone releasing IUDs has been shown to be associated with presence of anaerobic bacteria in the cervix (14).

Many studies over the last two decades have given conflicting results with regard to the association between chlamydial infection and OC use. For instance, Burns et al. found that of 287 women who were current users of OCs, 37 (12.9%) were positive for chlamydia, compared with 76 of 597 (12.7%) non-users of OCs (4). Oriel et al. also failed to establish a significant relationship between chlamydial infection and OC use (36). On the other hand, the studies of Hilton et al., Shafer et al., and Macaulay et al. reported that women using OCs were at greater risk of chlamydial infection compared to non-users (16,24,46). The mechanism through which OCs may increase risk of chlamydial infection has not been elucidated. Both chlamydia isolation and OC use has been shown to be associated with ectropion, as discussed above, which may suggest that the presence of OC-induced ectropion may facilitate chlamydial infection. However, chlamydia has been isolated in women with no evidence of ectropion or OC use (16,36).

Interruption of Menstrual Pattern

Menstrual bleeding may be important in the transmission of HIV infection in two ways. Menstrual blood provides a pool of lymphocytes and macrophages that are the targets of HIV. It is also possible that endometrial shedding leaves a "raw" area, which can facilitate viral entry. Any situation or condition that increases the duration of menstrual bleeding, or that causes intermenstrual bleeding, may theoretically contribute to increased risk of HIV infection.

Combination OCs (estrogen plus progestin) tend to make menstrual cycles regular. The amount of menstrual blood loss among OC users is usually less than it is among non-users. This effect could be protective against HIV infection. The progestin-only pill and the long-acting injectables and implants are associated with varying degrees of menstrual cycle disruption, leading to intermenstrual bleeding, spotting, and sometimes increased menstrual blood loss. Such a situation could theoretically increase the risk of HIV infection. The other contraceptive method that is associated with increased menstrual blood loss is the IUD (see below).

Immunological Changes

Literature on the interaction between hormonal contraceptives and immune response is limited. Some studies have suggested that sex steroids suppress immune response at the cellular level (1,28,29,51). Steroidal contraceptives, notably the combined OC, have been shown to lower humoral immunity in animals and in women (6,19,41), as well as cell-mediated immunity (CMI) in women (2,11,18,30). However, Tezabwala et al. were unable to show any depression of CMI in female OC users followed for up to 18 months of use (49). These investigators found that women using the progestogen pill only (0.35 mg of Norethisterone daily) showed significant suppression of CMI after 12-18 months of use, but this effect was not found among those using the method for less than one year. This seems to be in agreement with the findings of Collins et al., who found that norethindrone-containing combined OCs, but not those containing norgestrel, depressed humoral immunity, suggesting that different progestins in the pill may exert different effects on the immune system (6). The 1974 Royal College of General Practitioners Study (45) reported that there was an increased incidence of varicella and several other viral infections in

OC users, which was not confirmed by Keller et al. (20). In a study of malaria and OC use, Mati et al. (25) showed that a levonorgestrel-containing combined pill was not associated with increased prevalence of malarial parasitemia, and parasite densities were much less compared to non-users living in an endemic area for malaria. This suggests that this type of OC conferred some protection against malaria. Studies of the interaction between hormonal contraceptives and HIV infection should take into consideration the nature of the particular progestins used.

STUDIES ON HIV AND HORMONAL CONTRACEPTIVE USE

Studies on the association between OC use and HIV infection are few, and are summarized in Table 2. The first report linking OC use to an increased risk of HIV infection came from Nairobi, Kenya. In a cross-sectional study of low socio-economic status prostitutes, it was shown that OC use was an independent risk factor for HIV infection, with a multivariate OR of 2.0 (95% CI 1.2–3.4) (39,47). Since then, the same investigators have found a stronger association in a prospective study in the same population (Plummer et al., in press).

As this study is currently the only prospective study of this issue, it deserves careful consideration. 595 sex workers from a low socio-economic status area of Nairobi were enrolled in the first half of 1985. Of these women, only 196 were initially HIV seronegative, and thus eligible for

Table 2. Summary of studies of oral contraceptive use and HIV status.

First Author	Country	Study populat'n	Type	Sample size	Comparison	RR (95%CI)	Controlled
Plummer (1988)	Kenya	Sex worker	Prosp	124	Ever/never use	4.5(1.4-13.8)	Yes
Simonsen (1990)	Kenya	Sex worker	Case-C	418	Current/ non-current	2.2(1.2-3.4)	Yes
Darrow (1988)	USA	Sex worker	Case-C	640	?	1.0(0.4-2.2)	No
Carael (1988)	Rwanda	Couples	Case-C	288	OC in last 2 yrs/no use	4.3(1.4-15.4)*	No
Latif (1989)	Zimbabwe	Couples	Case-C	150	Current/ non-current	1.1(0.4-3.3)	No
European Study Group(1989)		Partners	Couples	308	OC/no method	1.4(0.4-5.9)	No
Siraprapasiri (1989)	Thailand	Sex worker	Case-C	238	OC use/ non-use	0.7(0.4-1.2)	No
Musicco (1990)	Italy	Partners	Couples (Case-C)	368	Current/ non-current	0.4(0.3-1.8)	Yes
Mati (1990)	Kenya	FP clients	Case-C	726	non-OC use	1.5(0.7-3.0)	Yes
Bulterys (1990)	Rwanda	Antenatal	Case-C	961	Ever/never use	5.0(2.1-11.3)	No

* Association not significant when controlled for confounders.

the prospective study of factors associated with seroconversion. 124 of these women were followed until seroconversion, or for at least 12 months; 72 were lost to follow-up. Given the transience of this population and the difficulties of conducting a prospective investigation among women engaged in activities that are still officially illegal, this degree of follow-up represents a considerable acheivement. However, as loss to follow-up is the most serious source of selection bias in a prospective study, the impact of the relatively high proportion of the initial cohort lost (36%) needs to be evaluated.

One way to conduct such an evaluation is to calculate odds ratios (ORs) that would obtain under assumptions about seroconversions that might have occurred in each group had follow-up been complete. The observed crude OR for OC use among those followed up is 3.1 (95% CI 1.1–8.6). If we recalculate this OR assuming that an equal proportion of the women lost to follow-up in each group would have seroconverted (seroconversion=2/3 among both OC users and non-users, i.e., there is no effect of OC use on seroconversion), the crude OR drops to 1.9 and is not statistically significant (95% CI 0.9–4.1). Thus, a plausible asummption about the observed loss to follow-up suggests that bias could have produced an observed relative risk that reached statistical significance.

The central condition for selection bias to have occurred is that OC users who were followed were more likely to have seroconverted than OC users who were not followed. This would require examining the joint distribution of other risk behavior by OC status by follow-up. (These data are not currently available.)

The authors did compare the initial characteristics of those followed with those not followed. Age, number of daily sex partners, and prevalence of genital ulcer disease at baseline were all very similar between the two groups. Duration of prostitution and prevalence of chlamydial cervicitis were higher among women who were followed, while the proportion using OCs was lower. These data suggest that women followed-up were not completely representative of the original cohort — consistent with, but by no means proving, the occurrence of selection bias.

Even if selection bias were absent, an elevation in risk could still be due to confounding by other risk factors among the women followed up. The authors have compared the distribution of confounding factors between OC users and non-users. The proportions experiencing genital ulcer disease and gonococcal and chlamydial infection were evenly balanced between the two groups. Women using OCs did report a higher number of sex partners per day (n=4.46 for OC users versus 3.63 for non-users, p=0.07); however, the authors state that OC use was still significantly positive in regression analyses including a term for number of sex partners. It is possible that this difference in number of sex partners underestimates the true difference (due to misclassification in reporting), or is an indication of underlying unmeasured risk behavior that could not be adequately controlled for.

A further concern that has been raised about this study is its generalizability. The study population, with high numbers of sexual partners and very high rates of STDs, is clearly not representative of most women who use OCs in developing countries. While this does not necessarily compromise the internal validity of the findings, the possibility exists that OC use may indeed be an independent risk factor for HIV, but only in association with other STDs or some other factor more prevalent among women in prostitution.

In summary, this study is consistent with an independant role for OC use in facilitating infection by HIV among exposed women. After a thorough and careful analysis of the data, the authors have not been able to explain this result as due to confounding, and offer several biological mechanisms through which the association might be causal. The high loss to follow-up and the possibility of unmeasured confounding are plausible alternative explanations. This study, like almost any first report of an exposure-disease relation in observational epidemiology, requires confirmation in other settings.

The other studies of this issue, all case-control, are summarized in Table 1. Carael et al. observed that use of OCs was significantly more frequent among HIV-seropositive mothers of children at an outpatient department in Rwanda than among those who were seronegative (5).

This relation was no longer significant after control for confounding factors. In a preliminary report also from Rwanda, Bulterys et al. also observed an elevation in the crude relative risk of being HIV-positive for ever-users of OCs (3). Three other relatively small studies have observed no association between OC use and HIV infection (7,8,23), although the confidence intervals of all these studies includes an OR of 2.0, compatible with the data of Plummer et al. (39) and Simonsen et al. (47). Two studies report inverse associations, and the upper confidence intervals for both these studies is less than 2.0 (33,48).

The study by Mati et al. (25) was designed to examine this association among women attending two family planning clinics in Nairobi who were believed to be at low risk for HIV infection. The majority of the women were married (89%), 7% were single and 4% divorced or widowed. Their reported number of lifetime sex partners was small: 70% reported up to three partners, and only 13% reported more than five partners. HIV seropositivity was significantly associated with increasing number of sex partners (17), however, the attributable risk for having more than 5 partners was low (due to the low self-reported prevalence of this risk factor). The prevalence of STDs was relatively low: 3% for gonorrhoea, 10% for chlamydia, and 2% for syphilis. The use of OCs was reported by 58% of the women. In preliminary data, a small, non-significant increase in risk associated with OC use (OR 1.5, 95% CI 0.7–3.0) was observed. Multivariate analyses controlling for age, marital status, education, sexual behavior, partner circumcision, STDs, and cervical ectropion did not materially alter these findings.

Summary of Findings

A formal meta-analysis of the case-control data would almost certainly conclude that there is little current evidence for an increase in risk of HIV transmission associated with OC use. The only prospective study, however, is the study with the second-highest highest relative risk for OC use. In the case-control study conducted at baseline in the same population (47), a positive, but smaller, relative risk was observed, consistent with a bias to the null due to misclassification of exposure relative to the time of transmission. More and better data are needed to evaluate the possible association between OCs and HIV infection.

INJECTABLE HORMONES

Injectable hormonal contraceptives could be associated with HIV transmission either through their physiologic effects or because of their route of transmission. Depo-provera, the most commonly used injectable, is a form of progesterone, and thus would not be expected to cause cervical ectropion. It may, however, cause menstrual irregularities, such as intermenstrual bleeding, which could theoretically increase risk.

It remains to be established definitively whether the re-use of unsterilized needles for intramuscular (IM) injection readily transmits HIV. This possibility, plus the unexplained outbreaks of nosocomial HIV transmission in hospitals in the U.S.S.R. (40), reinforces the need for the strict sterilization of needles, especially in high-prevalence areas. In many countries, depo–provera is provided in single-use, disposable syringe packs, which should eliminate the possibility that IM contraceptive administration could transmit HIV.

Few data are available on the relationship between injectable contraceptive use and HIV infection, partly because of the low prevalence of use in many studies. In some countries, injectables are only recommended for older women; thus, confounding by age or sexual behaviour must be carefully assessed. In the study of Carael et al. (5), use of injectable contraceptives was less prevalent among concordant seropositive couples than among seronegative couples. In the preliminary results of Mati et al. (25), depo-provera use was not associated with increased risk of HIV infection (OR 0.7, 95% CI 0.2–3.1), even after controlling for age, marital status, education, sexual behavior, partner circumcision, STDs, and cervical ectropion.

INTRAUTERINE DEVICES (IUDs)

IUDs have been associated consistently with higher risks of pelvic inflammatory disease and lower genital tract infections. Even in the absence of these infections, inflammation or increased bleeding associated with the use of an IUD could increase a woman's risk of HIV infection once exposed.

Little data are available on the specific relationship between IUDs and HIV transmission, mostly due to the low prevalence of IUD use compared with other contraceptive methods. In the case-control study of the European Study Group (8), a non-significant elevation in risk was observed (OR 2.0 relative to users of no method, 95% CI 0.4–10.9). Mati et al. observed an OR of 1.5 (95% CI 0.6–3.7) among current IUD users (25). Fathalla has suggested that, at least among women at high risk of HIV infection, the question of an association between IUDs and HIV is moot, as high-risk women should be counseled to avoid IUD use due to their risk of contracting other STDs (9).

SPERMICIDES

In vitro studies have demonstrated that spermicides, such as nonoxynol-9, are toxic to HIV and HIV-infected lymphocytes (15,50) and that both spermicides and the contraceptive sponge reduce the risk of gonorrhea and chlamydial infections (44). In addition, it appears likely that spermicide-lubricated condoms may still confer some protection against HIV transmission even after condom rupture (43). Data are very limited on the association of HIV and spermicides. In an intervention study among 98 prostitutes in Nairobi, women were randomly assigned to use of nonoxynol-9 contraceptive sponges or placebo vaginal suppositories. Acquisition of genital ulcers was significantly higher among sponge users; HIV seroconversion was also higher, though the increase was not significant (22). In a small survey of women in prostitution in Vancouver, 9 out of 24 women who had used nonoxynol-9-lubricated condoms stated that they experienced vaginal irritation after use (42). These data suggest that nonoxynol-9 may be of limited use by itself, or in conjunction with condoms, in preventing HIV transmission. As spermicides are one of the few contraceptive technologies that may protect against HIV, as well as one of the few methods under the control of women, the effectiveness of other spermicides needs urgent evaluation.

CONDOMS

Several studies have demonstrated that recently-manufactured latex condoms are impervious to HIV, even at HIV concentrations far higher than those likely to exist in semen (43). Thus, condoms would be expected to protect against male-female transmission of HIV by preventing passage of semen. It also seems likely that condoms would at least reduce female-male transmission probabilities by reducing exposure of the male urethral opening, prepuce, and penile shaft to cervical and vaginal secretions.

The weight of the evidence from epidemiologic studies confirms that condom use reduces HIV transmission. The question then becomes, By how much? Factors that may decrease the protection provided by condoms include incorrect fit and use; condom rupture (caused by suboptimal use, shelf-life, or storage); intermittent availability; or intermittent use.

Mechanical Factors

Data are sparse on condom failure rates in developing countries and the extent to which failures are determined by incorrect use or by mechanical factors. As all condoms used in sub-Saharan Africa are imported and frequently subjected to long delays and suboptimal storage, it is likely that condom failure as a result of latex deterioration is higher in this region than in developed countries. A higher frequency of failure not only reduces the protective efficacy of condoms, but undermines the faith of clients in condoms as a reliable method of both pregnancy and STD prevention.

Mathematical models of the protective potential of condoms

Mathematical models of the effect of increasing condom usage demonstrate that the degree of protection to an individual varies as a function of the number of sexual partners, the prevailing HIV prevalence, the risk of infection for each unprotected exposure, and the frequency of condom use (10). Because HIV transmission during a single sexual encounter results in lifetime infection, the protective effect of condoms can be nullified if one assumes a high enough rate of partner change among individuals in an area of high HIV prevalence. In lower-risk settings, however, protection afforded by condoms may be substantial, although the incremental decrease in risk of infection appears to be much higher for those moving from condom use in 50% of sexual encounters to 100% use than for those moving from 0% to 50% (in the latter instance a high proportion of sexual acts are still unprotected). Most studies of condom uptake among high-risk groups in sub-Saharan Africa have demonstrated that intermittent use of condoms increases in the short-term, but few individuals adopt condom use with all partners. More simulations would be useful, taking into account higher-order effects, such as the interaction of a varying probability of condom use with different partner pools.

Human evidence on the effect of condoms

Many studies, mostly of high-risk groups, have observed lower rates of HIV infection among users of condoms than among never users. In one of the few interventions studies reported to date, Ngugi et al. conducted a non-randomized evaluation of the effect of group AIDS education, with and without individual counseling, among sex workers in Nairobi (34). Increasing the availability of condoms apparently resulted in substantial increases in self-reported condom usage, while group and individual counseling provided further increments in use. Women reporting any condom use were at one-third the risk of HIV seroconversion of women reporting no condom use (OR 0.32, 95% CI 0.13–0.92). A trend of decreasing risk with increasing condom use was observed. In longer-term follow-up of this cohort and similar groups in Nairobi, the increase in condom use has been sustained, and declines in the incidence of other STDs observed (35). These and other studies clearly demonstrate that condoms have a major role to play in the prevention of HIV transmission, at least among high-risk groups for whom sexual partner reduction is not currently a feasible strategy for economic and social reasons.

Acceptability

Prior to the AIDS epidemic, condom use was generally promoted for family planning purposes rather than for STD prevention. Uptake varied widely around the world, being high in Japan and some other Asian countries, and very low in sub-Saharan Africa (<1% of currently married women reporting current use of condoms) (13,27). It is unclear to what extent these differences are attributable to differences in condom availability and promotion, or to cultural differences in acceptance of family planning in general, and condoms specifically.

Early in the AIDS epidemic in Africa, previous low rates of condom use for family planning purposes was cited as evidence that condoms were unlikely to be successfully promoted for the prevention of HIV. The limited evidence now available suggests, however, that acceptance of condoms for HIV and STD prevention can be high. In Zaire, public discussion of condoms has become more open, and "ever use" of condoms has increased, though "regular" or "always" users of condoms are still in the minority. Availability may be the major limiting factor (37,38). In Nairobi, self-reported condom use among sex workers increased substantially after a limited intervention, which can be tied to increased availability of condoms (34).

These data indicate that the concept of a generalized rejection of condoms in Africa is, like most generalizations about Africa, unlikely to be valid. Much more data are needed about specific cultural, religious, legal, and other barriers to condom use. More data are needed on the specific interpersonal contexts in which condom use is acceptable. For instance, a man may accept a condom from a sex worker, but be insulted by a similar offer from his wife.

Availability

Much anecdotal information suggests that lack of availability may be the major barrier to greater uptake of condoms in developing countries. Calculations of the number of condoms required to protect every sexual act in countries in which HIV is widely prevalent rapidly overwhelm both the mind and the condom production and distribution systems. This suggests that available supplies should be targetted to areas where they will be most effective, and that distribution schemes must be developed to serve these areas.

The groups most frequently cited for targetted distribution of condoms are prostitutes and their clients. Although data are sparse, it seems intuitively likely that condom distribution among high-risk groups would be a cost-effective use of limited resources. In one of the few specific studies to address this issue, Moses et al. calculated the cost of an STD/HIV prevention program, in which condom use was a central element, among approximately 1,000 women in prostitution in Nairobi, Kenya (31). After making a number of necessary assumptions, this group calculated that the intervention was preventing about 12,000 new HIV infections annually, at an average annual cost of $6 U.S. per capita. While the confidence intervals around this estimate are wide, the estimate suggests that condom distribution is cost-effective. At the same time, it indicates the enormity of the challenge for countries whose annual health budget may be $10 U.S. or less per capita.

FEMALE CONDOMS

The recent development and testing of designs for a female condom gives hope that a contraceptive method will be developed that is more easily controlled by women and requires less active consent by male partners. Pilot studies have indicated varying acceptability. Much more research is needed on design, acceptability, and promotion. A major limiting factor to female condom use will be the probable higher cost of female condoms compared with conventional condoms.

IMPLICATIONS OF THE HIV EPIDEMIC FOR FAMILY PLANNING SERVICES

There are at least two general reasons why family planning services must pay attention to, and become involved with, global efforts to limit the epidemic spread of HIV: necessity and opportunity.

Necessity

Any family planning service must counsel clients on method use according to the risk/benefit potential of each method for each client. For HIV seronegative women, the possibility that individual contraceptive methods may increase or decrease risk of STD or HIV acquisition should be considered in the light of a woman's (or couple's) circumstance. The current uncertainty associated with the effect of individual contraceptive methods on HIV transmission (with the exception of condoms) suggests that current recommendations should be guided by the better known factors, such as effectiveness in preventing pregnancy and other STDs. At the same time, it is important for the family planning community to monitor research on the relationship between different contraceptive methods and HIV transmission and to adapt recommendations as better data become available.

Certain theoretical routes of HIV infection, such as multiple use of needles or contamination of surgical intruments, are sufficiently plausible and preventable that the discovery of an epidemiologic link in a family planning setting should be regarded as a failure, not a precondition for action. The potential for HIV transmission is just another reminder that family planning personnel need to be provided with the equipment, training, and motivation to ensure that nosocomial spread of any infection is not facilitated by unsterile instruments.

Family planning services, particularly those in countries in which HIV is widespread, will increasingly have to counsel seropositive women on family planning choices. While a range of ethical and policy issues need to be considered, HIV-infected women must at least be offered effective contraception in order to prevent vertical transmission. Because the use-effectiveness of the condom results in an undesirable rate of unwanted pregnancy, the condom needs to be combined with other methods of contraception. This double contraceptive method will only be employed if adequate counseling is provided by family planning clinics.

Opportunity

Family planning services provide an opportunity for the prevention of HIV transmission, particularly in regions where the predominant mode of HIV spread is heterosexual. Family planning clinics cater to women (and occasionally men) of childbearing age, a period when individuals are also at increased risk of contact with STDs, including HIV infection. In some parts of Africa, there is increasing evidence that women are at greater risk of contracting HIV than men. In Uganda, women aged 15 to 24 years have been shown to have a risk 1.4 times higher than men in the same age range (21). Family planning services, especially those integrated with maternal and child health services, may provide the only outlet for health care, and thus prevention of HIV infection, for rural women.

In the initial phase of the HIV/AIDS epidemic, some members of the family planning community were worried that any integration of AIDS education into family planning services might "turn off" clients or compromise service delivery. The latter problem is still a real possibility in areas of contrained resources. However, the potential magnitude of the HIV/AIDS epidemic, combined with the links between HIV and sexuality, demand involvement from family planning services.

Ideally, family planning services should offer counseling about STDs and HIV. They should also provide simple facilities for diagnosis, treatment, and referral. Family planning managers need to recognize that adolescents are at increased risk of contracting STDs/HIV; therefore, special and appropriate programs need to be established for adolescents. Family planning researchers should direct their attention to the design and evaluation of cost-effective programs for the integration of AIDS education into family planning services. Such programs would permit the widespread communication and practical application of knowledge derived from studies on the relationship between different contraceptive methods and HIV transmission.

Acknowledgments
The authors wish to thank members of the AIDS and Reproductive Health Network for useful discussions, and Frank Plummer for sharing the manuscript of his paper before publication.

REFERENCES

1. Albin RJ, Bruns GR, Guinan P, Bush IM. The effect of estrogen on the incorporation of 3H-thymidine by PHA-stimulated human peripheral lymphocyte. *J Immunol* 1974; 113:705.
2. Barnes EW, MacCuish AC, Loudon NB, Jordan J, Irvine WJ. PHA-induced lymphocyte transformation and circulating autoantibodies in women taking oral contraceptives. *Lancet* 1974; i:898.
3. Bulterys M, Saah A, Chao A, Habimana P, Makafaranswa B, Kageruka M, Munyemana S. Is oral contraception use associated with prevalent HIV infection in Rwandan women? Abstract T.P.C.6. 5th Congress on AIDS and Associated Cancers in Africa, Kinshasa, October 1991.
4. Burns Macd. DC, Darougar S., Thin RN, Lothian L, Nico CS. Isolation of chlamydia from women attending a clinic for sexually transmitted disease. *Brit J Vener Dis* 1975; 51:314-318.
5. Carael M, Van de Perre PH, Lepage PH, Allen S, Nsengumuremyi F, Van Goethem C, Ntahorutaba M, Nzaramba D, Clumeck N. Human immunodeficiency virus transmission among heterosexual couples in Central Africa. *AIDS* 1988; 2:201-205. 6. Collins WE, Campbell CC, Berber A. The effect of oral contraceptives in malaria infections in rhesus monkeys. *Bull World Health Org* 1984; 62:627.
7. Darrow WW, Bigler W, Deppe D, French J, Gill P, Potterat J, Ravenholt O, Schable C, Sikes RK, Wofsy C. HIV antibody in 640 U.S. prostitutes with no evidence of intravenous (IV)-drug abuse. Abstract 4054, IV International Conference on AIDS, Stockholm, June 1988.
8. European Study Group. Risk factors for male to female transmission of HIV. *Brit Med J* 1989; 298:411-415.
9. Fathalla MF in *The Heterosexual Transmission of AIDS*. Alan R Liss, Inc. 1990, p. 235.
10. Fineberg HV. Education to prevent AIDS: prospects and obstacles. *Science* 1988; 238:592-596.
11. Fitzgerald PN, Pickering AF, Ferguson DN. Depressed lymphocyte response to PHA in long-term users of oral contraceptives. *Lancet* 1973; i:615.
12. Goldacre MJ, Loudon N, Watt B, Grant G, Loudon JDO, McPherson K, Vessey MP. Epidemiology and clinical significance of cervical erosion in women attending a family planning clinic. *Brit Med J* 1978; 1:748-750.
13. Goldberg HI, Lee NC, Oberle MW, Peterson HB. Knowledge about condoms and their use in less developed countries during a period of rising AIDS prevalence. *Bull World Health Org* 1989; 67:85-91.
14. Haukkamaa M, Stranden P, Jousimies-Somer H, Siitonen A. Bacterial flora of the cervix in women using different methods of contraception. *Am J Obstet Gynecol* 1986; 154:520-524.
15. Hicks DR, Martin LS, Getchell JP, Health JL, Francis DP, McDougal JS, Curran JW, Boeller B. Inactivation of HTLV-III/LAV-infected cultures of normal lymphocytes by nonoxynol-9 in vitro (letter). *Lancet* 1985; ii:1422-1423.
16. Hilton AL, Richmond SJ, Milne JD et al. Chlamydia A in the female genital tract. *Br J Vener Dis* 1984; 50:1-10.
17. Hunter D, Maggwa A, Mati J, Tukei P, Solomon M, Mbugua S, Bhullar V, Mohammedali Y. Risk factors for HIV transmission in women attending family planning clinics in Nairobi. Abstract Th.C.573, VI International Conference on AIDS, San Francisco, June 1990.

18. Irvine WJ, MacCuish AC, Barnes WE, Urbanik SJ, Loudon NB. Immunological function in OC users. *J Repd Fert* (Suppl) 1974; 21:33.

19. Joshi UM, Rao SS, Kora SJ, Dikshit SS, Virkar KD. Effect of steroidal contraceptives on antibody formation in the human female. *Contraception* 1971; 3:327.

20. Keller AJ, Irvine WJ, Jordan J, Loudon NB. PHA-induced lymphocyte transformation in oral contraceptive users. *Obstet Gynec* 1977; 49:83.

21. Konde-Lule JK, Berkeley SF, Downing R. Knowledge, attitudes and practices concerning AIDS in Ugandans. *AIDS* 1989; 3:513-518.

22. Kreiss J, Cameron DW, Ngogi E et al. Efficacy of the spermicide nonoxynol-9 (N-9) in preventing heterosexual transmission of HIV. IV International Conference on AIDS, Stockholm, Sweden, June 1988. Abstract 6525.

23. Latif AS, Katzenstein DA, Bassett MT, Houston S, Emmanuel JC, Marowa E. Genital ulcers and transmission of HIV among couples in Zimbabwe. *AIDS* 1989; 3:519-523.

24. Macaulay ME, Riordan T, James JM, Leventhall PA, Morris EM, Neal BR, Ellis DA. A prospective study of genital infections in a family planning clinic. *Epidemiol Infect* 1990; 104:55-61.

25. Mati JKG, Sinei SK, Mulandi TN, Ndaui PM, Mbwgua S, Mailu CK, Mungai JW. Oral contraceptive use and the risk of malaria. *E Afr Med J* 1986; 63:382-388.

26. Mati JKG, Maggwa A, Chewe D, Solomon M, Mbugua S, Bhullar V, Tukei P, Hunter D, Achola P. Contraceptive use and HIV infection among women attending family planning clinics in Nairobi, Kenya. Abstract Th.C.99, VI International Conference on AIDS, San Francisco, June 1990.

27. Mauldin WP, Segal SJ. Prevalence of contraceptive use in developing countries. The Rockefeller Foundation, New York, 1986.

28. Mendelshone JMM, Bernheim JL. Inhibition of human lymphocyte stimulation by steroid hormones: Cytokinetic mechanisms. *Clin Exp Immunol* 1977; 27:127.

29. Mori T, Kobayashi H, Nishimura T, Mori TS, Fuji G, Inou T. Inhibitory effect of progesterone on PHA-0induced transformation of human peripheral lymphocytes. *Immunological Commun* 1975; 4:519.

30. Morishima A., Henrich RT. Lymphocyte transformation and oral contraceptives. *Lancet* 1974; ii:646.

31. Moses S, Ngugi E, Nagelkerke NJ, Bosire M, Waiyaki P, Plummer FA. Cost-effectiveness of an STD/AIDS control programme for high-frequency STD transmitters in Nairobi, Kenya. Abstract F.D.837, VI International Conference on AIDS, San Francisco, June 1990.

32. Moss GB, D'Costa LJ, Ndinya-Achola JO, Plummer FA, Reilly MP, Kreiss JK. Cervical ectopy and lack of male circumcision as risk factors for heterosexual transmission of HIV in stable sexual partnerships in Kenya. Abstract Th.C.570. VI International Conference on AIDS, San Francisco, June 1990.

33. Musicco M. for The Italian Partners Study. Oral contraception, IUD, condom use and man to woman transmission of HIV infection. Abstract Th.C.584, VI International Conference on AIDS, San Francisco, June 1990.

34. Ngugi EN, Plummer FA, Simonsen JN, Cameron DW, Bosire M, Waiyaki P, Ronald AR, Ndinya-Achola JO. Prevention of transmission of human immunodeficiency virus in Africa: effectiveness of condom promotion and health education among prostitutes. *Lancet* 1988; ii:887-890.

35. Ngugi EN, Njeru EK, Karkuiki A, Plummer FA, Moses S, Muchunga EK. Impact of an STD/AIDS health education programme among four groups of women working as prostitutes in Kenya. Abstract 3033, VI International Conference on AIDS, San Francisco, June 1990.

36. Oriel JD, Johnson AL, Barlow D. Thomas BJ, Nayyar K, Reeve P. Infection of the uterine cervix with Chlamydia trachomatis. *J Infect Dis* 1978; 137:443-451.

37. Payanzo N, Mivumbi N, Kakera L. AIDS, STD's and condom acceptability in high risk grounds in Matadi, Zaire. Abstract Th.D.782, International Conference on AIDS, San Francisco, June 1990.

38. Payanzo N, Kakera L, Wahlmeier G. Condom usage and demand among Zaire river boat travellers. Abstract Th.D.783, International Conference on AIDS, San Francisco, June 1990.

39. Plummer F, Cameron W, Simonsen N, Bosire M, Maitha G, Kreiss J, Waiyaki P, Roland A, Ndinya-Achola J, Ngugi E. Co-factors in male-female transmission of HIV. Abstract 4554, IV International Conference on AIDS, Stockholm, June 1988.

40. Pokrovsky VV, Kuznetsova I, Eramova I. Transmission of HIV infection from an infected infant to his mother by breast-feeding. Abstract Th.C.48, VI International Conference on AIDS, San Francisco, June 1990.

41. Rangnekar KN, Joshi UM, Rao SS. Diminution in humoral antibodies to tetanus toxoid after ovulene therapy in mice. *Contraception* 1972; 6:5.

42. Reckart ML, Barnett JA, Manzon LM, Wittenberg L, McNabb A. Nonoxynol 9: its adverse effects. Abstract S.C.36, VI International Conference on AIDS, San Francisco, June 1990.

43. Reitmeijer CA, Krebs JW, Feorino PM, Judson FN. Condoms as physical and chemical barriers against human immunodeficiency virus. *JAMA* 1988; 259;1851-1853.

44. Rosenberg MJ, Rojanapithayakorn W, Feldblum PJ, Higgins JE. Effect of the contraceptive sponge on chlamydial infection, gonorrhea and candidiasis: a comparative clinical trial. *JAMA* 1987; 257:2308-2312.

45. Royal College of General Practitioners. Oral contraceptives and health: An interim report from the oral contraception study of the R.C.G. Pract. 1. Pitman Medical, New York, 1974.

46. Shafer M, Beck A, Blain B, Dole P, Irwin CE, Sweet R, Schachter J. Chlamydia trachomatis: Important relationship to race, contraception, lower genital tract infection, and Papanicolaou smear. *J Pediatr* 1984; 104:141-146.

47. Simonsen JN, Plummer FA, Ngugi EN, Black C, Kreiss JK, Gakinya MN, Waiyaki P, D'Costa LJ, Ndinya-Achola JO, Piot P, Roland A. HIV infection among lower socioeconomic strata prostitutes in Nairobi. *AIDS* 1990; 4:139-144.

48. Siraprasiri T, Thanprasertsuk S, Rodklay A, Srivanichakorn S, Teerathan C, Labsomtob A, Sawanpanyalert P, Temthanaluk J. Study of risk factors for HIV infection among prostitutes in Chiengmai, Thailand. Presented at Field Epidemiology Training Program, 2nd International Conference, Puebla, Mexico, January 1990.

49. Tezabwala BU, Hedge UC, Joshi JV, Jaswaney VL, Rao SS. Studies on cell-mediated immunity in women using different fertility regulating methods. *J Clin Lab Immunol* 1983; 10:199-202.

50. Voeller B. Nonoxynol-9 and HTLV-III (letter). *Lancet* 1986; i:1153.

51. Wyle FA, Kent JR. Immunosuppression by sex steroid hormones. I. The effect upon PHA and PPD stimulated lymphocytes. *Clin Exp Immunol* 1977; 27:407.

HUMAN SEXUALITY AND AIDS:
THE CASE OF MALE BISEXUALITY

Richard G. Parker

State University of Rio de Janeiro

Manuel Carballo

World Health Organization

INTRODUCTION

The rapid spread of the international AIDS pandemic has forced us to confront the limitations in our understanding of a whole range of social and behavioral factors linked to infection with HIV (11). Nowhere has this been more evident than in studies of sexual behavior, the single most important mode of HIV transmission in almost every society. Yet, in spite of its obvious importance, human sexuality has suffered a long history of scientific neglect, leaving us largely unprepared to deal with many of the most important issues raised by the sexual transmission of HIV (1).

The general lack of interest in and attention to the study of sexual behavior has been especially evident in many of the fields or disciplines most immediately charged with responding to the HIV/AIDS pandemic. In public health, population science, epidemiology, and a range of other related fields, the theoretical paradigms and research methodologies used to interpret and understand sexual experience have been characterized less by openness and innovation than by restrictiveness. The study of sexual life has traditionally focused almost exclusively on reproductive relations, and more complex patterns or variations in human sexual behavior have been largely excluded from attention (1,49).

These longstanding limitations have become all too obvious in the wake of HIV and AIDS. Even in the earliest phase of the epidemic, the urgent need for baseline data on the previously unstudied practices of homosexual men had become painfully evident (e.g., 49). In just a few years, as the heterosexual transmission of HIV became pronouced in many parts of the world, the no less pressing need for a fuller understanding not only of reproductive behavior, but of sexual relations more broadly, became equally apparent (e.g., 12,49). It is now impossible to ignore the extent to which a more rapid and effective response to the HIV/AIDS pandemic has been inhibited by largely unexamined and uncriticized limitations in existing knowledge and conceptual frameworks, particularly in relation to sexual behavior.

No area of human sexuality relevant to HIV/AIDS underscores these dilemmas as forcefully as does bisexuality (e.g., 8,37,48). While bisexual behavior has remained a relatively secondary and poorly defined issue in emerging AIDS research agendas, it may actually present a greater challenge than does any other domain of human sexuality in terms of its potential implications for HIV transmission. Although it is difficult to estimate the exact size of the population at risk, there is increasing evidence that the number of men who have sex with men as well as with women may be quite significant, and is certainly larger than previously assumed. In addition to carrying the health risks associated with some same-sex sexual practices, male bisexual behavior may contribute to the spread of HIV beyond the population of men involved in bisexual contacts, potentially affecting the health of the female sexual partners of bisexual men and the health of their children. It is also possible that at least some patterns of female bisexual behavior (even less a focus of attention than male bisexuality), such as occasional sexual contacts between lesbians and gay men, may increase the risk of HIV transmission in some populations previously thought to be largely protected from infection through sexual contact.

In spite of the potential importance of bisexuality in relation to HIV and AIDS, a fuller understanding of bisexual behavior, like human sexuality in general, has been inhibited by our conceptual paradigms (48). Preconceived notions about the nature of human sexual life, and an essentially dichotomous view of homosexuality and heterosexuality as polar opposites, have failed to permit the exploration of more complex variations in human sexual experience (8,32,38).

In this chapter, we begin to move beyond these limitations by examining bisexuality as a key issue for AIDS research and an important point of intersection between AIDS and reproductive health. Focusing principally on male bisexuality, we will explore the social and cultural construction of sexual experience from a comparative perspective in order to suggest the wide range of settings in which bisexual behaviors are present, as well as the complex factors that must be taken into account in seeking to understand these behaviors. Building on this discussion, we will analyze some of the ways in which bisexual behaviors may be linked to the risk of HIV transmission in different settings, and suggest how a better understanding of bisexuality might lead to more effective strategies for intervention. In examining bisexuality, we hope to suggest at least some ways in which it might be possible to develop a fuller understanding of human sexual behavior in general, and consequently, a more adequate response to HIV and AIDS in the future.

CULTURAL DETERMINANTS OF BISEXUAL BEHAVIOR

While a number of perspectives are useful in seeking to understand patterns of human sexual behavior, it has become increasingly clear that more attention needs to be given to the social construction of gender and sexuality. Findings from a variety of different disciplines and a number of distinct intellectual traditions suggest that sexual life is as much a construct of history and culture as a function of human nature or biology. While sexual desire may be among the strongest and most basic of human drives, the shapes that it takes and the behaviors that it gives rise to are molded within a much wider social universe. It is this socio-cultural, political, and legal environment that requires further study in order to approach an understanding of human sexual experience (e.g., 10,24,51).

In the study of homosexuality, this focus on the construction of sexual life has already gone far in drawing attention to the many forces that shape and structure sexual life in specific settings (25). Among other things, it has led to an important historical analysis of homosexuality in many industrialized societies where sexual relations between individuals of the same sex have become more open and research more possible (e.g., 19,43,50). Studies in this area have shown that, in societies such as Great Britain and the United States, the emergence of homosexual subcultures was closely linked to a series of social and political changes that not only permitted, but may have promoted lifestyles other than those revolving around traditional patterns of family organization and reproduction (19,50).

The gradual construction of homosexuality as a distinct sexual identity in these societies thus gave rise to relatively well-defined and sharply bounded gay communities characterized by their own social institutions and cultural traditions. It was this configuration that made possible the early and rapid transmission of HIV, yet also produced an organized, collective, community-based response to the threat of HIV infection (4).

The homosexual experience in industrialized societies may bear little resemblance to the organization of same-sex relations in different social contexts or in other parts of the world, however (e.g., 7,26,28). In industrialized societies, the homosexual experience was clearly the product of specific historical events linked to the emergence of a new social and economic order. But in other societies that did not go through similar processes of social change, other factors will have shaped the homosexual experience.

While homosexual behavior has been documented in almost all periods of history and all parts of the world, the forms that it has taken, the ways in which it is conceptualized, and the social responses it elicits vary significantly by place and time. For example, where cultural values associated with family life and reproduction have been strong and procreation has been idealized, the dominant patterns of sexual organization have been quite distinct from those that have emerged recently in industrialized contexts. Where homosexuality may have been eclipsed by more dominant heterosexual themes, bisexuality may have assumed the functional role of permitting both societal expectations regarding family life and personal sexual preferences to be satisfied at one and the same time.

In many parts of the world, it is clear that the choice of sexual partner (whether male or female) is conceptually less important than the specific roles that individuals play during the sexual act. In a variety of cultural settings, the distinction between active and passive partners in same-sex interactions appears to determine the definition of gender and sexuality much more than does any Western notion of homosexuality or heterosexuality. Notions of sexuality linked to culturally defined concepts of masculinity and femininity appear ultimately more important than categories such as homosexuality or heterosexuality. Ethnographic research suggests, for example, that in some societies the male gender identity need not necessarily be threatened by homosexual interactions because only the passive partner in receptive anal intercourse is perceived to assume the female role and is, hence, definable as homosexual. Distinctions of this order have been observed in Mexico (14,15,16,18,39,47); Brazil (21,22,32-36,40); Nicaragua (29); Peru (5); and in other parts of the Latin and Mediterranean world (9,20,52), as well as in parts of Africa (2,45), and Asia (28,31).

In much the same way, similar conceptions of gender and sexual roles may function in situations where heterosexual contacts have to be postponed and where there is a need to legitimize same-sex interactions as a form of sexual release. The institutionalized segregation of males in prisons, military establishments, and migrant labor camps, for instance, may contribute to the construction of new gender definitions that permit same-sex interactions (e.g., 54). Similarly, the widespread segregation of young people along gender lines may result in extensive bisexual behavior during adolescence. This may result, in part, from a lack of opposite-sex partners, but also, and perhaps no less importantly, because of the socially and culturally defined importance of adolescence as a period of sexual exploration and experimentation crucial to the formation of sexual identities (17,23,27,34).

Thus, in a wide range of different contexts and in a variety of different ways, the social and cultural construction of gender and sexuality in different settings seems to open up the possibilities for same-sex, as well as opposite-sex, sexual contacts along lines that differ significantly from those found in the gay communities of many industrialized societies. Even in the complex, pluralistic, and multi-ethnic societies in which gay communities are present, notions of homosexuality and heterosexuality may actually be less significant among some segments of the population, or in certain circumstances or situations, than are more local and popular definitions of sexual roles or practices. Among some ethnic minorities and socio-economic groups, the construction of same-sex interactions may have more in common with persisting cultural patterns and local social contexts than with the sexual lifestyles that have emerged in the predominantly white, middle-class sectors of the gay community (3,41,44).

BISEXUAL BEHAVIOR AND THE RISKS OF HIV TRANSMISSION

The differences that appear to exist in the social and cultural construction of same-sex sexual interactions in different settings should, perhaps, be enough to suggest the importance of examining bisexuality within the broader framework of human sexuality and reproductive health. The urgency of this becomes all the more evident in thinking about the potential relation of bisexuality to HIV infection and AIDS. Indeed, had the AIDS epidemic not brought to light bisexual contacts and the ways in which they clearly increase risk of HIV infection, they might not otherwise have been acknowledged.

In seeking to evaluate the risk of HIV transmission in relation to bisexuality, special emphasis should be given to the potential risks faced by behaviorally bisexual men themselves. This is especially important precisely because, in many settings, bisexual behavior is considered relatively unproblematic by those involved. Actively bisexual men rarely appear to indentify their bisexual behavior as a health concern. Even in settings where information about HIV infection and AIDS is quite widely disseminated, many behaviorally bisexual men may be unaware of the risks they may face as both receptors and vectors of HIV infection.

Just as cross-cultural differences may influence the ways in which behaviorally bisexual men perceive themselves, the social and cultural construction of same-sex interactions may also structure their risk of HIV infection in important, although still poorly understood, ways. It has been suggested, for example, that strict active/passive role separation in same-sex anal intercourse may actually offer some degree of protection for active (insertive) partners, and, by extension, for the female partners of exclusively insertive bisexual men (53). Where there appears to be more flexibility in active and passive roles, the risks involved for behaviorally bisexual men, as well as for their sexual partners (male or female), may be more significant. In these cases, bisexual men may be more efficient vectors in HIV transmission.

Ultimately, a fuller understanding of the risks involved in bisexual contacts depends upon expanding scientific knowledge of the dynamics of HIV transmission in relation to specific sexual practices (such as insertive as opposed to receptive anal intercourse). This, in turn, might point to the study of bisexual behavior as a key to broadening and deepening our understanding of HIV transmission more generally.

A fuller understanding of the risks involved for behaviorally bisexual men will be the first step toward a more accurate appraisal of the risks that may be faced by their male and female sexual partners. Because male bisexual behavior is so often clandestine or hidden from female partners, much of the attention given to bisexuality in relation to HIV and AIDS understandably has focused on the role of bisexual behavior as a "bridge" between high-prevalence groups, such as homosexual men, and the heterosexual population. The risks to female sexual partners have been seen as especially worrisome precisely because these partners are so often unaware that they may in fact be at risk, and are, thus, unlikely to take any precautions to reduce risk. This is all the more true in cultural contexts that largely deny women power within reproductive relations, and that limit the possibilities for negotiating sexual and reproductive practices (e.g., 3).

The specific risks involved in heterosexual relations involving behaviorally bisexual men have only begun to be explored. Evidence has clearly shown that high-risk practices, such as anal intercourse, play an important role in raising the risk of transmission to the female sexual partners of bisexual men (46); yet it is unclear whether or not such practices play a more significant role in the sexual experience of bisexual men and their partners than they do in the behavior of exclusively heterosexual couples (8). The poverty of our knowledge concerning bisexual behavior in general has limited our ability to evaluate HIV-related risks because we have almost no empirical data on the actual sexual practices involved, and, perhaps more importantly, the meanings they hold for their participants (8,32,55).

If little is known about the dynamics of HIV transmission or the degrees of risk involved in the heterosexual practices of behaviorally bisexual individuals (the one area that has received at least some limited attention in AIDS research thus far), even less is known about the more unexpected consequences of HIV infection in relation to bisexuality. It is becoming increasingly apparent, for example, that bisexual behavior may play an important role in the vertical transmission of HIV. In Brazil, roughly 20% of the reported cases of pediatric AIDS are in children with bisexual fathers (6). It has been suggested that, among ethnic minorities in the United States, the incidence of vertical transmission linked to intravenous drug use may be significantly overstated, at least in part as a result of the hidden nature of much bisexual behavior in the black and Latino communities (3).

As we seek to evaluate the risks of HIV transmission that may arise, either directly or indirectly, in relation to bisexual behavior, we are confronted at almost every turn with vague assumptions and limited evidence. The relatively widespread practice of bisexual behavior clearly opens up the possibility of HIV transmission in a variety of different directions, but the clandestine nature of such behavior continues to limit our ability to evaluate such risks. Our failure to make bisexual behavior a significant issue on the research agendas in both the HIV/AIDS and reproductive health fields accentuates the lack of information and leaves open a gap in our knowledge of human sexuality that may seriously limit our ability to control the spread of HIV through more effective AIDS prevention programs and policies. Addressing bisexual behavior more effectively may be a key issue for health promotion in relation to both AIDS prevention and reproductive health.

RISK REDUCTION AND AIDS PREVENTION

To date, most AIDS health promotion activities, particularly the more successful ones, have been directed to relatively well-identified sexual minority groups or communities that have usually actively participated in AIDS prevention efforts. Because bisexual behavior has remained hidden and apparently unacknowledged as a potential problem in relation to AIDS, the task of responding to the risk of HIV transmission through bisexual contacts is likely to be more difficult than has been the task of responding to other HIV-related risk behaviors. Neither bisexual men nor their female sexual partners constitute clear epidemiological or sociological categories. In many respects, they have little or no social reality as members of identifiable groups. Almost nowhere has there been extensive, collective mobilization on the part of bisexual men, and few if any bisexual "communities" have emerged that could be utilized in developing and diffusing targeted HIV/AIDS risk-reduction messages. Furthermore, because AIDS prevention and education messages have tended to focus on risk groups rather than on risk behaviors, bisexual men may not see themselves as potential receptors or vectors of HIV.

Existing AIDS education messages targeted principally to gay men are inappropriate in contexts in which local social and cultural norms are so opposed to sex between men that the bisexual male finds it necessary to maintain highly public and socially acceptable heterosexual relationships. Dualism of this type may make such AIDS prevention messages seem irrelevant to bisexuals. From a purely psychological perspective, the bisexual male may be neither prepared to receive, nor capable of receiving, HIV-related information that introduces disequilibrium into a series of symbiotic male/female relationships that have been carefully created, balanced, and fostered over time.

In light of these concerns, current methods and approaches to AIDS education may have only limited value in reaching bisexual men and their male or female sexual partners. If HIV/AIDS prevention strategies are to be successful with regard to bisexuality, it will probably be necessary to develop new techniques that meet the special needs of a population group that has previously remained invisible and well outside the attention of public health officials (48). This will require a wide set of changes in the ways in which bisexual behavior is treated within the context of both the HIV/AIDS and reproductive health fields.

The first step in this direction is a fairly simple one: begin to focus on bisexuality as a key issue that must be incorporated into AIDS prevention activities and national AIDS programs, even where the extent of bisexual behavior may be unknown or publicly denied. This will demand a commitment to basic social and behavioral research aimed at developing greater understanding of the patterns of bisexual behavior in different settings, of the ways in which these behavioral patterns are socially constructed, and of the meanings that they hold for their participants. In different settings, different behavioral patterns may be found, or the same patterns may be invested with different meanings. AIDS education and prevention in relation to bisexual behavior will depend to a great extent on research aimed at responding to the silences that have so often surrounded bisexuality (3,37,48).

With a fuller understanding of the patterns of bisexual behavior found in different settings, it may become possible to develop AIDS education and information programs that integrate health promotion activities into a fuller understanding of the ways in which sexuality is lived and experienced in diverse social settings. In order to meaningfully reach what may superficially appear to be a relatively undifferentiated population, it will be necessary to distinguish between the behavior of long-term adult bisexual men, situationally specific and temporary bisexuality, the bisexual behavior of adolescents, the bisexual behavior of male prostitutes, and so on. Building a fuller understanding of the social and cultural construction of sexual experience and the meaningful patterns of sexual behavior in different settings will require innovative educational strategies that can be used to develop forums and formats for AIDS education that is both culturally appropriate and sensitive to the specific dynamics of bisexuality within distinct populations (e.g., 30).

Because of the often clandestine nature of bisexual behavior, and, thus, the difficulty of addressing it in more impersonal health promotion activities, counseling programs may play a key role in effectively addressing the issue of bisexuality (e.g., 13). The discussion of male bisexual behavior has been largely absent from the counseling agenda in both the HIV/AIDS and reproductive health communities. Yet in many cultural situations, behaviorally bisexual men are members of heterosexual families and have offspring and parental responsibilities, making the question of bisexuality in the context of the AIDS epidemic not only important, but also sensitive. Counseling behaviorally bisexual men on the health implications of HIV must necessarily address a much broader sphere than counseling for exclusive homosexual men, as there are social, economic, and ethical dimensions of the HIV/AIDS problem that are unique to relationships involving women, mothers, and children, as well as other men. Indeed, few areas of HIV-related human behavior warrant the degree of counseling attention and skills as does bisexuality and the welfare of the individuals and families involved. Counseling on the complex issues involved in bisexual behavior should be developed as a key component in the design of AIDS prevention and risk reduction programs.

CONCLUSION

Despite the relatively rapid advances made in understanding the virology and immunological aspects of AIDS, there still remain major lacunae in knowledge about the social epidemiology of the disease. In the early stages of the epidemic, it was generally held that AIDS was a problem primarily associated with high-risk homosexual behaviors and intravenous drug use. It soon became apparent, however, that transmission of HIV between heterosexual partners was not only possible, but was apparently the main route of HIV infection throughout major parts of sub-Saharan Africa, Latin America, and, increasingly, Western Europe, North America, and Australasia (42). To date, most prevention and research activities have focused on high-risk homosexual and heterosexual sexual practices and intravenous drug use, themselves highly complex areas of behavior that are difficult to study.

But over the course of a number of years, it has become increasingly evident that male bisexual behavior has also played an important role in the epidemiology of AIDS in many parts of the world. While usually covert, and invariably denied for a variety of reasons, bisexual behaivor is apparently far more widespread than previously appreciated. Its relative contribution to the spread of HIV may have been, and may continue to be, considerable. The failure to make bisexual behavior a significant issue within HIV/AIDS and reproductive health research agendas has meant that, at the end of the first decade of a rapidly accelerating epidemic, there is a major gap in our knowledge about human sexuality and our understanding of how to respond to the spread of HIV with more effective AIDS prevention programs and policies (48).

The relative lack of attention directed to the question of bisexual behavior in relation to HIV/AIDS is indicative of the limitations that have characterized the scientific investigation of human sexuality in general. Sadly, these limitations have been especially evident in many of the disciplines most directly involved in responding to the problems posed by HIV and AIDS. The rapid spread of the HIV/AIDS pandemic has underscored the urgent need for new theoretical paradigms, more innovative methodological strategies, and a radically expanded vision of the entire field of human sexuality. The diversity that exists in the construction of perceptions and definitions of sexual life in different social and cultural settings makes the study of human sexuality in general, like the study of bisexuality in particular, indispensable to HIV/AIDS prevention. Our ability to respond to the spread of HIV more effectively in the future will be critically dependant upon our willingness to move beyond the limitations of the past to broaden and deepen our understanding of sexual behavior. Integrating studies of human sexuality in all of its dimensions must be a key part of the research agenda for public health.

Acknowledgments

We would like to thank Joseph Carrier and Rob Tielman for comments that have been useful in developing this paper. Richard Parker would like to acknowledge the Foundation for the Support of Research in the State of Rio de Janeiro for their support of research on the social dimensions of AIDS.

REFERENCES

1. Abramson PR and Herdt G. The Assessment of Sexual Practices Relevant to the Transmission of AIDS: A Global Perspective. *The Journal of Sex Research* 1990; 27(2):215-232.
2   Aina T. Nigeria. In: Tielman R, Carballo M, Hendriks A, eds. *Bisexuality and HIV/AIDS*. Amherst, N.Y.: Prometheus Books, 1987.
3. Alonso AM and Koreck MT. Silences: "Hispanics," AIDS, and Sexual Practices. *Differences* 1989; 1:101-124.
4. Altman D. *AIDS in the Mind of America*. New York: Anchor Press, 1987.
5. Arboleda M. Social Attitudes and Sexual Variance in Lima. In: Murray SO, ed. *Male Homosexuality in Central and South America*. New York: Gai Saber Monographs, 1987.
6. Bergamaschi D et al. Pediatric AIDS in Brazil: Description and Analysis of Trends. V International Conference on AIDS, Montreal, Canada, 1989; Abstract Th.G.O. 50.

7. Blackwood E, ed. *Anthropology and Homosexual Behavior*. New York: Haworth Press, 1985.
8. Boulton M. Review of Literature. In: Tielman R, Carballo M, Hendriks A, eds. *Bisexuality and HIV/AIDS*. Amherst, N.Y.: Prometheus Books, 1991.
9. Brandes S. Like Wounded Stags: Male Sexual Ideology in an Andalusian Town. In: S. Ortner and H. Whitehead, eds. *Sexual Meanings: The Cultural Construction of Gender and Sexuality*. New York: Cambridge University Press, 1981; pp. 216-239.
10. Caplan P. *The Cultural Construction of Sexuality*. New York: Tavistock Publications, 1987.
11. Carballo M. International Agenda for AIDS Behavioral Research. In: Kulstad R, ed. *AIDS 1988: AAAS Symposia Papers*. Washington, D.C.: American Association for the Advancement of Science, 1988; pp. 271-273.
12. Carballo M et al. A Cross National Study of Patterns of Sexual Behavior. *The Journal of Sex Research* 1989; 26:287-299.
13. Carballo-Dieguez A. Hispanic Culture, Gay Male Culture, and AIDS: Counseling Implications. *Journal of Counseling and Development* 1989; 68: 26-30.
14. Carrier JM. Participants in Urban Male Homosexual Encounters. *Archives of Sexual Behavior* 1971; 1(4):279-291.
15. Carrier JM. Cultural Factors Affecting Urban Mexican Male Homosexual Encounters. *Archives of Sexual Behavior 1976*; 5:103-124.
16. Carrier JM. Mexican Male Bisexuality. *Journal of Homosexuality* 1985; 1(1/2):75-85.
17. Carrier JM. Gay Liberation and Coming Out in Mexico. *Journal of Homosexuality* 1989; 17(1/2):225-252.
18. Carrier JM. Sexual Behavior and Spread of AIDS in Mexico. *Medical Anthropology* 1989; 10(2/3):129-142.
19. D'Emilio J. *Sexual Politics, Sexual Communities: The Making of a Homosexual Minority in the United States, 1940-1970*. Chicago: The University of Chicago Press, 1983.
20. Dundes A et al. The Strategy of Turkish Boys Verbal Dueling Rhymes. *Journal of American Folklore* 1970; 23:225-249.
21. Fry P. *Para Inglês Ver*. Rio de Janeiro: Zahar Editores, 1982.
22. Fry P. Male Homosexuality and Spirit Possession in Brazil. *Journal of Homosexuality* 1985; 11(3/4):137-153.
23. Gagnon JH. Sexuality Across the Life Course in the United States. In: Turner CF, Miller HG, Moses LE, eds. *AIDS, Sexual Behavior, and Intravenous Drug Use*. Washington, D.C.: National Academy Press, 1989; pp. 500-536.
24. Gagnon JH. and William S. *Sexual Conduct: The Social Sources of Human Sexuality*. Chicago: Aldine, 1973.
25. Greenberg DE. *The Construction of Homosexuality*. Chicago: The University of Chicago Press, 1988.
26. Herdt G. *Guardians of the Flutes: Idioms of Masculinity*. New York: MacGraw-Hill, 1981. 27. Herdt G. Introduction: Gay Youth, Emergent Identities, and Cultural Scenes at Home and Abroad. *Journal of Homosexuality* 1989; 17(1/2):1-42.
28. Jackson PA. *Male Homosexuality in Thailand*. New York: Global Academic Publishers, 1989.
29. Lancaster RN. Subject Honor and Object Shame: The Cochon and the Milieu-Specific Construction of Stigma and Sexuality in Nicaragua. *Ethnology* 1988; 27:111-125.
30. Magaña JR et al. A Pedagogy for Health: AIDS Education and Empowerment. Unpublished manuscript.
31. Nanda S. The Hijras of India: Cultural and Individual Dimensions of an Institutionalized Third Gender Role. *Journal of Homosexuality* 1985; 11(3/4):35-54.
32. Parker RG. Acquired Immunodeficiency Syndrome in Urban Brazil. *Medical Anthropology Quarterly* 1987; 1(2):155-175.

33.   Parker RG. Sexual Culture and AIDS Education in Urban Brazil. In: *AIDS 1988: AAAS Symposia Papers*. Kulstad R, ed. Washington, D.C.: The American Association for the Advancement of Science, 1988; pp. 169-173.

34.   Parker RG. Youth, Identity, and Homosexuality: The Changing Shape of Sexual Life in Brazil. *Journal of Homosexuality* 1989; 17(1/2):267-287.

35.   Parker RG. *Bodies, Pleasures, and Passions: Sexual Culture in Contemporary Brazil.* Boston: Beacon Press, 1991.

36.   Parker RG. Responding to AIDS in Brazil. In: *Action on AIDS: National Policies in Comparative Perspective*. Moss D and Misztal B, eds. Westport, CT: Greenwood Press, 1990; pp. 51-77.

37.   Parker RG and Tawil O. Bisexual Behaviour and HIV Transmission in Latin America. In: Tielman R, Carballo M, and Hendriks A, eds. *Bisexuality and HIV/AIDS*. Amherst, N.Y.: Prometheus Books, 1991.

38.   Paul JP. Bisexuality: Reassessing Our Paradigms of Sexuality. In: Klein F and Wolf TJ, eds. *Bisexualities: Theory and Research*. New York: The Haworth Press, 1985; pp. 21-34.

39.   Paz O. *The Labyrinth of Solitude*. New York: Grove Press, 1961.

40.   Perlongher N. *O Negócio do Michê*. Sao Paulo: Editora Brasiliense, 1987.

41.   Peterson JL and Marin G. Issues in the Prevention of AIDS among Black and Hispanic Men. *American Psychologist* 1988; 43:871-875.

42.   Piot P et al. An International Perspective on AIDS. In: *AIDS 1988: AAAS Symposia Papers*. Kulstad R, ed. Washington, D.C.: The American Association for the Advancement of Science, 1988; pp. 3-18.

43.   Plummer K, ed. *The Making of the Modern Homosexual*. Totowa, New Jersey: Barnes & Noble Books, 1981.

44.   Rogers M and Williams W. AIDS in Blacks and Hispanics: Implications for Prevention. *Issues in Science and Technology* 1987; 3(3):89-94.

45.   Sheperd G. Rank, Gender, and Homosexuality: Mombasa as a Key to Understanding Sexual Options. In: Caplan P, ed. *The Cultural Construction of Sexuality*. New York: Tavistock Publications, 1987; pp. 240-270.

46.   Sion FS et al. Anal Intercourse: A Risk Factor for HIV Infection in Female Partners of Bisexual Men, Rio de Janeiro, Brazil. V International Conference on AIDS, Montreal, Canada, 1989; Abstract T.A.P. 117.

47.   Taylor C. Mexican Male Homosexual Interaction in Public Contexts. *Journal of Homosexuality* 1985; 11(3/4):117-136.

48.   Tielman R, Carballo M, Hendriks A, eds. General Introduction. In: Tielman R, Carballo M, Hendriks A, eds. *Bisexuality and HIV/AIDS*. Amherst, N.Y.: Prometheus Books, 1991.

49.   Turner CF, Miller HG, Moses LE, eds. *AIDS, Sexual Behavior, and Intravenous Drug Use*. Washington, D.C.: National Academy Press, 1989

50.   Weeks Jeffrey. *Coming Out: Homosexual Politics in Britain from the 19th Century to the Present*. New York: Horizon Press, 1977.

51.   Weeks J. *Sexuality and its Discontents: Meanings, Myths, and Modern Sexualities*. London: Routledge & Kegan Paul, 1985.

52.   Wikan U. Man Becomes Woman: Transsexualism in Oman as a Key to Gender Roles. *Man* 1977; 12:304-319.

53.   Wiley JA and Herschkorn JS. Homosexual Role Separation and AIDS Epidemics: Insights from Elementary Models. *The Journal of Sex Research* 1989; 26:434-449.

54.   Wooden W and Parker J. *Men Behind Bars: Sexual Exploitation in Prison*. New York: Plenum Press, 1982.

55.   de Zalduondo BO. Culture, Sex, and Science: Anthropological Perspectives for AIDS Prevention and Care. V International Conference on AIDS, Montreal, Canada, 1989; Abstract M.G.O.7.

MOTHER-TO-FETUS/INFANT TRANSMISSION OF HIV-1: SCIENTIFIC EVIDENCE AND RESEARCH NEEDS

Olav Meirik

World Health Organization

INTRODUCTION

In less than two decades, the HIV virus has spread throughout the world, with virtually every country reporting cases of HIV infection to the World Health Organization (WHO) by 1990. It is remarkable how quickly researchers identified the HIV virus and its basic characteristics and structure, major modes of transmission, pathogenic mechanisms, and the symptoms and signs of HIV infection. But only recently has transmission from infected mothers to their fetuses and infants attracted the attention it deserves from the scientific community.

While HIV infection among infants sometimes results from transfusions of blood from HIV-infected donors, or from the use of unsterilized syringes, it now appears that most HIV-infected infants are infected intra-uterinely via placenta or at birth (5,9,13,14,16,27). This chapter outlines current knowledge on mother-to-fetus/infant HIV-1 transmission. It will discuss research questions that may lead to a better understanding of the mechanism of mother-to-infant transmission, and factors that may modify the risk of HIV transmission to fetuses and infants.

In this chapter we are mainly concerned with clinical and epidemiological research and with measures to reduce the risk of HIV infection in fetuses and infants. Our focus is not on basic research questions addressed by immunologists and molecular biologists — though research in these areas may ultimately generate the knowledge needed to halt the HIV epidemic in infants.

MOTHER-TO-FETUS HIV TRANSMISSION ACROSS THE PLACENTA

Evidence of intra-uterine transmission of HIV from mother to fetus can be obtained in two ways: 1) the presence of the virus in fetal tissue can be demonstrated directly; and 2) infection can be identified in the newborn infant and indirectly attributed to intra-uterine transmission after examination has excluded alternative transmission routes.

To demonstrate intra-uterine mother-to-fetus transmission, one would ideally obtain blood or tissue samples (or both) directly from the live fetus. Procedures for sampling the live fetus *in*

AIDS and Women's Reproductive Health
Edited by L.C. Chen *et al.*, Plenum Press, New York, 1991

utero are currently available, but the technologies are invasive and therefore carry the risk of viral transmission from an infected mother to a non-infected, healthy fetus. In this light, it does not seem ethical to carry out intra-uterine sampling of live fetuses to determine whether or not HIV transmission has occurred.

In the case of a legal abortion in which an intra–amniotic injection of abortifacient has been used, a sample of amniotic fluid could be obtained and examined for the presence of HIV or markers of HIV infection in the fetus. Studies in which the presence of HIV is determined by examining tissues of aborted fetuses of varying gestational age seems to be the only feasible method at present to determine whether fetal HIV infection occurs during pregnancy. At least four published studies of this sort have claimed that transmission of HIV can occur in the first and second trimesters of pregnancy. In two studies, positive HIV polymerase chain reactions (PCR) on tissue of aborted fetuses was demonstrated in fetuses of HIV-positive mothers and, in a third study, in thymic cells of the fetus (17, 19, 28). The fourth study demonstrated HV antigens and nucleic acid in tissues from fetuses aborted by HIV-positive mothers at eight weeks of pregnancy (20). It should be noted that, although precautions were taken in these studies to avoid contaminating the fetal samples with HIV of maternal origin, one cannot preclude the possibility that such contamination may have occurred.

Other evidence for transplacental transmission of HIV comes from clinical findings that suggest established HIV infection in newborn infants, and from research claiming to show a specific embryopathy resulting from HIV infection (21). The early onset of HIV-related diseases in some infants may also be taken as evidence for intra-uterine infection. It is unclear whether findings of shorter pregnancy duration, lower birth weight, and increased stillbirth rate among infants of HIV-seropositive mothers are attributable to maternal or fetal infection (13,14, 22, 24, 27).

It is not unjustified to assume that HIV is transmitted across the human placenta; transplacental transmission has been documented for a number of other viruses, including rubella virus, cytomegalovirus, varicella zoster virus, and parvo virus (3). Some viruses, such as the herpes viruses, are of particular interest in the context of mother-to-fetus/infant transmission of HIV; like HIV, these viruses remain latent following primary infection (10). This is also the case for human T-cell leukemia virus I (HTLV-I) and, to some extent, for hepatitis B virus (HBV).

Typically, primary infections with herpes viruses during pregnancy may lead to fetal infection (though the rate of fetal infection is different for the different herpes viruses). Activation of a latent herpes virus infection may also lead to fetal infection, but the risk is lower compared to the risk of fetal infection as a result of primary infection of the mother. Effects of fetal infection are more serious and more readily observed when transmission occurs in the first trimester of pregnancy. The retrovirus HTLV-I is transmitted through breast-feeding; there does not appear to be any firm evidence supporting the hypothesis that this virus is transmitted across the placenta (1, 23). Transplacental transmission of the hepatitis B virus occurs only occasionally among mothers with chronic hepatitis B infection (11).

MOTHER-TO-FETUS/INFANT TRANSMISSION AT BIRTH

Transmission of HIV from the mother to the fetus/infant during delivery is plausible, as the fetus/infant is usually extensively exposed to maternal cervical and vaginal secretions and maternal blood. However, in observational clinical studies (as opposed to experimental study situations), it is technically difficult to distinguish the passage of virus (or provirus, or both) from the mother to fetus during pregnancy from passage during delivery. If transmission of HIV from mother to fetus/infant takes place during delivery, the lesson learned from mother-to-infant transmission of HBV may be applicable to HIV.

Mother-to-fetus/infant HBV transmission appears to occur mainly at birth. This became evident in trials of passive immunization, in which hepatitis B immune globulin were given at birth (e.g., 2). The trials revealed that the sooner immune globulin was given after birth, the lower the infection rate in infants. The trials also revealed that passive immunization was equally effective in infants with HBV-antigen-positive cord blood and in those without antigen. This latter observation suggests that antigen-positive cord blood is a reflection of maternal-fetal blood exchange taking place during delivery, and is not necessarily evidence of established fetal infection. Rapidly changing intra-uterine pressure and compression of the placenta due to uterine contractions during delivery is a probable explanation for this maternal-fetal exchange of blood.

The bimodal distribution of clinical manifestations of HIV infection and mortality among infants infected with HIV by their mothers may be a reflection of infection at different time periods in pregnancy/birth. Alternative explanations for this phenomenon would include varying amounts of HIV engaged in transmission; repeated or continuous transmission of the virus through pregnancy; or different strains of HIV with varying pathogenicity.

POSTNATAL MOTHER-TO-INFANT HIV TRANSMISSION

There are now several reports of mother-to-infant HIV transmission in cases where mothers were infected in the postpartum period via blood transfusions. The majority of these cases were reviewed by Oxtoby (25). The plausible route of transmission in these cases is breast-feeding, as this represents the most intimate bodily contact and interchange of bodily secretions between mother and infant. Although these cases provide strong evidence for HIV transmission via breast-feeding, they reflect situations in which infants were exposed to infected mothers lacking antibodies for a period of time. The relevance of these cases is uncertain with respect to the majority of HIV-infected mothers, who become infected before pregnancy and have varying amounts and types of circulating HIV antibodies during pregnancy and breast-feeding.

Because reliable methods for ascertaining HIV infection in newborn infants are still not available, it has generally not yet been possible to distinguish between infants who become infected during pregnancy or delivery, and those infected shortly after birth. Observational studies have so far not shown any important differences in the proportion of infants infected at age 18 months (when infection can be ascertained) between those who were breast-fed and those who were not. An exception is a French study that suggests there is a higher infection rate among breast-fed infants than among those bottle-fed (5). It is noteworthy that the main route of transmission from mother to infant for another human retrovirus, HTLV-I, appears to be breast-feeding, according to data from epidemiological cohort studies (1, 18, 23).

Current data on mother-to-infant HIV transmission via breast-feeding among mothers with chronic HIV infection suggest that breast-feeding is not a major route of transmission. According to the WHO, the advantages of breast-feeding in developing countries most probably outweigh any small risk for HIV transmission that breast-feeding may carry (32).

RESEARCH NEEDS FOR PREVENTION AND RISK REDUCTION OF MOTHER-TO-FETUS/INFANT HIV TRANSMISSION

Since mother-to-fetus/infant HIV transmission is secondary to parental and maternal infection, an obvious way to halt fetal and infant infection is to institute general measures to reduce further spread of HIV in the adult population. Although such efforts must be given highest priority, an intermediate goal would be to advise HIV-positive women of childbearing age to abstain from having children if they are found to be at risk of infecting their infants in pregnancy or infancy. Some HIV-positive women will understandably want to bear children despite the risk of infecting their offspring; these mothers will need information on optimal timing of pregnancies with regard to their chances of bearing a healthy child.

Maternal characteristics that can quantify the risk of transmission from a mother to her fetus and infant must be identified. Such data are urgently needed to provide effective counseling to HIV-seropositive mothers, which would include substantive advice regarding childbearing. Improved counseling, which would inform mothers about the probability of having a healthy or infected infant, would not only be important in itself, but would probably increase the motivation of couples and women of childbearing age to seek HIV screening in areas where HIV infection is now prevalent, such as Central and East Africa (7). The current, crude recommendation that HIV-infected women not become pregnant does not encourage couples and women to undergo screening for HIV infection. Optimally, screening for HIV infection, risk evaluation, and counseling would take place in family planning settings prior to pregnancy. Pre-pregnancy screening in family planning clinics could have the added benefit of reinforcing the motivation and behavior of HIV-negative couples and women to remain HIV-negative.

Further data on mother-to-infant/fetus HIV transmission could also be of value in evaluating the treatment of HIV-positive pregnant mothers with respect to reducing the risk of fetal transmission. The drug Zidovudine (azidothymidine) and passive and active immunization have been proposed for this purpose. Zidovudine has a number of side effects and is potentially teratogenic. It can be assumed that other virucidal drugs could also be teratogenic, as most will interfere with cell metabolism and replication. Therapeutic trials with drugs such as Zidovudine could be directed to pregnant mothers for whom a high risk of fetal transmission can be predicted. Mothers whose probability of bearing an uninfected, healthy infant is high should probably be excluded from such treatment trials until the safety and efficacy of the treatments have been established.

Clinical characteristics have so far not proved very useful as determinants of mother-to-fetus/infant HIV transmission. It has been reported that mothers with advanced disease are at higher risk for transmission, but this determinant is too crude and insensitive for practical clinical use (27). CD4 enumeration, which is of considerable importance for prognostic purposes, especially when repeated in the same individual, was claimed to be associated with risk of mother-to-fetus/infant transmission in one study, but not in another (12, 27). Rossi et al. found that maternal antibodies to certain epitopes of the gp120 of HIV were associated with decreased risk of mother-to-fetus/infant transmission (26). Similar findings were reported shortly thereafter by Goedert et al., and recently by Devash et al. (8, 12). These observations point to the possible importance of antibodies to gp120 as a predictor for maternal transmission to the fetus/infant.

The results of the studies on the importance of gp120 as a marker of HIV infectivity are promising not only for the purpose of identifying determinants of transmission, but also for the development of active and passive immunization. The studies on gp120 antibodies have been undertaken in developed countries; similar studies should be repeated in developing countries, preferably Central and East Africa, where the problem of mother-to-fetus/infant transmission is greatest.

While several studies have implicated advanced HIV disease (measured as viremia, low CD4 cell count, and p24 serum antigen levels) with fetal/infant transmission, few studies have been concerned with the influence of pregnancy per se as a factor affecting the course and possible progression of HIV infection in women. Admittedly, the possible influence of pregnancy on the course of HIV infection is only indirectly associated with mother-to-fetus/infant transmission. But disease progression in the mother has implications for infant health and survival, and may have impact on the risk of transmission in subsequent pregnancies. One prospective study has suggested that the physiological CD4 suppression that occurs in healthy women during pregnancy also takes place in HIV-seropositive women who already have low CD4 counts (4). Postpartum recovery of CD4 cells to pre-pregnancy levels did not occur among women infected with HIV, however. This finding indicates that full-term pregnancy may accelerate the loss of CD4 cells in HIV-positive women.

Two relatively small follow-up studies (6, 29) found no conclusive evidence of disease progression in pregnant, HIV-positive women related to completion of pregnancy, although one of the studies did give some evidence of a trend of worsening disease among women completing their pregnancies. Further studies are needed on this subject, as it will have important implications for counseling HIV-positive women with respect to family planning and management of unplanned pregnancies. Studies on the possible effects of pregnancy on the course of HIV infection should preferably be done in sub-Saharan African countries, as the problem of HIV infection is greatest in these areas. Diseases complicating pregnancy and HIV infection are also prevalent in these countries and differ from those in developed countries.

HIV infection is often associated with other intercurrent and chronic infections. Some infectious diseases have been claimed to be independently associated with progression of HIV infection, but conclusive evidence for the direction of causality is lacking (15, 30). If intercurrent infections are, in fact, associated with disease progression and viremia (a sign of disease progression), they may be related to increased risk of mother-to-fetus/infant transmission of HIV. Infectious diseases during pregnancy should be studied further to assess not only their possible association with HIV transmission to the fetus, but also their potential impact on the progression of HIV infection in the mother.

As indicated above, it is unclear whether HIV is transmitted via breast-feeding from mothers who became infected prior to pregnancy. If it occurs, it appears to be at a low rate. The lack of data on HIV transmission through breast-feeding is not only a problem for individual mothers, but has also given rise to a public health controversy. While most developed countries advise HIV-seropositive mothers not to breast-feed their infants because of the possible risk of HIV transmission, mothers in developing countries continue breast-feeding irrespective of HIV serological status. In these settings, according to current knowledge, breast-feeding protects infants against other serious diseases and premature death, overshadowing the possible risk of HIV transmission through breast-feeding (31). This situation is very unsatisfactory; research on HIV transmission via breast-feeding in cases of chronic HIV infection must be given high priority.

It is unlikely that the breast-feeding issue can be resolved by means of observational studies alone. Some form of experimental trial design must be considered as part of the effort to answer the questions surrounding this issue. To facilitate the determination of the role of breast-feeding in HIV transmission, the WHO has recommended that priority be given to developing clinical methods to ascertain HIV infection in newborn infants. This should be reiterated. Our current inability to demonstrate infection in newborn infants is a serious hindrance in clinical epidemiological research on mother-to-fetus/infant transmission and clinical management of infants of HIV-seropositive mothers.

This reviewer has been unable to find data to answer the question of whether maternal HIV-infected white blood cells that enter the circulatory system of the fetus or newborn are functional in terms of viral replication, or are neutralized by immunological mechanisms (and, if so, at what gestational stage such mechanisms develop). If maternal lymphocytes and monocytes are functionally neutralized by the fetus or the newborn, then in order for HIV infection to be established in the fetus/infant, transmission would have to occur by cell-free virus. This, in turn, implies that HIV-neutralizing antibodies (immunoglobulins) given to the mother may be a feasible modality for the reduction of fetal and perinatal HIV transmission. By way of analogy to HBV, immunoglobulins given to the infant immediately after birth may reduce the risk of HIV infection from any possible viral transmission during delivery. If questions about the functional properties of maternal leukocytes after entering the fetal/newborn circulatory system are not yet answered, research should be undertaken to resolve them.

It is needless to point out that research on active and passive immunization must continue to have high priority. In the context of mother-to-fetus/infant transmission, it is worth considering that the time period elapsing between a possible intervention (such as active immunization to boost immunoresponse in a HIV-seropositive mother) and outcome in terms of infant infectivity is relatively short. Given safety clearance and ethical acceptance and approval, pregnant HIV-positive women and nonpregnant HIV-positive women who are considering childbirth may be the first to benefit from therapeutic trials of vaccines and drugs to prevent fetal/infant HIV transmission and extend the asymptomatic period of HIV infection.

Because the vast majority of mother-to-fetus/infant HIV transmissions currently take place in sub-Saharan Africa, priority should be given to strengthening the infrastructure in this area for clinical and epidemiological research that will enable the development of clinical management guidelines for the care of HIV-infected patients (according to prevailing social and cultural conditions). Clinical trials of treatment modalities, such as drugs and vaccines, are also needed in sub-Saharan Africa. In parallel, institutions in this region should be given the capability to develop and produce drugs and vaccines for intervention that are tailored towards locally and regionally prevalent strains of HIV. In this way, the first steps can be taken toward reducing mother-to-fetal/infant transmission of HIV in the geographic region where such a reduction is needed most.

REFERENCES

1. Ando Y, Nahano S, Saito K et al. Transmission of adult T-cell leukemia retrovirus (HTLV-I) from mother to child: comparison of bottle- with breast-fed babies. *Jpn J Cancer Res* 1987; 78:322-324.
2. Beasley RP, Hwang L-Y, Lin C-C et al. Hepatitis B immune globulin (HBIG) efficacy in the interruption of perinatal transmission of Hepatitis B virus carriers state. *Lancet* 1981; ii:388-393.
3. Best JM & Banatvala JE. Congenital virus infections. *Brit Med J* 1990; 300:1151-1152.
4. Biggar RJ, Pahwa S, Minkoff H et al. Immunosuppression in pregnant women infected with human immunodeficiency virus. *Am J Obstet Gynecol* 1989; 161:1239-1244.
5. Blanche S, Rouzioux C, Moscato M-LG et al. A prospective study of infants born to women seropositive for human immunodeficiency virus type I. *N Engl J Med* 1989; 320:1643-1648.
6. Bledsoe K, Olopoenia L, Barnes S et al. Effect of pregnancy on progression of HIV infection. Sixth International Conference on AIDS, San Francisco, CA, June 1990; Abstract Th.C.652.
7. Chin J. Current and future dimensions of the HIV/AIDS pandemic in women and children. *Lancet* 1990: ii:221-224.
8. Devash Y, Calvelli TA, Wood DG et al. Vertical transmission of human immunodeficiency virus is correlated with the absence of high-affinity/avidity maternal antibodies to the gp120 principal neutralizing domain. *Proc Natl Acad Sci* 1990; 87:3445-3449.
9. European Collaborative Study. Mother-to-child transmission of HIV infection. *Lancet* 1988; i:1039-1043.
10. Freij BJ and Sever JL. Herpesvirus infections in pregnancy: Risk to embryo, fetus and neonate. *Clin perinatal* 1988; 15:203-230.
11. Ghendon Y. Perinatal transmission of Hepatitis B virus in high incidence countries. *J Viral Methods* 1987; 17:69-79.
12. Goedert JJ, Mendez H, Drummond JE et al. Mother-to-infant transmission of human immunodeficiency virus type 1: Association with prematurity or low anti-gp120. *Lancet* 1989; ii:1351-54.
13. Hira SK, Kamanga J, Bhat GJ et al. Perinatal transmission of HIV 1 in Zambia. *Brit Med J* 1989; 299:1250-1252.
14. Halsey NA, Boulos R, Holt E et al. Transmission of HIV1 infections from mother to infants in Haiti. *JAMA* 1990; 264:2088-2092.
15. Holmberg SD, Stewart JA, Gerber AR et al. Prior Herpes Simplex Virus 2 infection as a risk factor for HIV infection. *JAMA* 1988; 259:1048-1050.
16. Italian Multicentre Study. Epidemiology, clinical features, and prognostic factors of paediatric HIV infection. *Lancet* 1988; ii:1043-46.

17. Jovaisas E, Koch MA, Schaafer A et al. LAV/HTLV-III in 20-week fetus. *Lancet* 1985; ii:1129.

18. Kusuhara K, Sonoda S, Takahashi K et al. Mother-to-child transmission of human T-cell leukemia virus type I (HTLV-I): A fifteen-year follow-up study in Okinawa, Japan. *Int J Cancer* 1987; 40:755-757.

19. Lapointe N, Michaud J, Perovic D et al. Transplacental transmission of HTLV-virus. *N Engl J Med* 1985; 312:1325-1326.

20. Lewis SH, Reynolds-Kohler C, Fox H et al. HIV-1 in trophoblastic and villous Hofbauer cells, and heamatological precursors in eight-week fetuses. *Lancet* 1990; 335:565-68.

21. Marion RW, Wiznia AA, Hutcheon RG et al. Fetal AIDS syndrome score: Correlation between severity of dysmorphism and age at diagnosis of immunodeficiency. *Am J Dis Chil* 1987; 141:429-431.

22. Mok JQ, Giaquinto C, DeRossi A et al. Infants born to mothers seropositive for human immunodeficiency virus: preliminary findings from a multicentre European study. *Lancet* 1987; i:1164-68.

23. Nakano S, Ando Y, Saito K et al. Primary infection of Japanese infants with adult T-cell leukemia-associated retrovirus (ATLV): evidence for viral transmission from mothers to children. *J Infect* 1986; 12 205-212.

24. Olness K, personal communication, 1990.

25. Oxtoby MJ. Human immunodeficiency virus and other viruses in human milk: placing the issue in broader perspective. *Pediatr Infect Dis J* 1988; 7:825-835.

26. Rossi P, Moschese V, Broliden PA et al. Presence of maternal antibodies to human immunodeficiency virus 1 envelope glycoprotein gp120 epitopes correlates with the uninfected status of children born to seropositive mothers. *Proc Natl Acad Sci* 1989; 86:8055-8058.

27. Ryder RW, Nsa W, Hassig SE et al. Perinatal transmission of the human immunodeficiency virus type I to infants of seropositive women in Zaire. *N Engl J Med* 1989; 320:1637-1642.

28. Sprecher S, Soumenkoff G, Puissant F et al. Vertical transmission of HIV in 15 week fetus. *Lancet* 1986; ii: 288-289.

29. Terragna A, Anselmo M, Camera M et al. Influence of pregnancy on disease progression in 31 HIV infected patients. Conference on the Implications of AIDS for Mother and Children, November 27-30, 1989, Paris, France; Abstract E2.

30. Webster A, Grundy LE, Lee CA et al. Cytomegalovirus infection and progression to AIDS. *Lancet* 1989; ii: 681.

31. World Health Organization. Statement from the consultation on breast-feeding/breast milk and Human Immunoefficiency virus (HIV). World Health Organization, Geneva, 1987.

Note

The views expressed by the author do not necessarily represent those of the WHO.

HIV PERINATAL TRANSMISSION AND REPRODUCTIVE HEALTH

Phyllis J. Kanki

Harvard School of Public Health

Mbowa Kalengayi

University of Kinshasa Medical School, Zaire

Souleymane M. Boup

University of Dakar, Senegal

HIV-1 infection in risk groups such as intravenous drug abusers, their sexual partners, and sexually active women in many developing countries has resulted in an increased number of HIV-infected women of childbearing age. In most parts of the world, where blood bank screening for HIV-1 is now in effect, mother-to-child transmission of the virus will be the major mode of infection to infants. Several prospective studies of infants born to infected mothers have shown a perinatal transmission rate of approximately 25-40% in both developed and developing countries (1-5). The actual mechanisms of mother-infant transmission are not yet known; data is supportive of trans-placental spread (6-8), birth canal transmission at delivery (9), and breast feeding (1,10).

Difficulties in diagnosing HIV infection in infants during the first few months of life have complicated natural history studies of pediatric populations. Nonetheless, it is apparent that the majority of HIV-infected infants will present with clinical signs between 5 months and 2 years of age. The clinical latency period of HIV-1 infections is, thus, very different for children and for adults. Early clinical findings in HIV-infected children include failure-to-thrive, hepatosplenomegaly, adenopathy, Pneumocystis pneumonia, lymphocytic interstitial pneumonitis, and loss of developmental milestones (11-14). Early immunologic alterations include depressed T4 lymphocytes, hypergammaglobulinemia and circulating immune complexes (11). The earlier clinical and immunologic alterations appear in children, the higher the observed mortality (15). Current studies concerning AIDS in infants indicate a 12-month survival rate of 50% and a 24-month survival rate of 25% (4,11-16).

HIV-1-infected children show a shorter incubation period as compared to HIV-1-infected adults. Unlike infected adults, infected children often do not present initially with T cell defects, though B cell defects are often presenting signs (6). Infected children may have poor *in vitro* lymphocyte response to B cell mitogens and poor *in vivo* antibody responses to protein and carbohy-

Table 1. Summary of the CDC classification of HIV infection in children under 13 years of age.

Class	Classification
P-0	**Indeterminate infection**
P-1	**Asymptomatic infection**
Subclass A	**Normal immune function**
Subclass B	**Abnormal immune function**
Subclass C	**Immune function not tested**
P-2	**Symptomatic infection**
Subclass A	**Nonspecific findings**
Subclass B	**Progressive neurologic disease**
Subclass C	**Lymphoid interstitial pneumontis**
Subclass D	**Secondary infectious disease**
Category D-1	Specified secondary infectious diseases listed in the CDC surveillance definition for AIDS
Category D-2	Recurrent serious bacterial infections
Category D-3	Other specified secondary infectious diseases
Subclass E	**Secondary cancers**
Category E-1	Specified secondary cancers listed in the CDC surveillance definition for AIDS
Category E-2	Other cancers possibly secondary to HIV infection
Subclass F	**Other diseases possibly due to HIV infection**

Adapted from Centers for Disease Control: Classification system for human immunodeficiency virus (HIV) infection in children under 13 years of age. MMWR 1987; 36:227.

drate antigens (17). This situation may preclude specific antibody production to HIV-1, thereby giving rise to false-negative serologic results; it may also raise concerns about responses to immunizations for childhood diseases. Altered humoral immunity gives rise to a propensity for recurrent or specific bacterial infections, in addition to the specific clinical syndromes that have been incorporated in the CDC revised or expanded definition of HIV-related disease in children (Table 1).

The surveillance of AIDS in the pediatric age group in developing countries has utilized clinical surveillance definitions, since diagnostic facilities for serologic or other testing may not be readily available. The World Health Organization (WHO) proposed a clinical case definition (Table 2) focusing on the general, major signs of abnormally slow growth, chronic diarrhea, and prolonged fever.

A major difficulty in studying perinatal HIV-1 transmission has been the identification of large numbers of HIV-1-infected pregnant women who are available for such studies. American and European studies of HIV-1 have focused on high-risk groups, such as intravenous drug

Table 2. World Health Organization clinical case-definition of AIDS in pediatric populations proposed at World Health Organization Workshop on AIDS in Central Africa, Bagui 1985.

Pediatric AIDS is suspected in an infant or child presenting with at least two major signs associated with at least two minor signs in the absence of known cases of immunosuppression.

Major Signs
Weight loss or abnormally slow growth
Chronic diarrhea > 1 month
Prolonged fever > 1 month

Minor signs
Generalized lymphadenopathy
Oropharyngeal candidiasis
Repeated common infections (Otitis, pharyngitis, etc.)
Presistent cough
Generalized dermatitis
Confirmed maternal HIV infection

abusers, or relied on large-scale multicenter screening. Data on infants born to drug-abusing mothers is frequently difficult to interpret, as drug abuse may significantly increase infant morbidity/mortality independent of HIV status. In Africa, these difficulties may be more easily overcome because HIV prevalence is often higher, and risk groups for infection are more representative of the general population.

HIV-2 PERINATAL TRANSMISSION AND DISEASE ASSOCIATION IN INFANTS

HIV-2 is believed to be transmitted via routes similar to HIV-1. However, a large prospective study of HIV-2 perinatal transmission has yet to occur. Scattered case reports indicate that similar to HIV-1, passive transfer of maternal antibodies is a problem with HIV-2 diagnosis in infants (18); furthermore, low numbers of reported perinatally-acquired HIV-2 infection makes even approximate estimates of transmission difficult. A better understanding of this mode of transmission is critical in geographic areas where the virus is known to be infecting sexually active adults at high rates (2-40%). Data from such studies will be important in projections of the impact of HIV-2 infection on the population in general and will aid in targeting interventions to prevent the spread of this virus.

The published literature provides some early data on HIV-2 perinatal transmission. Two recently reported prospective perinatal studies present preliminary data on 16 children born to HIV-2-seropositive mothers who were followed for over 9 months; 0/16 infants were found to have persistent HIV-2 antibodies after 9 months (19,20). Other studies have sought to evaluate perinatal transmission indirectly by evaluating children born to mothers currently known to be HIV-2-seropositive. In a study by Poulson et al., 18 children (<3 years of age) born to 15 mothers currently HIV-2-seropositive were evaluated; none of the 18 children were found to be HIV-2-seropositive (21). This, of course, does not preclude the possibility that seropositive infants were born and died prior to the survey, nor the possibility that the mothers were infected subsequent to giving birth. Nonetheless, the lack of seropositivity among the 18 children is noteworthy and may imply a low perinatal transmission rate of HIV-2.

A recent cross-sectional study of children and their mothers in Abidjan, Ivory Coast may reveal differences in rates of transmission of HIV-1 and HIV-2 (22). All infants (15 months of age) found to be seropositive had mothers who were also currently seropositive. Although passive antibodies would still be present in many of these infants, it was still of interest to note that 66% (35/53) of infants born to HIV-1-seropositive mothers were HIV-1-seropositive, whereas only 30% (3/10) of infants born to HIV-2-seropositive mothers were HIV-2-seropositive. Among children (ages 15-71 months), 14 of 30 (47%) HIV-1-seropositive children were concordant with their mothers, whereas 1 of 12 (8%) children of HIV-2-seropositive mothers was HIV-2-seropositive. Again, although this study does not directly measure transmission rates, it does provide support for other studies suggesting that the efficiency of perinatal transmission may be lower for HIV-2 than for HIV-1.

Scattered case reports can only suggest actual disease association of HIV-2 in infants and children. Most identified HIV-2-seropositive children have been healthy (18,23). Two related cases have shown clinical abnormalities, including generalized lymphadenopathy (7- year-old girl), or generalized lymphadenopathy and diarrhea (her 20-month-old brother) (24). The sparsity of case reports and lack of any case-control or prospective studies makes further conclusions difficult at this time. As can be seen, the transmission and natural history of HIV-2 in pediatric populations are areas in need of further study. In as much as HIV-1 infection in pediatric populations is distinct and more progressive than in adults, the study of HIV-2 infection in these infants may contribute to our overall understanding of the pathobiology of HIV-2 versus HIV-1.

USE OF VIROLOGIC MARKERS FOR DIAGNOSIS AND PROGNOSIS OF PEDIATRIC HIV INFECTION

Studies of the natural history of HIV-1 infection in perinatally acquired infection are complicated by the difficulty of distinguishing true infection from passively acquired maternal HIV-1 antibodies. Most perinatal transmission studies have shown that passively acquired maternal antibodies usually are non-detectable after 18 months of age. As an alternative to standard serology, methods for detecting HIV infection in the newborn have included alternate serologic markers or techniques (25,26), *in situ* hybridization (27), the presence of HIV-1 antigenemia (28,29), polymerase chain reaction (PCR) (30-32), and HIV-1 viral culture (32). None of these alternate techniques give uniformly positive results in the presence of known or subsequently determined infection. The performance characteristics of the techniques, especially PCR, are still under evaluation. The presence of a seronegative, virus-positive state suggested by some PCR studies indicates a potential underestimation of HIV-1 perinatal transmission.

HIV-1 and HIV-2 share a number of unique properties when compared to other known human and animal retroviruses, including a complex genetic structure that encodes the structural proteins of the virus and at least six regulatory genes. Present data suggests that these genes function by way of positive and negative feedback loops affecting viral replication, transcription, and translation. It appears that, with appropriate serologic assays, specific antibodies to all of the known HIV-1 gene products in infected individuals can be detected, although at varying rates (33-38). It is not known if differential responses to these viral antigens are important in the pathogenesis of HIV infection, or if they can be utilized as prognostic markers for disease progression.

The regulatory gene products common to both HIV-1 and HIV-2 include: vif (p23), tat (p14), rev (p19), nef (p27), and vpr (p18). In addition, HIV-1 has a unique regulatory gene product, vpu (p15), and HIV-2 has a unique regulatory gene product, vpx (p16). The immunogenicity and/or coding origin of the HIV-1 vif, nef, vpr, and vpu antigens and the HIV-2 vpx antigen were first described (in the cases of HIV-1 vif and nef) or reported by members of our laboratory (35,36,39,40). All of these regulatory gene products are recognized by some proportion of HIV-1-infected individuals. The regulatory gene products of HIV-2 have been identified by sequence analysis (50), and in many cases can be assayed in conventional immunoblot or RIP-SDS/PAGE (e.g., nef, tat, and vpx). In some cases, recombinant expressed proteins can be used in immunoblot assays as a screening test. We have employed this method for the detection of vpx (HIV-2) and vpu (HIV-1).

Studies using HIV-1-seropositive serum samples, classified by health status using the Walter Reed Staging system, show an increase in antibodies to the rev and vpu proteins with increased severity of disease (42). Antibodies to vif, nef, vpr, and tat do not appear to be associated with health status (42). Little is known regarding the immunogenicity of HIV-2 regulatory proteins. Our preliminary data suggests that, similar to the HIV-1 system, they will be less uniformly immunogenic. These less immunoreactive serologic markers may not be useful for serodiagnosis, but may be useful in distinguishing active from passive antibodies in mother-infant studies. In many cases, discordance between antibodies to these regulatory gene products may be useful in distinguishing passive antibodies from an active virus infection in babies born to infected mothers (43). We are hopeful that we will be able to adapt this to the HIV-2 system and assess this technique for detecting early HIV infection in infants.

The env-encoded proteins of HIV-1 and HIV-2 are known to be the most immunogenic proteins of the virus and are readily detected in virtually all infected individuals. The variable genetic constitution of this gene also confers the type specificity of the major env protein, the gp120, allowing for distinction of infection with HIV-1 from other cross-reactive viruses such as HIV-2 (44-46). Dr. Tun-Hou Lee and coworkers have shown that two antigenic domains exist on the gp120 molecule of HIV-1 (47). One domain requires the "native" conformation (normal spatial configuration) of gp120; the other is defined by the "reduced" conformation of gp120 (in which disulfide bonds required for the spatial configuration of the protein have been broken during the processing of the antigen). The reduced conformation of gp120 is less consistently immunogenic when compared to the native, non-reduced configuration. This differential immunogenicity may explain the less frequent production of antibodies to gp120 by certain Western blots that utilize a reduced antigen source, as compared to the RIP-SDS/PAGE assay that utilizes a non-reduced antigen preparation.

A number of studies that distinguish the antibody response to these two domains of gp120 have indicated that these may be important prognostic markers of HIV-1 infection. Patients in the later stages of the Walter Reed Staging Classification System are much less likely to have antibodies detected to the reduced gp120 than to the native, non-reduced gp120, which is present in virtually all infected individuals. Furthermore, this lack of antibody to the reduced configuration of gp120 in late-stage AIDS is not due to a loss of antibody titer. In an analysis of samples of the Multi-center AIDS Cohort Study (MACS) after 18-24 months of follow-up, a significantly lower rate of antibodies to the gp120-reduced domain was seen in individuals who developed AIDS as compared to matched controls that remained asymptomatic in the same time period (47). At least a portion of the gp120-reduced domain has been identified and expressed in bacteria. The resulting peptide demonstrates the same reactivity as was previously described with gp120-reduced virus antigen preparations. A major portion of the gp120-reduced domain has been mapped to the carboxyl-terminal region of gp120 (48).

A recent report by Goedert et al. examined the antibody profiles of seropositive mothers who were subsequently followed to determine if their infants demonstrated HIV infection after 15 months (49). The study demonstrated that certain high-affinity antibodies to gp120 may provide protection to infants born to HIV-infected mothers. On commercial immunoblot antigen (presumably in reduced form), 9 of 16 transmitting mothers lacked antibodies to gp120, compared to 7 of 35 nontransmitting mothers (p = 0.008). Rossi and coworkers conducted a similar study of mother-infant pairs in which they evaluated reactivity to synthetic peptides representing the major b-cell immunodominant regions of env, gag, and pol. Their results also indicate that select epitopes of the carboxyl terminus region of gp120 may be recognized by seropositive mothers who fail to transmit HIV to their infants (p = 0.016) (50). At least one interpretation of both of these studies would support the hypothesis that antibodies directed to the gp120-reduced form may confer immunologic protection against HIV infection when passively transferred to infants.

Table 3. Prevalence of HIV in pregnant women.

CITY	n	HIV-2%	HIV-1%
KAOLACK	317	0.3%	0.0%
PIKINE	220	0.4%	0.0%
LOUGA	180	1.1%	0.0%
DAKAR	175	1.1%	1.1%
ZIGUINCHOR	173	2.3 %	0.0%

The question of whether an infant is infected with HIV or seropositive as a result of maternal passive transfer of antibodies could eventually be answered by the periodic assessment of the infant's serostatus after 12-18 months. However, earlier identification of active infant infection would allow for more accurate evaluation of the early pathogenic effects of HIV on perinatally exposed infants. At present, our ability to discern these effects in infants born to seropositive mothers who die prior to definitive viral diagnosis is presumptive and highly dependent on our ability to distinguish this mortality from that of highly comparable negative mother-infant pairs. The study of serologic markers of infection over the course of infection may indicate their utility as prognostic markers in pediatric HIV pathogenesis.

Seroepidemiologic studies conducted in West Africa over the last four years have frequently included pregnant women who are readily accessible for such cross-sectional surveys. Populations of pregnant women from various urban centers in Senegal (Table 3) indicate slight differences in the proportion of HIV seropositivity, with a predominance on HIV-2 antigens. These were samples taken from consecutive women visiting major gynecology/obstetric services in the cities indicated, during 1987-89. All samples were analyzed by immunoblot of HIV-1 and HIV-2. The data demonstrate some variation in HIV-2 prevalence by city, which parallels differences in HIV-2 prevalence in high-risk groups from the same cities. Evidence for HIV-1 is sparse, except in Dakar, the capital city, where higher rates of HIV-1 have been demonstrated in registered female prostitutes, as compared to other urban centers.

In 1987 we evaluated 92 mother-infant pairs visiting the perinatal-maternity service. Heel-prick blood samples dried on filter paper were obtained from all infants (age = 1-24 months). 1.5 cm diameter circles of blood soaked filter paper were eluted in PBS and 2% Tween. Infant eluates and maternal serum samples were analyzed on standard immunoblot for antibodies to HIV-2 and HIV-1 (Table 4).

All three HIV-2-positive mothers identified were paired to the three HIV-2-positive infants.

Table 4. HIV prevalence in mother/infant pairs.

	n	HIV-2+	HIV-1+
Mothers (serum)	92	3	0
Infants (filter-paper eluate)	92	3	0

Irrespective of whether the antibodies found in these infants was passive or active, it appears that infant blood sampled by way of the filter-paper eluate technique was well correlated with maternal serum antibodies (51). All three infants, resampled two years after the initial study, were found to be seronegative, healthy, and without signs or symptoms of AIDS or related disorders, indicating that their previous seropositivity was due to maternal antibody transfer. Because these studies were conducted to test the feasibility of the sampling techniques, the data are too sparse to draw any reasonable conclusions regarding HIV-2 perinatal transmission.

CONCLUSION

The transmission of HIV by adults in their reproductive years has a significant effect on the reproductive health of child-bearing women. To date, only fragmentary and isolated data have been reported on the HIV seroprevalence among Zairean pregnant women attending antenatal clinics at the Mama Yemo Hospital in Kinshasa. In a 1987 survey, 18% seroprevalence was found in this population (52). This may be a highly selected hospital population, however, given that pregnant women at the University of Kinshasa Hospital have only shown a 2-3% seroprevalence for HIV-1 (Lomami Kashala & Kalengayi, unpublished data).

In a perinatal transmission study conducted by Projet Sida, over 50% perinatal transmission of HIV-1 was found by cord blood isolation or detectable IgM antibodies. Poor immunologic status of the infected mother appeared to be highly predicative of transmission (5). Our preliminary studies also indicated that HIV carrier status and AIDS in pregnant women results in inflammatory damages to the placenta, which could subsequently impair the course of the pregnancy (53). These studies certainly indicate the severe effect HIV infection may have on reproductive health. But these data are scanty and limited almost exclusively to very select female populations of Kinshasa. Much is yet to be learned about the perinatal effects of HIV infection.

Sociologic and behavioral factors will have to be taken into account in future studies of perinatal HIV transmission. Most of the Zairean population (>85%), for example, live in rural areas, where, according to preliminary data, HIV seroprevalence is quite low compared to the country's urban areas. Pregnant women studied in a rural village in Goma showed a 0.3% seroprevalence rate for HIV-1 (Kanki, unpublished data) as compared to 18% in pregnant women at the Mama Yemo Hospital in Kinshasa (52). The sociologic and behavioral characteristics of these rural populations and their interaction with urban populations, thought to be complex, has hardly been addressed in AIDS studies to date. It is urgent that studies be conducted in rural areas, not only to assess the magnitude of the problem in these areas, but also to compare rural data with data from urban populations. A better understanding of HIV infection in rural populations will improve the design of prevention and control programs for HIV, benefitting not only reproductive-age adults, but their children as well.

REFERENCES

1. Blanche S, Rouzioux C, Guihard Moscato, ML et al. A Prospective Study of Infants Born to Women Seropositive for Human Immunodeficiency Virus Type 1. *New Engl J Med* 1989; 320:1648.
2. The European Collaborative Study. Mother-To-Child Transmission of HIV Infection. *Lancet* 1988; 2:1039-43.
3. Andiman WA, Simpson J, Dember L et al. Prospective Cohort of 50 Infants Born to HIV Seropositive Mothers. IV International Conference on AIDS, Stockholm, Sweden, June 1988.
4. Italian Multicentre Study. Epidemiology, Clinical Features, and Prognostic Factors of Paediatric HIV Infection. *Lancet* 1988; ii:1043-1045.
5. Ryder RW, Nsa W, Hassig SE, Behets F, Rayfield M, Ekungola B et al. Perinatal Transmission of the Human Immunodeficiency Virus Type 1 to Infants of Seropositive Women in Zaire. *New Engl J Med* 1989; 320:1637-1642.

6. Sprecher S, Soumenkoff G, Puissant F, Degueldre M. Vertical Transmission of HIV in 15-Week Fetus. *Lancet* 1986; 2:288.

7. Marion RW, Wiznia AA, Hutcheon G, Rubinstein A. Human T-Cell Lymphotropic Virus Type III (HTLV-III) Embryopathy: A New Dysmorphic Syndrome Associated with Intrauterine HTLV-III Infection. *Am J Dis Child* 1986; 140:638-640.

8. Qazi AH, Sheikh TM, Fikrig S, Menikoff H. Lack of evidence for craniofacial dysmorphism in perinatal human immunodeficiency virus infection. *J Pediatr* 1988; 112:7-11.

9. Wofsy CB, Cohen JB, Hauer LB et al. Isolation of AIDS-associated retrovirus from genital secretions of women with antibodies to the virus. *Lancet* 1986; i:527-529.

10. Thiry L, Sprecher-Goldberger S, Jonckheer T et al. Isolation of AIDS c=virus from cell-free breast milk of three healthy virus carriers. *Lancet* 1985; ii:891-892.

11. Scott GB, Buck BE, Leterman JG et al. Acquired Immunodeficiency Syndrome in Infants. *New Engl J Med* 1984; 310:76-81.

12. Pahwa S, Kaplan M, Fikrig S et al. Spectrum of human T-cell lymphotropic virus Type III infection in children. *JAMA* 1986; 255:2299-2305.

13. Oleske J, Minnefor A, Cooper R et al. Immune deficiency syndrome in children. *JAMA* 1983; 249:2345-2349.

14. Belman AL, Ultmann MH, Horoupian D et al. Neurological complications in infants and children with acquired immune deficiency syndrome. *Annals of Neuro* 1985; 18:560-6.

15. Scott GB, Hutto C, Makuch RW, Mastrucci MT, O'Connor T, Mitchell CD, Trapido EJ, Parks WP. Survival in children with perinatally acquired human immunodeficiency virus type 1 infection. *New Engl J Med* 1989; 321:1791-1796.

16. Novick BE, Rubinstein A. AIDS – The paediatric perspective. *AIDS* 1987; 1:3-7.

17. Bernstein LJ, Rubinstein A. Acquired immunodeficiency in infants and children. *Prog Allergy* 1986; 37:194-206.

18. Matheron S, DeMaria H, Dormont D, Rey MA, Courpotin C, Couland JP, Saimot AG, Brun-Vesinet F. HIV-2 Infection in mother-infant couples. IV International Symposium on AIDS, Stockholm, Sweden, June 1988.

19. Andreasson P-A, Dias F, Goudiaby JMT, Naucler A, Biberfield G. HIV-2 Infection in prenatal women and vertical transmission of HIV-2 in Guinea-Bissau. IV International Conference on AIDS in Africa, Marseilles, France, October 1989.

20. Hojlyng N, Kvinesdal BB, Molbak K, Aaby P. Vertical Transmission of HIV-2; Does It Occur? IV International Conference on AIDS in Africa, Marseilles, France, October 1989.

21. Poulsen A-G, Aaby P, Frederiksen K, Kvinesdal B, Molbak K, Dias F, Lauritzen E. Prevalence of and Mortality from Human Immunodeficiency Virus Type-2 in Bissau, West Africa. *Lancet* 1989; i:827-830.

22. Ouattara SA, Gody M, Rioche M et al. Blood transfusions and HIV infections (HIV1, HIV2/LAV2) in Ivory Coast. *J of Tropical Medicine and Hygiene* 1988; 91:212-215.

23. Veronesi R, Mazza C, Santos Ferreira MO, Lourenco MH. HIV-2 in Brazil. Lancet 1987; ii:402 (letter).

24. Gnaore E, De Cock KM, Gayle H et al. Prevalence and Mortality from HIV Type 2 in Guinea Bissau, West Africa. *Lancet* 1989; ii:513 (letter).

25. Johnson JP, Nair P, Alexander S. Early Diagnosis of HIV Infection in the Neonate. *New Engl J Med* 1987; 316:273-274.

26. Pyun KH, Ochs HD, Dufford MTW, Wedgwood RJ. Perinatal Infection with Human Immunodeficiency Virus. *Med Intellig* 1987; 317:611-614.

27. Harnish DG, Hammerberg O, Walker IR, Rosenthal KL. Early detection of HIV infection in a newborn. *New Engl J Med* 1987; 316:272-271.

28. Borkowsky W, Paul D, Bebenroth D, Krasinski K, Moore T, Chandwani S. Human-immunodeficiency-virus infections in infants negative for anti-HIV by enzyme-linked immunoassay. *Lancet* 1987 i:1168-1170.

29. Monforte AA, Novati R, Marchisip et al. Early Diagnosis of HIV Infection in Infants. *AIDS* 1988; 3:391-395.

30. Laure F, Rouzioux C, Veber F et al. Detection of HIV-1 DNA in infants and children by means of the Polymerase Chain Reaction. *Lancet* 1988; ii:538-541.

31. Rogers MF, Ou CY, Rayfield M et al. Use of the Polymerase Chain reaction for early detection of the proviral sequences of human immunodeficiency virus in infants born to seropositive mothers. *New Engl J Med* 1989; 320:1649-1654.

32. Dormont D, DiMaria H, Courpotin C et al. Virology and Immunology Follow-Up of Newborns from Positive Mothers: Diagnostic and Prognostic Value of HIV Positive Cell Culture During the Neonatal Period. IV International Symposium on AIDS, Stockholm, Sweden, June 1988.

33. Wong-Staal F. Human Immunodeficiency Viruses and Their Replication. In: *Virology*, 2nd Edition, eds, Fields DM et al. Raven Press, Ltd., 1990, pp. 1529-1540.

34. Essex M, Allan J, Kanki P, McLane MF, Malone G, Kitchen L, Lee TH. Antigens of Human T-Lymphotropic Virus Type III / Lymphadenopathy-Associated Virus. *Ann Int Med* 1985; 103:700-703.

35. Lee TH, Coligan JE, Allan JS, McLane MF, Groopman JE, Essex M. A New HTLV-III/LAV Protein Encoded by a Gene Found in Cytopathic Retroviruses. *Science* 1986; 231:1546-1549.

36. Allan JS, Coligan JE, Lee TH, McLane MF, Kanki PJ, Groopman JE, Essex M. A New HTLV-III/LAV Encoded Antigen Detected by Antibodies from AIDS Patients. *Science* 1985; 230:810-813.

37. Arya SK, Gallo RC. Three Novel Genes of Human T-Lymphotropic Virus Type III: Immune Reactivity of Their Products with Sera from Acquired Immune Deficiency Syndrome Patients. *Proc Natl Acad Sci* 1986; 83:2209-2213.

38. Franchini G, Robert-Guroff M, Aldovini A et al. Spectrum of Natural Antibodies Against Five HTLV-III Antigens in Infected Individuals: Correlation of Antibody Prevalence with Clinical Status. *Blood* 1987; 69:437-441.

39. Matsuda Z, Chou MJ, Matsuda M, Huang JH, Chen YM, Redfield R, Mayer K, Essex M, Lee TH. Human Immunodeficiency Virus Type 1 has an additional coding sequence in the central region of the genome. *Proc Natl Acad Sci* 1988; 85:6968-6972 (1988).

40. Yu XF, Ito S, Essex M, Lee TH. A Naturally Immunogenic Virion-Associated Protein Specific for HIV-2 and SIV. *Nature* 1988; 335:262-265.

41. Guyader M, Emerman M, Sonigo P, Clavel F, Montagnier L, Alizon M. Genome Organization and Transactivation of the Human Immunodeficiency Virus Type 2. *Nature* 1987; 326:662-669.

42. Essex M, Kanki PJ, Barin F, Chou MJ, Lee TH. Immunogenicity of HIV-1 and HIV-2 Antigens and Their Relationship to Disease Development. 2nd Colloque des Cent Gardes 1987, ed. Girard M and Vallette L, 1988, pp. 219-220.

43. Allan JS, Essex M. Unpublished data.

44. Barin F, McLane MF, Allan JS, Lee TH, Groopman J, Essex M. Virus Envelope Protein of Human T-cell Leukemia Virus Type III (HTLV-III) Represents Major Target Antigen for Antibodies in AIDS Patients. *Science* 1985; 228:1094-1096.

45. Allan J, Coligan JE, Barin F, McLane MF, Rosen C, Sodroski J, Haseltine WA, Lee TH, Essex M. Major Glycoprotein Antigens that Induce Antibodies in AIDS Patients are Encoded by HTLV-III. *Science* 1985; 228:1091-1094.

46. Barin F, M'Boup S, Denis F, Kanki P, Allan JS, Lee TH, Essex M. Serological Evidence for a Virus Related to Simian T-Lymphotropic Retrovirus III in Residents of West Africa. *Lancet* 19485; ii:1387-1390.

47. Lee TH, Redfield RF, Chou MJ, Huang TH, Saah A, Hsieh CC, Yu XF, McLane MF, Marlink R, Burke DS, Essex M. Association Between Antibody to Envelope Glycoprotein

gp120 and the Outcome of HIV Infection. In: *Vaccines 1988: New Chemical and Genetic Approaches to Vaccination*, eds. Ginsberg H et al. Cold Spring Harbor Press, 1988, pp. 373-377.

48. Lee TH, Syu WJ, Chou MJ, Essex M. Immunodominant Epitopes of HIV-1 gp120: A Possible Obstacle for Vaccine Development. In: *Vaccines 89 Modern Approaches to New Vaccines Including Prevention of AIDS*, eds. Lerner RA, Ginsberg H, Chanock RM, Brown F. Cold Spring Harbor Press, 1989, pp. 191-194.

49. Goedert JJ, Drummond JE, Minkoff HL, Stevens R, Blattner WA, Mendez H, Robert-Guroff M, Holman S, Rubinstein A, Willoughby A, Landeman SH. Mother-to-Infant Transmission of Human Immundeficiency Virus Type 1: Association with Prematurity or Low Anti-gp120. *Lancet* 1989; ii:1351-1354.

50. Rossi P, Moschese V, Broliden PA, Fundaro C, Quinti I, Plebani A, Giaquinto C, Tovo PA, Ljunggren K, Rosen J, Wigzell H, Jondal M, Wahren B. Presence of maternal antibodies to human immunodeficiency virus type 1 envelope glocoprotein gp epitopes correlates with the uninfected status of children to seropositive mothers. *Medical Sciences* 1989; 86:8055-8058.

51. Kanki P, Ricard D, M'Boup S, Essex M. Perinatal Transmission of HIV-2. IV International Conference on AIDS, Stockholm, Sweden, June 1988.

52. Ryder RW and Hassig SE. The epidemiology of perinatal transmission of HIV. *AIDS 2* (suppl) 1988; S83-S89.

53. Nelson AM, Anderson V, Ryder R et al. Placental pathology as a predictor of perinatal HIV infection in infants born to HIV seropositive women in Kinshasa, Zaire. IV International Conference on AIDS, Stockholm, Sweden, 1988. Abstract 6585.

METHODS FOR DECREASING HIV TRANSMISSION TO INFANTS

Sally Jody Heymann

Harvard School of Public Health

INTRODUCTION

AIDS poses a potentially devastating threat to children's health internationally. The World Health Organization (WHO) estimates that in areas where the seroprevalence of HIV infection in women of childbearing age ranges from 10 to 25%, AIDS will lead to "an increase in child mortality by at least 25%; the gains achieved with difficulty by child survival programs over the past two decades may be nullified"(1). These tragically high seroprevalence rates already hold true for some areas in central Africa, as do the infant mortality rates associated with being born to a seropositive mother. In Zaire, the infant mortality rate of children born to seropositive mothers was 21%, compared to 3.8% for infants born to seronegative mothers. Of the infants born to seropositive mothers who survived the first year of life, an additional 7.9% had developed clinical AIDS, thereby presumably contributing to higher 1-to-4-year child mortality rates (2).

Ideally, the way to prevent perinatal transmission to infants would have been to prevent the initial infection of reproductive-age adults. But with an estimated 5 to 10 million people already infected worldwide, this is no longer an option in many regions. The prevalence of HIV infection in young adults is so high that we must face the problem of how to limit the spread of the virus to infants effectively.

METHODS

In this chapter, decision analysis is used to examine the question of how best to decrease the child morbidity and mortality associated with AIDS. Data for this chapter were gathered from a review of current literature, and from a series of interviews with officers of international development organizations and medical and social science researchers working with AIDS. An analysis of current options for decreasing transmission to infants prenatally, at birth, and postnatally is based on these data.

Decision trees are used here to model current approaches of international organizations to decreasing transmission of HIV to infants. The trees are used to show which courses of action current programs follow to decrease transmission; what alternative courses of action they have ignored; and what assumptions these choices are based upon (Figures 1-2).

AIDS and Women's Reproductive Health
Edited by L.C. Chen *et al.*, Plenum Press, New York, 1991

The question of how to decrease postnatal transmission of HIV is also considered. Methods for decision analysis are used to model the risks and benefits of breast-feeding and alternative infant feeding practices (Figure 3). Each feeding practice is associated with different risks of mortality from HIV infection and from other causes such as malnutrition and diarrheal disease.

Important problems arise in modeling infant feeding practices. There is a substantial degree of uncertainty surrounding the central parameter: the probability of transmission of HIV via breast-feeding. Several of the parameters vary significantly between regions, such as the practicality of screening for HIV and the prevalence of HIV infection. Graphical sensitivity analyses are performed around each of these variables (Figures 4-6).

Modeling interventions in fields such as AIDS, where both our knowledge of the problem and available interventions are increasing rapidly, is most useful when the models are adaptable to new information and programs. To this end, the issue of infant feeding practices is also modeled with hypothetical changes in variables such as the probability of survival with HIV and child mortality from other causes (Figures 7,8).

DECREASING PRENATAL AND CONATAL HIV TRANSMISSION TO INFANTS

Current Efforts to Limit Vertical Transmission

Current efforts to prevent the spread of HIV infection to infants have focused on preventing new infections in adults. UNICEF summarizes this view in their position paper: "changing high-risk sexual behavior of adults in developing countries is currently the most effective means to stop the spread of HIV infection to children" (3). Efforts to change high-risk behavior of adults currently consist primarily of mass media and mass education campaigns promoting condom use and limited sexual partners.

While such efforts are crucial for decreasing transmission among adults, and can contribute to limiting the spread of HIV to children, they represent efforts to change only what occurs at the first decision point in a tree of choices and chance events that leads to the ultimate infection of infants. There are several subsequent decisions and chance events that health programs may be able to influence (Figure 1).

Alternative program options include screening reproductive-age women and offering them individual counseling regarding the risks to themselves and their children posed by their HIV status and the status of cofactors found to be important in transmission. Many women are not yet educated about the risk of transmitting HIV infection to their unborn children (4). The relative efficiency of mass education and of individual counseling will depend on the costs and efficacy of each and the relative importance given to preventing adult and infant cases. Currently available data neither support nor refute the conclusion that mass education is the most cost-effective prevention approach.

A Broader Approach to Limiting Vertical Transmission

What can be done about vertical transmission in the future? Ideally, interventions to decrease prenatal and conatal transmission would be aimed at each of three stages until a vaccine or cure has eliminated the need for further prevention efforts. The goals of this three-part intervention would be to decrease the incidence of new infection among adults; give infected adults the information and means to make their own reproductive choices; and decrease the HIV transmission rate from infected pregnant women to their infants. Decision analysis can help illustrate the considerations involved in choosing between alternative programs in a setting of limited resources.

The most effective means currently available for preventing new infections in adults is the use of condoms. Other methods of birth control, such as the oral contraceptive, are more effective

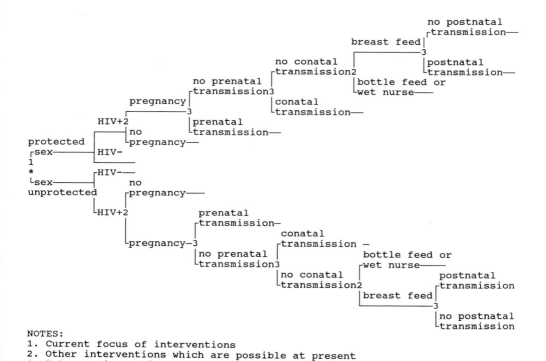

NOTES:
1. Current focus of interventions
2. Other interventions which are possible at present
3. Interventions which may be available in the future

Figure 1. Steps in vertical transmission.

in preventing pregnancy in women who are HIV-infected.* Many international organizations have not considered setting up screening programs because of the complexity of implementing such programs in an ethically sound manner. The fact that the best method of decreasing HIV transmission is different for seropositive and seronegative adults raises the question, Should adults in high-prevalence areas who are considering contraception be offered voluntary testing?

A decision tree can be used to model the question of whether mass education or individual screening and counseling would be more cost-effective, and to place a value on the screening test. The tree in Figure 2 takes the viewpoint of the project planner and evaluates two different recommendations: whether to screen for HIV and whether to provide individual counseling or mass media education.

Following the decision regarding what to recommend, the next branches give the probabilities that the individual chooses a barrier method of contraception, a non-barrier method, or no method. These probabilities will vary depending on whether individual counseling or a mass media campaign is used. The probabilities depend both on the prior probability of a given method being used in the population and on how efficacious a particular intervention is at changing behavior. The outcome measures used combine HIV and pregnancy status.

---

*There is limited data that has raised the question of whether oral contraceptives increase the risk of becoming infected with HIV. While the data is controversial, and the observed effect may have been due to confounding factors related to sexual activity, the suggestion of an increased risk has raised concern about prescribing oral contraceptives for HIV-negative women. This should not raise any concerns about prescribing oral contraceptives for HIV-positive women.

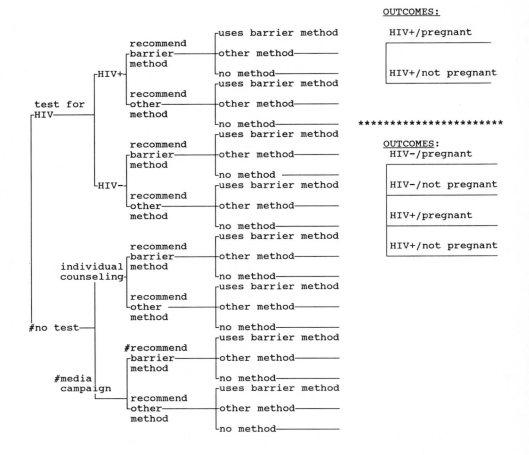

OUTCOMES:

HIV+/pregnant

HIV+/not pregnant

****

OUTCOMES:
HIV-/pregnant

HIV-/not pregnant

HIV+/pregnant

HIV+/not pregnant

NOTES:
1. Decision tree is from point of view of PVO
2. Tree can be expanded to include the possibility that an individual uses two means of birth control simultaneously (one for STD prevention, one for pregnancy prevention
3. Majority of current programs follow # path

Figure 2. Choices regarding screening, individual counseling, and media campaigns.

In comparing the values of the different decision tree branches, results will depend on the prevalence of HIV infection. In regions with high rates of infection, the best policy may be to screen all reproductive-age adults and then perform individual counseling, recommending that those who are seronegative use barrier methods of contraception and that couples in which both adults are seropositive use more effective means of preventing pregnancy if they choose not to take the risk of having an HIV-infected child.

The per person cost of screening and counseling individuals and couples would clearly be greater than the per person cost of a mass media effort. However, per person exposed, individual screening and counseling frequently has a higher success rate of changing behavior than do mass media campaigns. Thus, the individualized method might prove to be less expensive per case of AIDS averted.

The decision tree helps highlight the fact that screening and individual counseling may be a cost-effective intervention even in a setting of limited resources. But the tree does not address two important issues: 1) the question, What is the relationship between mass education and individual counseling? (Is there an interaction term? Does the existence of a mass media campaign make individual counseling more effective?); and 2) the fact that mass education and individual counseling each avert a different proportion of adult and infant infections.

Future Options

We are now beginning to identify cofactors that affect prenatal and conatal transmission. For example, the stage of a pregnant woman's HIV infection may change the probability of vertical transmission and the probability of the pregnancy adversely affecting the woman's health. There is also initial evidence that higher levels of anti-GP120 correlate with lower probabilities of HIV transmission (5,6).

As more information becomes available, improved guidance for HIV-infected women considering pregnancy should become available. Progress is being made in developing and trying therapies that may decrease the rate of transmission from a known HIV-positive mother. Future options may include such immunotherapies as CD4 immunoglobulin (7).

DECREASING POSTNATAL TRANSMISSION OF HIV

Infant Feeding Alternatives: Risks and Benefits

The risk of breast-feeding is that the infant may become infected with HIV. Current predictions are that nearly 100% of infants who become infected with HIV will eventually develop and die from AIDS. (Estimates of the time it takes for HIV-infected children to develop AIDS have been made for the United States but not for Africa, where the disease may progress more rapidly in children [8].)

Several sources of evidence suggest that HIV can be transmitted via breast milk. First, HIV has been isolated in breast milk (9). Second, there are documented cases of transmission to infants whose mothers received infected blood products after the birth of their child and prior to breast-feeding (10,11,12). Third, a recent, prospective, collaborative study by French researchers showed a significant increase in transmission to infants who were breast-fed (13).

Despite the good evidence that HIV can be, and has been, transmitted via breast milk, the extent of transmission to infants through breast-feeding remains unclear. Because children are often breast-fed until two years of age in many parts of the world, even a very low rate of transmission per exposure to breast milk could result in a significant incidence of breast-feeding-related AIDS.*

The wide range of estimates and confidence intervals around the estimates of breast-feeding transmission in currently published data make it clear that we can not yet be confident that breast-feeding will not prove to be a significant route of transmission. Studies range from those unable to show a statistically significant effect to the statistically significant French collaborative study cited above in which five out of six breast-fed infants, compared with 25 out of 99 bottle-fed infants, were HIV-seropositive at 18 months (13).

---

*Let $p2$ = the probability of infection occurring each time the infant is breast-fed. Let $p1$ = the probability of infection occurring during two years of breast-feeding. Let n = the number of times the infant is breast-fed over the course of two years. If the probability of infection each time the infant is breast-fed is found to be independent, then $p1 = 1 - (1-p2)^n$. Even for a very small $p2 = .0001$, $p1 = .25$. (This assumes the probabilities for infection at each subsequent exposure are independent and remain constant. In a multihit model, the rate of increase could be exponential.)

The recent data pointing to an overall perinatal transmission rate ranging from 25% to 45% make it unlikely that breast-feeding will play a role in the majority of cases, but does not rule it out as a clinically significant route. For example, if 25% of infants were infected prenatally and conatally, and 20% of the remaining were infected postnatally via breast-feeding, then a total of 40% of breast-fed infants and 25% of alternative-fed infants would become infected. These results would fall within the range of observed cases of vertical transmission. While the 83%-infected breast-fed children in the French study would be an outlier compared to the bulk of studies showing under 50% of children of HIV-positive mothers infected with HIV, the study still raises the serious threat that breast-feeding may turn out to be a significant route of transmission.

The advantages of breast-feeding have been well demonstrated in women not infected with HIV. Breast-feeding by an uninfected mother offers several advantages to a newborn infant. First, breast milk contains maternal antibodies that provide the infant with passive immunity against many diseases. Second, breast milk is nutritionally complete; the infant does not need any supplemental food for the first months of life. This fact helps protect the newborn from many of the water-borne and food-borne causes of diarrhea associated with high infant mortality rates in developing countries. (Frequently, infant mortality is due to the interaction between malnutrition and diarrheal or other diseases. A guaranteed source of a balanced diet is critical to infant survival.) Third, breast milk does not have to be purchased (and is, in this sense, "free"), so even the poorest families have enough to feed their newborns.

While the advantages of breast milk from HIV-negative mothers have been well documented in the literature, it is not clear that breast milk from all HIV-positive mothers would offer the same advantages. First, if a mother is significantly immunocompromised, then the breast milk may not confer significant passive immunity on the infant. Second, the milk may not be truly "free" because of the toll it may take on the mother's health: When a mother is malnourished, as AIDS patients frequently are after a long course of illness, the mother's nutritional status is sacrificed to produce milk for the newborn.

One alternative to breast-feeding by the natural mother is bottle-feeding. The advantage of bottle-feeding for HIV-infected mothers is that there is no associated risk of transmitting HIV infection to the infant. The disadvantages of bottle-feeding are that it confers no passive immunity to the infant, is currently expensive, and is often unavailable in rural areas of developing countries. To prepare the powdered formula that is available, water must be added. This process introduces two problems: 1) given poor sanitary conditions, water often carries organisms that cause diarrheal disease; and 2) families with insufficient incomes to pay for the amount of formula needed to meet an infant's nutritional requirements frequently are forced to overdilute the formula. These disadvantages are life-threatening in developing countries. A survey conducted in an urban hospital in Egypt found a relative risk of death of 3.9 in infants who were "never breast-fed" as compared to infants who were "ever breast-fed" (95% CI 3.1-5.0) (14).

Wet nursing provides a potential intermediate course. If a wet nurse is found who has never been exposed to HIV, then wet nursing would present no risk of HIV transmission to the newborn. (In reality, the best one could do in determining HIV exposure of the proposed wet nurse would be to screen for HIV. Given that all screening tests have false negatives, it will be important to look at the probability of the wet nurse having a false negative and the mother having a false positive result in any given setting). If it turns out that HIV-infected mothers' breast milk lacks components that effectively provide immunity, then wet nursing performed by an immuno-competent woman would also offer the advantage of providing passive immunity to the infant.

The principle disadvantage of wet nursing is that, depending on the circumstances, the wet nurse may not be able to produce sufficient milk to meet all the infant's nutritional needs, such as when relactation is required (15). The infant would then need supplemental feeding. Wet nursing will have a similar risk profile for non-HIV infections as partial breast-feeding and partial bottle-feeding. Many studies have shown that infants whose feeding is divided between breast and bottle have higher mortality rates from causes other than HIV infection than do purely breast-fed infants, but have lower mortality rates than do purely bottle-fed infants (16). A study in Brazil showed that the relative risk of mortality due to diarrhea alone was 5.7 for infants who were breast- and bottle-fed, and 18.3 for infants who were purely bottle-fed compared to infants who were exclusively breast-fed (17).

Using Decision Analysis to Model Postnatal Options

Decision analysis can be used to compare the survival outcomes of children of HIV-infected women who are breast-fed, bottle-fed, and wet-nursed. The goal of the decision tree, algebraic calculations, and graphic sensitivity analysis is to provide a flexible framework that can be reused as better estimates of transmission risks and probabilities of survival become available.

The decision tree in Figure 3 can be used to evaluate the three different feeding practices. Note the current absence of screening programs and the recommendation that all mothers breast-feed regardless of HIV status. Whether or not this strategy should dominate depends on the relative risk of the three feeding practices and the transmission rate of HIV via breast-feeding.

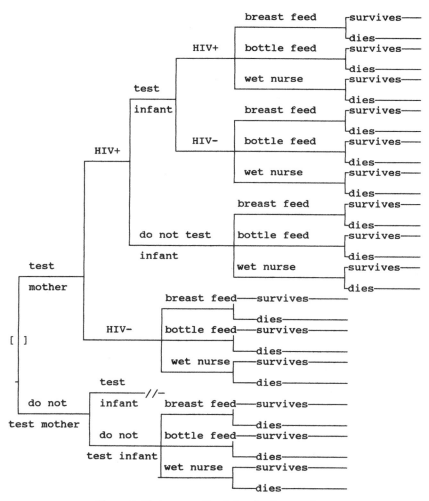

Figure 3. Choices regarding infant feeding practices.

The question of which feeding practice to recommend can be simplified. In any given setting, the choice will be between breast-feeding, with its protection against malnutrition and infectious diseases, and the next best alternative, wet nursing or bottle-feeding, with their protection against HIV transmission. Wet nursing by an uninfected woman and bottle-feeding both avoid the risk of HIV transmission but increase the risk of infant mortality due to other causes. Wet nursing has a significantly lower risk of infant mortality from non-HIV causes than does bottle-feeding and, thus, will always be the preferable alternative to breast-feeding in any setting in which a wet nurse who is not infected with HIV is available.

Algebraic calculations were performed to determine the critical transmission rate of HIV via breast-feeding for a given relative risk of a feeding practice alternative to breast-feeding that would make breast-feeding and an alternative feeding practice equally recommendable. Such an

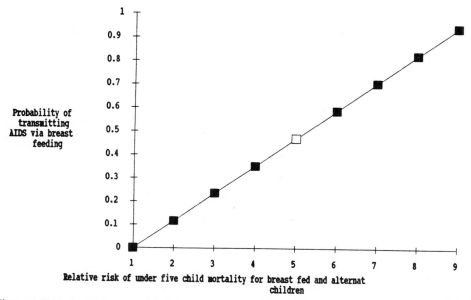

Figure 4. Critical transmission probability for case in which mother is known to be HIV-infected, CMR=.1, P(die/AIDS)=.95.

analysis establishes the critical transmission rate above which the best available alternative feeding practice will be associated with the lowest child mortality rate and below which breast-feeding will have the lowest child mortality rate.

To find the critical transmission rate (expressed here in probabilities), one sets the outcomes of the alternative and breast-feeding branches equal and solves for the transmission probability. The results are shown graphically in Figures 4-8. These graphs plot the critical transmission probability (y-axis) against the relative risk of child mortality for the alternative feeding practice compared to breast-feeding (x-axis). The line drawn is the "indifference line" above which the alternative feeding practice will be recommended and below which breast-feeding will be recommended.

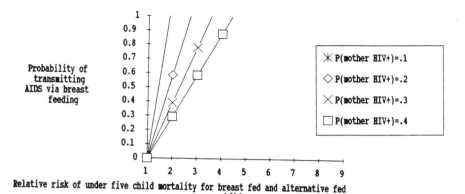

Figure 5. Critical transmission probability for case in which screening is unavailable, baseline CMR=.1, P(die/AIDS)=.95.

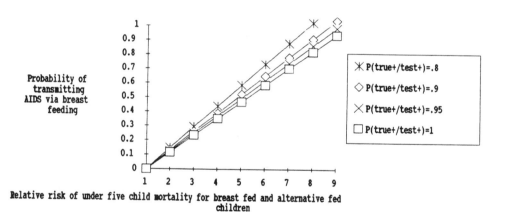

Figure 6. Critical transmission probability for case in which an imperfect HIV screening test is available, baseline CMR=.1, Pdie/AIDS)=.95.

Working Through the Model: Five Cases

Case 1: HIV-infected mother. Figure 5 depicts the case in which the mother is known with certainty to be HIV-infected and the question is posed, Is it best for her to breast-feed or use an alternative method of feeding her infant? The graph assumes a child mortality rate for 0-to-5-year-olds of 100 per 1000 live born infants and a 5% probability of surviving HIV infection for more than 5 years.

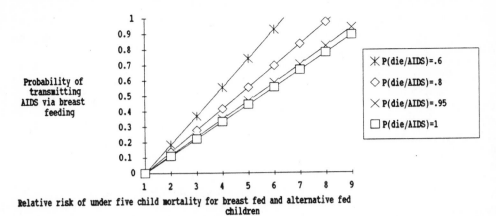

Figure 7. Critical transmission probability for case in which mother is known to be HIV-infected, baseline CMR=.1, P(die/AIDS) varies because a treatment becomes available.

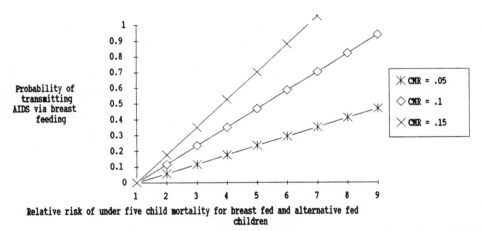

Figure 8. Critical transmission probability for case in which mother is known to be HIV-infected, baseline CMR varies, P(die/AIDS)=.95.

What does the graph tell us, using currently available data on the transmission rates and relative risk of alternative feeding practices? First, in the many settings in developing countries in which the relative risk of alternative feeding practices is very high (5 or greater), we already have enough data to support the continued recommendation of breast-feeding. If breast-feeding turns out to be a clinically significant route of transmission, then we will need to provide safer alternatives before this recommendation could be changed. Second, in settings in developed countries in which the relative risk approaches one (i.e., where a safe alternative to breast milk is available), even small degrees of transmission make it advisable not to breast-feed. Third, the most difficult decisions at present may occur in second world settings where a relative risk of 2 or 3 would lead to different recommendations within the range of possible rates of transmission. Combining this graph with available data on relative risk and transmission rate, we should be convinced that the question of breast-feeding cannot be put to rest, particularly in countries and regions where the relative risk of alternative feeding practices is intermediate.

Case 2: HIV status of mother unknown; screening unavailable. Figure 5 shows the graph for this case. The most striking feature of this case is how much less likely one is to recommend an alternative feeding practice when the maternal status is unknown than when the mother is known to be HIV-infected (as in the first case). For communities with a prevalence of 100 cases of HIV infection per 1000 reproductive-age women where screening is unavailable, one would almost never recommend against breast-feeding. Even if p (transmission/HIV+ mother breast-feeds) = 1, and the relative risk of wet nursing to breast-feeding were only 2:1, one would recommend that mothers of unknown HIV status breast-feed.

Case 3: imperfect screening test available. A sensitivity analysis can also be conducted around the specificity of the screening text. The graph in Figure 6 shows how the "indifference curve" between breast-feeding and alternative feeding practices shifts as the p (true+/test+) ranges from 1.0 to .8. What is most striking is that, even with a relatively high number of false positives for a high-risk population (e.g., 20%), the circumstances in which one should recommend a particular feeding practice do not shift greatly.

Case 4: AIDS treatment available; Case 5: child mortality from other causes changes. Not surprisingly, if a treatment becomes available that increases the survival rate for HIV infection, then one would recommend breast-feeding for higher HIV transmission rates and lower relative risks of wet nursing than at present. Conversely, the lower the infant mortality from other causes such as diarrhea and malnutrition against which breast-feeding protects, the more attractive alternative feeding practices become.

Ethical Issues

The consideration of infant feeding practices raises several important ethical issues. While different people will respond differently to these ethical dilemmas, the dilemmas are raised here because they effect how outcomes of the decision analysis should be weighted.

How should the needs of the mother and child be balanced? Conspicuously absent from most discussions of the policy options is the possibility that, at times, infant and maternal health promotion may be in conflict. If, in future studies, the risk of HIV infection from breast-feeding turns out to be lower than the excess mortality associated with partial or complete bottle-feeding of babies of HIV-positive women, then it would be better for the infant of the HIV-positive mother to be breast-fed. Yet, in advanced stages of AIDS, it may prove difficult at best for the mother to take on the physically exhausting task of breast-feeding; at worst, breast-feeding may prove detrimental to the mother's nutritional and health status. A woman does not and should not be asked to give up her rights and needs as an individual when she becomes a mother.

How should averted cases of HIV transmission to infants and to adults be weighed against each other? Because programs that are most effective for infants and adults may differ, and because resources available for health programs in many countries are extremely limited, choices made in allocating resources inherently will place relative weights on infant and adult lives saved. Economic analyses of the impact of AIDS on Africa have looked at productive years lost, often inherently weighting the death of a young adult as more serious than the death of an infant. Should this practice be followed for health programs as well because of the great poverty in many HIV-affected countries and the central role productive adults play in survival in these countries? Or should health programs be evaluated on the basis of years of life saved, which inherently weights benefits to infants more than to adults? Should all lives be treated equally, as they are in certain religious laws and formulations of justice?

How do we feel about bringing new people into the risk pool? An episode of possible HIV transmission from infants to mothers was reported in the Soviet Union. The infants had a known exposure to HIV in the hospital. The HIV antibody status of the mothers prior to birth was unknown. The mothers had a variety of exposures to the infants' body fluids including, but not limited to, infant saliva during breast-feeding. If this report turns out to have credibility, then it will raise questions about the safety of wet-nursing HIV-infected infants. While infants could be screened at birth and only seronegative infants recommended for wet nursing, the current limited predictive value of infant screening would make this process imperfect at best. If there is a small risk to the wet nurse, should this risk be weighted more heavily than the risk to the infant because the risk to the wet nurse is in some sense more "avoidable" or "voluntary"?*

In considering policies with respect to HIV-seropositive parents, one has to worry about the spillover effects of policies on the general population. How do you make sure that uninfected mothers keep breast-feeding while convincing infected mothers to stop? How do you keep it from appearing "healthier" not to breast-feed? From the opposite side, how do you keep women who do not breast-feed from being stigmatized as carriers of the AIDS virus? (If they were stigmatized they might well be unwilling to have a wet nurse or to bottle-feed.) While spillover effects on the healthy population would be far less for recommendations involving individual screening than for those requiring changes in national policies, policies should still anticipate and address all negative spillover effects.

CONCLUSION

AIDS poses an immediate threat to infant health. Because neither vaccines nor cures are currently available for AIDS, our most effective means of limiting the impact of AIDS is to limit its transmission. In the case of vertical transmission to infants, this means limiting the number of infected parents who transmit the virus to their newborns before and at birth, and limiting postnatal transmission via breast-feeding.

At present, most educational campaigns are aimed at promoting condom use among adults. While condoms are an effective means of decreasing transmission to HIV-negative adults, they are not one of the most effective means of limiting transmission from infected adults to children. With well over a million reproductive-age women already infected according to the World Health Organization's Global Programme on AIDS estimates, we can no longer afford to focus exclusively on ways to prevent adult cases and believe that this will take care of infant cases.

To avoid further tragedy, research needs to focus on determining the most effective means of limiting the transmission of HIV to infants before, during, and after birth. Until further preventive and therapeutic interventions are available, counseling that communicates the risk of transmitting HIV to children must be made available to infected parents. Such counseling must offer infected parents effective birth control measures should they choose not to bear additional children.

While this analysis supports previous reports recommending breast-feeding in areas where the relative risk of alternative feeding practices is high, available data make it impossible to generalize worldwide for the mother who is known to be infected with HIV. We need to determine how efficiently HIV infection is transmitted via breast milk. If the transmission is significant, we must help HIV-infected mothers find safe feeding alternatives so that their infants who are not infected at birth can remain that way.

---

*This case differs from the more commonly discussed case of vaccines. In the case of vaccines, an individual is at risk if they are not vaccinated, as they may develop a preventable disease, and at risk if they are vaccinated, as they may develop vaccine complications. In this case, the wet nurse may be at risk from west nursing, but would not be at risk from not nursing.

Acknowledgments

I am indebted to Dr. Timothy Brewer of Massachusetts General Hospital for his wise and patient advice at every stage of this project. I would like to thank Richard Zeckhauser and Tom Schelling of the Kennedy School of Government for their invaluable suggestions on earlier drafts.

REFERENCES

1. Mann JM, Chin J, Piot P, Quinn TC. The International Epidemiology of AIDS. *Scientific American* 1988; 259:82-89.
2. Ryder RW, Nsa W, Hassig SE et al. Perinatal Transmission of the Human Immunodeficiency Virus Type 1 to Infants of Seropositive Women in Zaire. *NEJM* 1989; 320 (25): 1637-1642.
3. Review of the Impact of Acquired Immunodeficiency Syndrome (AIDS) on Women and Children and the UNICEF Response. United Nations Children's Fund, 1988.
4. Carme B, Samba-Lefevre MC, Giovachinni AM et al. Knowledge of and attitude towards AIDS (young educated Brazzavillians) – Congo. International Conference on AIDS, Stockholm, Sweden, 1988; Abstract 5097.
5. Devash Y, Calvelli TA, Wood DG et al. Vertical Transmission of Human Immunodeficiency Virus is Correlated with the Absence of High-affinity/avidity Maternal Antibodies to the GP120 Principal Neutralizing Domain. *Proc Natl Acad Sci USA* 1990; 87 (9): 3445-9.
6. Goedert JJ, Mendez H, Drummond JE et al. Mother-to-Infant Transmission of Human Immunodeficiency Virus Type 1: Association with Prematurity or Low Anti-GP120. *Lancet* 1989; 2(8676):1351-4.
7. Byrn RA, Mordenti J, Lucas C et al. Biological Properties of a CD4 Immunoadhesin. *Nature* 1990; 344 (6267): 667-70.
8. Auger I, Thomas P, De Gruttola V et al. Incubation periods for paediatric AIDS patients. *Nature* 1988; 336 (8): 575-577.
9. Thiry L, Sprecher-Goldberger S, Jonekheer T et al. Isolation of AIDS virus from cell-free breast milk of three healthy carriers. *Lancet* 1985; 2 (8460): 891.
10. Weinbreck P, Loustaud V, Denis F et al. Postnatal transmission of HIV infection. *Lancet* 1988; 1(8583): 482.
11. Lepage P, Van de Perre P, Carael M et al. Postnatal transmission of HIV from mother to child. *Lancet* 1987; 2 (8555):400.
12. Ziegler JB, Cooper DA, Johnson R, Gold J. Postnatal transmission of AIDS associated retrovirus from mother to infant. *Lancet* 1985; 1 (8434): 896-899.
13. Blanche S, Rouzioux C, Moscato ML et al. A prospective study of infants born to women seropositive for human immunodeficiency virus type 1. *NEJM* 1989; 320 (25): 1643-8.
14. Janowitz B et al. Breast feeding and child survival in Egypt. *J Biosoc Sci* 1981; 13: 287.
15. Brown RE. Relactation with Reference to Application in Developing Countries. *Clinical Pediatrics*; 17 (4): 333-337.
16. Jason J, Nieburg P, Marks JS. Mortality and infectious disease associated with infant feeding practices in developing countries. *Pediatrics* 1984; 74 (4 supplement): 702-727.
17. Huffman SL and Combest C. Breastfeeding: a prevention and treatment necessity for diarrhea. Presented at UNICEF/NCIH meeting, December 1988.

AN OVERVIEW OF AIDS INTERVENTIONS IN HIGH-RISK GROUPS: COMMERCIAL SEX WORKERS AND THEIR CLIENTS

Peter Lamptey

AIDSTECH/Family Health International

INTRODUCTION

Although the epidemiological features of the AIDS epidemic vary throughout the world, HIV infection has followed a set pattern (1). Initially, HIV infection is introduced into a relatively small group of people who are at most risk of getting infected because of their behavior. This group spreads the infection to other groups. In time, the epidemic is a risk to everyone in the population.

Those at high risk of acquiring or spreading HIV sexually can be divided into two specific groups: the primary risk group and the secondary risk group. The primary risk group consists of prostitutes, clients of prostitutes, and people who frequently change sexual partners, such as homosexual and bisexual men. In addition, sexually active IV drug users (IVDUs), especially in developed countries and certain developing countries, such as Thailand, fall into this group. Most often, persons in these primary risk groups are found among truckers, traders, businessmen, military personnel, fishermen, prisoners, sailors, or young unmarried adults living in urban areas. However, it should be emphasized that it is behavior and not vocation, age, or marital status that puts an individual at risk of acquiring infection. For example, prostitutes and clients who regularly and consistently practice safer sex (non-penetrative sex or penetrative sex using a condom properly) reduce their risk of HIV infection considerably.

All persons who practice risky behaviors need intervention; however, it is more efficient and effective to identify the groups who most often practice high-risk behavior, and develop specific interventions for reaching these groups. Prostitutes remain at high risk at least in part because of their societal status. One of the factors that makes AIDS a "political" as well as a public health problem is the fact that primary risk groups, such as prostitutes, often live on the fringes of society. Decision-makers do not always find it easy to mobilize society's resources to meet fringe-group needs. Furthermore, in some cases, the high-risk behaviors and other activities of primary risk groups may be contrary to a nation's statute law, and are nearly always outside the traditions of majority custom. However, officially ignoring the spread of HIV infection within primary risk groups who appear to live on society's fringe is exceedingly shortsighted, as the HIV virus is bound to spread from people in primary risk groups to people in secondary risk groups and to the general population.

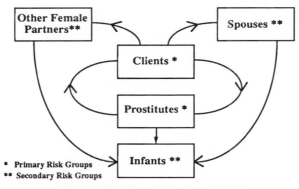

Figure 1. Prostitution and the spread of HIV.

The secondary risk group of concern for the practical targeting of AIDS interventions consists of individuals who do not actively practice behaviors that put them at risk of acquiring infection, but who are infected by individuals in the primary risk group. Sexual partners of individuals who practice high-risk behavior are within this group, including regular, non-paying partners of female prostitutes (spouses, boyfriends); regular sexual partners of clients of prostitutes (spouses, girlfriends); and sexual partners of IVDUs. Infants of infected mothers also constitute a secondary risk group. An understanding of the difference between primary and secondary risk groups is essential for prevention programs. Most current AIDS prevention efforts are directed at changing the high-risk practices of primary risk groups. Individuals in secondary risk groups who do not practice high-risk behavior are often not aware of their risk; therefore, they may not initiate any behavior change to reduce their risk of infection.

The size of primary and secondary risk groups and their interaction with the rest of the population is an important determinant of how quickly the HIV infection spreads within a country. Figure 1 illustrates the interaction between primary and secondary risk groups.

EPIDEMIOLOGY OF AIDS IN HIGH-RISK GROUPS

Although HIV infection follows a set a pattern, the global problem is complicated by epidemiologic characteristics that vary by geographic location. Worldwide, the most important and largest primary risk groups are prostitutes, clients of prostitutes, and other persons who frequently change sexual partners (2). Prostitution varies by location; in Africa, for example, virtually all prostitutes are women. African prostitutes enjoy somewhat more autonomy and are not likely to be controlled by male "pimps". These prostitutes provide vaginal intercourse to nearly all clients, and, to date, they have rarely used condoms.

The two most important behavioral factors that put these individuals at high risk of HIV infection are frequency of sexual partner change and multiplicity of sexual partners. A number of other risk factors have been identified in HIV transmission, including: genital ulcer disease caused by chancroid, syphilis, and herpes; lack of circumcision in males; and the presence of other STDs, including genital chlamydia infection and trichomoniasis (3).

The Center for International Research, U.S. Bureau of the Census, has compiled a comprehensive HIV/AIDS Surveillance database that contains over 4,300 data entries for Africa. Figure 2 shows the HIV-1 surveillance for high-risk urban populations, such as prostitutes, in Africa. The highest rates are concentrated in the high-risk groups of central Africa. Rates of 50-90% are common among prostitutes in the major urban centers of Tanzania, Uganda, Malawi, Rwanda, and

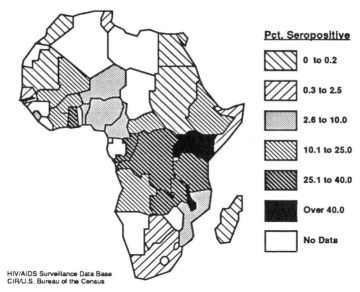

HIV/AIDS Surveillance Data Base
CIR/U.S. Bureau of the Census

Figure 2. African HIV-1 seroprevalence for high-risk urban populations. (HIV/AIDS Surveillance Data Base CIR/U.S. Bureau of the Census)

Kenya. Moderately high rates of HIV-1 infection are found in high-risk groups in the urban areas of other parts of Africa, including Ethiopia (18.1%), Gambia (30.0%), Togo (31.1%), and Mali (48.0%). Figure 3 shows the distribution of HIV-2 in high-risk groups in Africa. French West Africa has the highest seroprevalence levels, although the virus has also spread to urban areas of Angola and Mozambique.

Prostitution is also playing a major role in the spread of HIV in Asia. In Thailand, which has an estimated commercial sex worker population of over 100,000, HIV prevalence rates as high as 30% have been reported among some prostitute groups (4). Cultural practices in Thailand are likely to contribute to the rapid spread of HIV from the primary risk group of prostitutes to secondary risk groups and the general population. The recruitment of young women from the countryside to provide urban prostitution, followed by their eventual return to the countryside to settle socially, provides a route of spread to the rest of the country. The practice of young urban males "starting" their sexual life with prostitutes is also likely to provide a ready access route for HIV infection into the general population.

Prostitution is likely to play a significant role in the epidemiology of HIV in other Asian countries as well, such as India, the Philippines, and Indonesia. In India, HIV prevalence rates as high as 30% have been reported in some urban areas (4). In the Philippines, the current HIV seroprevalence is low in all populations; but the Philippines has a very large commercial sex industry that represents a potential time bomb for a devastating HIV/AIDS epidemic.

In the Americas, various primary risk groups have already been infected to a considerable degree. In the U.S., HIV rates are high among homosexuals and IVDUs, and relatively low among prostitutes who do not use IV drugs. In Haiti and the Caribbean, HIV prevalence rates among prostitutes range from 0% to 60% (5). In Central and South America, the epidemic is shifting within primary risk groups from the homosexual and IVDU population to the female prostitute population (6).

There is a paucity of data on the prevalence of HIV in the partners of prostitutes, but one of the most important and consistent risk factors in HIV-positive men is contact with prostitutes. Figure 4 shows the comparative HIV prevalence rates in various segments of the population in

153

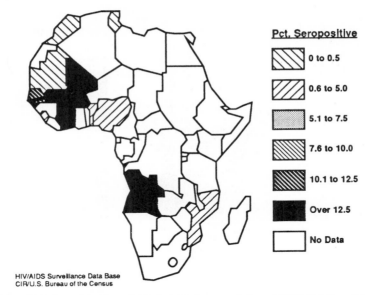

Pct. Seropositive

▨	0 to 0.5
▨	0.6 to 5.0
▨	5.1 to 7.5
▨	7.6 to 10.0
▨	10.1 to 12.5
■	Over 12.5
□	No Data

HIV/AIDS Surveillance Data Base
CIR/U.S. Bureau of the Census

Figure 3. African HIV-2 seroprevalence for high-risk urban populations. (HIV/AIDS Surveillance Data Base CIR/U.S. Bureau of the Census)

Rwanda. Prostitutes and clients of prostitutes have the highest prevalence rates (88% and 28%, respectively) (7). Studies of STD patients have shown that contact with prostitutes is an important risk factor for HIV and other STDs. In some parts of Africa, from 30% to 70% of STD patients are reported to be HIV positive (8). Clients of prostitutes and STD patients constitute an important primary risk group that needs to be reached with targeted AIDS intervention.

STRATEGIES FOR TARGETED INTERVENTION

Prevention of the spread of HIV/AIDS using targeted interventions has two primary prevention goals: preventing high-risk groups from becoming infected in the first place; and preventing infected primary risk groups from spreading the infection to secondary risk groups and to the rest of the population. It also has the secondary prevention goal of preventing disease progression in those already infected with HIV. This chapter focuses only on the primary prevention of HIV;

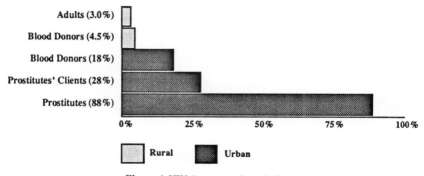

Figure 4. HIV-1 seroprevalence in Rwanda.

however, it must be emphasized that the prevention of STDs and disease progression in HIV-infected individuals may be an extremely important and significant component of prevention of HIV infection within the general population.

Targeting interventions to high-risk groups is important for a number of reasons, but three reasons are primary: first, high-risk groups are (by definition) at high risk of acquiring and transmitting HIV infection; second, despite what some health providers believe, high-risk groups can be identified and reached with intervention programs; and third, targeted interventions are a very cost-effective approach to containing the HIV/AIDS epidemic, or at least reducing further spread of the disease. Mathematical models that have looked at prostitution suggest that interventions directed at prostitutes and their partners could have a dramatic and cost-effective impact on HIV transmission.

The first targeted interventions carried out by Family Health International (FHI, a USAID-funded project that provides technical assistance and funding for AIDS prevention and contraceptive research in developing countries) were limited to three pilot studies in Ghana, Cameroon, and Mali. To date, FHI has developed over 40 interventions directed at prostitutes and their partners in 21 countries in Africa, Asia, Latin America, and the Caribbean. From our experience, we have determined that intervention strategies directed at high-risk groups should usually contain the following components: behavior research; AIDS education; STD control and prevention; condom distribution; evaluation; and capacity building.

Behavior Research

Studies on the behavior of high-risk groups have been extremely limited. These groups have been ignored not only by the society-at-large, but also by health care providers. Attempts to design interventions aimed at changing high-risk group behaviors are likely to fail or be short-lived unless there is a better understanding and appreciation of the groups' behaviors, knowledge, attitudes, and practices, as well as other facets of their subcultures. For example, in order to get prostitutes and their clients to use condoms, the subculture of prostitution and the particular environment of each prostitute group needs to be understood.

Behavior research needs to examine the following issues: 1) What are the relevant demographics of a prostitute or a client, such as age, level of education, ethnic origin, access to health care? 2) What are the health-related behaviors that affect HIV transmission, such as condom use and recognition and treatment of STDs? 3) What socio-economic variables are likely to affect risk reduction behavior? 4) What are the social and economic costs of risk reduction to the client or prostitute? 5) Are there existing organizational and social structures for the target group? 6) What psycho-social variables are likely to impede initiation and sustainability of behavior change? 7) In a society where multiple partners is an accepted norm, what is the social cost to an individual for reducing the number of partners? 8) What are the perceived benefits to the client and prostitutes (if any) for low-risk behavior?

A number of different strategies have been used to obtain relevant information on target groups, including: Knowledge, attitudes, behavior and practices (KABP) surveys; focus group discussions; and ethnographic studies. This research should be relevant, confidential, and non-invasive. It should be accomplished quickly and should provide information that is useful for the design of an appropriate intervention.

AIDS Education

The goal of the educational component is to modify high-risk behaviors in order to reduce the transmission of HIV. This requires: 1) informing the target group about AIDS and the modes of transmission within that community; 2) motivating the group to change behavior in order to reduce risk of infection; 3) motivating the group to use condoms correctly and consistently; and 4) teaching the group to recognize common symptoms of STDs and the importance of obtaining prompt treatment.

Different strategies have been used to reach target groups with education. These have included diffusion models (such as peer education) within the target group; clinical or clinic-based approaches that use existing infrastructures (such as STD and family planning clinics) to provide services to target groups; institutional strategies that target interventions to institutions associated with individuals who are at high risk of HIV infection (such as hotels, brothels, factories, the military, and prostitutes' collectives); and social marketing approaches to reach both high-risk groups and the general population (discussed in more detail in the next section).

The peer education strategy begins with the identification and recruitment of natural leaders within the target group to serve as health educators and condom distributors to their peers. Where possible, existing organizations are used to identify leaders and to involve the target population in the planing and implementation of such programs. The effectiveness of peer health educators has been enhanced by other health education and condom distribution efforts, such as periodic community meetings led by peer health educators where dramatic presentations, condom demonstrations, and educational messages are given to a large group. In Cameroon and Zaire, groups of prostitutes formed a drama troupe that provides AIDS education and condom promotion activities in a play format to the prostitutes' peers and customers. On-site AIDS education and condom distribution programs carried out in the places prostitutes and clients work and socialize, such as bars, nightclubs, and hotels, have also proven useful. Workshops have helped sensitize hotel and bar managers to the danger AIDS presents to customers and employees. This sensitization has, in turn, helped in the development of employer-assisted AIDS prevention programs. This approach has been used for high-risk group intervention programs in Zimbabwe, Zaire, and Nigeria (see Table 1).

The clinical approach to AIDS education features the use of current STD service providers, outreach workers, and contact traces to educate individuals at risk of HIV infection when they come to health facilities for treatment of STDs. This strategy is particularly useful in countries where prostitutes are required to visit a STD clinic regularly. Programs in Mexico, Barbados, Trinidad, Zambia, and Kenya have used this approach. Components of the STD clinic-based strategy include: 1) improving the attitudes of STD clinic staff toward all clients, but especially toward prostitutes; 2) educating health care providers about AIDS and how to promote condom use; 3) training clinic staff on how to educate their patients to recognize symptoms of common STDs; and 4) developing educational materials for use in the STD clinic.

Condom Distribution

The goal of a condom distribution component is to increase condom accessibility primarily to target groups, but also to the general population. This requires developing and implementing a system to increase condom demand and use among the target population; implementing a system that will provide easy access to affordable condoms for members of the target population; and assuring sustainability of condom distribution programs. Target groups have been supplied with condoms using a variety of distributors and techniques. These have included: peer health educators; trained STD clinic staff; work-site employees; and family planning providers. In each case, important management and implementation issues for the condom distribution program must be resolved. These include: providing storage and distribution of condoms from a central storehouse to the STD clinic or health educator and to the prostitutes and their partners; training condom distributors; coordinating education and condom distribution efforts; monitoring the number of condoms supplied to and distributed by each condom outlet; and ascertaining whether condoms will be sold, at what price, and by whom. Health providers, such as STD clinic staff and family planning workers, can be trained to promote condom use, and should have supplies of condoms available to provide to patients; however, these staff cannot be relied upon as the sole supplier of condoms to members of high-risk groups: health providers see only those members of the target population who are patients and come to the health clinics.

Condoms are the single most expensive component of AIDS intervention programs for pros-

Table 1. Targeted intervention programs in selected countries.*

Prostitutes' and Clients' Programs

Location	Target Population	Approach	Program Manager
Ouagadougou, Burkina Faso	Prostitutes Clients	Peer education; condom social marketing planned	Dr. Guy Yoda Division of Education for Health and Hygiene
Yaounde, Douala, Maroua, Cameroon	Prostitutes Clients	Peer education; condom social marketing	Dr. Marcel Mony-Lobe National AIDS Control Service
Mombasa, Kenya	Prostitutes Clients	Peer education; outreach to community women; STD clinic; bars/hotels	Dr. H. W. Waweru Coast Province STD/AIDS Committee
Nairobi, Kenya	Prostitutes Clients	Community-based; health workers	Mr. Mohamed Hanif Cresent Medical AID
Nairobi, Kenya	Truckers Partners	Peer education	Dr. David Nyamwaya AMREF/Kenya
Bamako, Mali	Prostitutes Clients	Peer education	Mme. Oumou Fofana Ministry of Public Health & Social Affairs
Calabar, Nigeria	Prostitutes Clients Proprietors	Peer education; hotel/bar proprietors	Dr. Eka Williams Cross River State AIDS Committee
Dar es Salaam, Tanzania	Truckers Partners	Peer education	Dr.Ulrich Laukamm-Josten AMREF/Tanzania
Goma, Matadi, Zaire	Prostitutes Clients	Condom social marketing	Mr. Carlos Ferreros Population Services International
Bulawayo, Zimbabwe	Prostitutes Clients Taxi drivers	Peer education; bar/hotel proprietors	Dr. Barnet Nyathi Bulawayo City Health Dept.
Ghana	Military personnel	General education; condom social marketing	Dr. Frank Apeagyei

*AIDSTECH/Family Health International funded targeted AIDS Prevention Programs in Africa.

titutes and their partners; therefore, efforts must be made to recover at least part of the cost of the condoms. To this end, subsidies from employers, bar and hotel owners, or unions may be available. Even if condoms are initially provided free of charge as part of a marketing strategy to increase demand, an effort should be made to determine whether men and women are willing to pay for condoms, and at what price, after free condoms are distributed.

In some programs, social marketing of condoms has been used to reach large segments of both high-risk groups and the general population. Social marketing distributes a branded product through established retail channels backed by professional advertising. The price can be adjusted to subsidize use and achieve maximum health benefits. Social marketing programs have been developed in Zaire, Cameroon, and Burkina Faso to reach prostitutes, their clients, and the general population.

STD Control and Prevention Programs

The goal of the STD services component of a targeted intervention is to reduce STDs as a risk factor of transmission for individuals in primary target groups. This requires improving STD prevention activities (e.g., health education and condom distribution); improving diagnosis of STDs; providing affordable treatment of STDs; and providing prevention counseling services. The strategy for accomplishing these objectives involves strengthening current programs at general health facilities or at designated STD clinics. Development of the program usually includes a needs assessment of the STD health facility in terms of supplies and equipment, training, educational programs, and counseling. After the needs assessment, a plan is developed for implementing activities to meet the highest priority needs. STD control should be a vital component of any AIDS prevention program for two major reasons: STDs are important risk factors for HIV transmission, and individuals who get STDs are often at risk of HIV infection as well. (See Section II in this volume for more on STDs and HIV.)

Program Monitoring and Evaluation

The objectives of program monitoring and evaluation are to estimate program impact; identify program strengths and weaknesses; and identify resources needed to sustain the program. Monitoring and evaluating intervention programs must not be burdensome and should provide a meaningful and practical assessment of how well a program is meeting its objectives. The best indicators are those offering a demonstrable decrease in HIV incidence that can be linked to the program. The ideal methodology is to follow cohorts of the target population that have been exposed to the intervention and a control group not exposed to the intervention and compare the estimated difference in HIV seroconversion rates over time. This approach raises serious ethical, practical, financial, and logistical issues, however. First, it requires a significant amount of data; second, it is expensive, and particularly difficult to implement with highly mobile individuals such as prostitutes; and third, a lethal disease cannot be randomly allotted, and the mere attempt to identify control cohorts may open the opportunity for some negative or counterproductive interventions.

Two other indicators have proved to be more practical and useful in behavior change: changes in reported condom use and changes in STD incidence in the target population. Changes in reported condom use are estimated on the basis of pre- and post-intervention surveys of knowledge, attitudes, and behavior among prostitutes exposed to the intervention and, where possible, similar surveys of a control group. Activities necessary for implementation of KABP surveys include: developing a survey protocol; pretesting the questionnaire; training interviewers; editing and coding questionnaires; preparing data for analysis; and analyzing data. Of course, there may be a disparity between reported and actual condom use. Validation of reported condom use, where possible, is recommended. Changes in STD incidence in the target population is an objective and practical measure of program effectiveness. Programs may include baseline and follow-up examinations of a sample of men or women for evidence of selected STDs, such a gonorrhea, syphilis, and genital ulcer disease. Clinic-based programs can be evaluated by means of pre- and post-program surveys of knowledge and attitudes among clinic staff, and through monitoring STD clinic statistics on the number of patients seen, tests provided, condoms distributed, and women counseled.

Capacity Building

The goal of capacity building is to ensure that a targeted intervention program can be sustained in terms of both human and fiscal resources. This requires ensuring appropriate infrastructure development to support the program; providing adequate training for program staff including technical and managerial skills; planning for the institutionalization of the program; and planning for financial sustainability. The current availability of donor resources for AIDS programs has not encouraged adequate long-term planning for monitoring and supporting these programs. Some of the issues that have not been adequately addressed by most National AIDS Control Programs include: projected costs of programs beyond the mid-term plan (MTP); support for programs when donor assistance declines; cost-recovery strategies; and involvement in the private sector for intervention programs.

The development of an infrastructure to support targeted intervention programs is critical for the maintenance of these relatively new activities. Pilot projects involving dedicated and motivated program staff and external donor support do not necessarily lead to infrastructure development. Allocation of space is essential, but brick and mortar development is expensive and should be kept to a minimum. Planning the purchase of essential equipment and supplies is critical. This may include basic equipment for diagnosing STDs, condom dispensing machines where appropriate, office equipment, and even computers. Project managers should carefully plan the projected needs of the program and how these needs will be met.

An important component of capacity building is the training of staff. Targeted interventions for prostitutes and clients are relatively new. Most health personnel are not trained for it, many are uncomfortable or not interested, and some may even be opposed to it. Training should include: upgrading the knowledge of health personnel in biomedical facts about AIDS; upgrading health personnels' skills in the diagnosis and treatment of STDs; providing prevention counseling; and training staff in the management of programs.

The success of intervention programs depends on adequate training of community-based personnel, such as peer educators, community volunteers, and hotel and bar proprietors and managers. Technical assistance should be obtained if needed. Staff needs and training for a larger program should be carefully planned. Project managers should realize that managing a large, targeted intervention program is not a part-time job and can not be combined with other work.

Most early targeted intervention projects were carried out outside the formal health system and were designed as operations research studies to test various approaches. In order to expand and sustain these intervention programs, they must be integrated into existing institutions. Support could come from Ministries of Health or city health programs, the private sector, or community-based institutions. In all instances, close involvement with a country's National AIDS Control Program and the Ministry of Health is essential.

One of the most important ways of ensuring the acceptance and sustainability of AIDS intervention programs is to involve the target population in the planning, design, and implementation of the intervention. Often, prostitute groups and organizations such as unions can be contacted. In most instances, natural or opinion leaders are willing to be involved in such programs. In some locations, organizations of hotel, bar, and brothel owners exist and can be mobilized to support intervention programs. It is vital for capacity building that such community-based organizations be identified and strengthened (if feasible) as partners in the intervention program.

Planning for financial sustainability is critical if programs are to have a long-term impact on reducing HIV transmission. There are several sources for ensuring the financial sustainability of such programs: 1) External donor support: This support is currently available but may not last forever. Programs in some countries may not survive without such support. 2) National or local government support: Continuing financial government support may wane as the epidemic worsens and government resources become stretched further. 3) Private sector involvement: This is one of the more promising avenues for resources. It includes the involvement of hotel/bar proprietors and owners, employer-supported workplace education, transportation workers' unions, and the private sector social marketing of condoms. 4) Community-based support from organizations such as prostitute collectives: These are an invaluable resource and essential for the sustainability of these programs.

Some of the costs of AIDS intervention programs, such as the cost of condoms or STD diagnosis and treatment, may have to be recovered from program beneficiaries. The cost of condoms constitutes the most expensive component of a targeted intervention program. Partial or full recovery of the cost of the condoms from prostitutes and/or clients should be explored. Cost recovery for STD diagnosis and treatment is one way to improve health services in some developing countries, especially in Africa, where most free health services are under-funded and of poor quality.

CASE STUDIES OF TARGETED INTERVENTION PROGRAMS

Figure 5 shows examples of targeted intervention programs for prostitutes and clients in Africa. The following case studies illustrate a variety of approaches and innovative combinations used to reach high-risk groups.

Zaire

The goal of the program in Zaire is to reduce the incidence of HIV infection and other STDs in prostitutes and their clients in Goma and Matadi, two commercial cities in Zaire. A secondary goal is to reduce unwanted pregnancies. The program uses social marketing strategies similar to those used for mass consumer goods, such as soft drinks (although mass media brand advertising for condoms is thus far prohibited in Zaire). Point-of-purchase advertising, brand-name advertising, and AIDS education are available at pharmacies, medical centers, and other non-traditional outlets, such as hotels, bars, and taxis. The project pays for consumer promotion activities such as "rapping" by disc jockeys and night club singers, condom use demonstrations, and consumer giveaways. Peer educators are also used to reach prostitutes.

During the first 12 months of the project, more than 1.5 million condoms were sold in over 70 pharmacies and 40 bars/hotels. Pharmacies accounted for 75% of sales, hotels for 11%, and all other outlets for the remaining 14%. Nearly 90% of the pharmacies, 49% of the medical centers, and 45% of the bars and hotels in the cities participated in the project. It is estimated that condom distribution reaches 70% of the targeted high-risk group. Several hotels now include condoms along with the usual amenities normally provided in the rooms.

Philippines

This program is targeted at high-risk groups in Olangapo and Angeles City in the Republic of the Philippines. These cities are hosts to two U.S. military bases: Olangapo is the site for the Subic Naval Base and Angeles City is the site of the Clark Air Force Base. There are an estimated 9,000 registered sex industry workers (female and male prostitutes) and almost the same number of unregistered prostitutes working in these areas. The clientele of the prostitutes are primarily military personnel.

The program has conducted a survey of over 1,000 female prostitutes, 150 male prostitutes, and 50 "Mama-sans" and managers. Survey data is currently being analyzed. A local AIDS Prevention Task Force has been organized to coordinate the efforts of the project staff and includes representatives of the local sex industry, city government, the media, project staff, and the U.S. Navy.

Nearly 6,000 prostitutes have been targeted for AIDS education, instruction on condom use, and promotion of non-penetrative sex, and 215 establishments have been involved in program activities. Program activities have included training sessions organized for 220 managers and Mama-sans during which an AIDS intervention plan was developed that could be implemented in the various represented establishments. Training has also been provided for 170 peer counselors, each of whom is expected to reach 30 individuals. Utilizing the local AIDS Prevention Task Force, program organizers were able to convince city officials to pass an ordinance requiring condoms to be available in various establishments. Condoms were distributed to: STD clinics (free); 400 bars/clubs (free); and 50 tailor shops, barber shops, beauty shops, and billiard halls (distributed at cost to be sold at market value).

Zimbabwe

The goal of this program is to reduce the sexual transmission of HIV in prostitutes and their clients in Bulawayo, Zimbabwe's second largest city (population 700,000). Baseline research was conducted among prostitutes, their clients, STD patients, and the general population to provide ethnographic and psycho-social data. A number of interventions were designed, including: 1) a training program for nursing and health education professionals, and for community personnel, including prostitutes and client peer educators, hotel security personnel, reception and bar personnel and taxi drivers; 2) a community outreach component that included meetings with prostitutes and clients at prostitute residences, hotels, and bars, with hotel security personnel and peer educators also conducting outreach activities in their networks; 3) a condom distribution program that supplements the national contraceptive distribution program (the best in Africa); and 4) the strengthening of the STD services of the city by offering training in diagnosis, treatment, and prevention counseling.

This program has employed a multiplicity of approaches in reaching prostitutes and clients. For example, it uses non-conventional personnel, such as hotel security personnel, receptionists, bar personnel, and taxi drivers, as well as other community-based workers, such as prostitutes and client peer educators; and it is one of the few programs that directly uses professional medical staff, indicating the commitment of the city health services to the program.

The Zimbabwe program emphasizes a community-based approach, with community meetings and condom distribution at prostitute residences, hotels, and bars. The commitment of the Bulawayo City Council is remarkable and is likely to lead to a long-term sustainable program.

Nigeria

The goal of the program in Nigeria's Cross River State is to reduce STD rates in prostitutes and their partners and to keep HIV seroprevalence rates low (currently less than 2%). Targeted groups include: prostitutes, prostitutes' clients, and hotel managers and proprietors (who may also be non-paying partners of prostitutes). To date, activities have begun in two towns: Calabar and Ikom. Programs have been established in 24 intervention sites, and have reached 750 prostitutes and approximately 2,500 clients.

Program activities include: health education activities, with on-site education sessions in hotels and compounds for prostitutes and clients; focus group discussions; distribution of educational materials; AIDS films shown in night clubs; outreach by the project's male (hotel manager) and female (prostitute) peer health educators; and periodic workshops involving prostitutes and hotel managers. Promotion and distribution of condoms to prostitutes and clients (partners) has also been undertaken. Peer health educators and the managers, chairladies, or supervisors of full-time prostitutes carry out these activities. Regular condom users have also been enlisted in promotional activities. In order to provide services to the target population, an STD clinic was established. Patients are self-referred or referred by prostitutes or, sometimes, hotel managers. Services include: diagnosis and treatment of STDs; health education and prevention counseling; follow-up of patients; condom distribution; and voluntary HIV testing.

This program has involved key members of the target population in planning and implementation. Hotel proprietors and owners, managers, chairladies, and motivated peer/natural prostitute leaders representing the various intervention sites have been involved in all stages of the project. The program offers a good example of the need for flexibility in program design. The original design called for the extensive use of peer health educators; but results of focus group discussions, KABP surveys, and practical field experience have shown that the existing structure in hotels and compounds is not compatible with this strategy. The strength of the program in this setting relies on the use of managers and chairladies, with peer health educators being better utilized to reach part-time prostitutes. Additional flexibility has been shown in the willingness of program staff to respond to other problems: they have assisted in resolving issues ranging from police detention to sanitation.

Official support from the State Ministry of Health and the Cross River AIDS Committee has been a key feature for the success and sustainability of this program; the Commissioner of Health has officially opened project workshops and the STD clinic. This is especially important to this group of women who, up until this time, had only identified government officials with harassment.

DISCUSSION

What lessons have been learned from current targeted interventions? What are some of the urgent research needs of these programs? Through these programs we have learned about prostitution and the behaviors that put prostitutes and their clients at risk of HIV infection. We have learned, for example, that, despite the common denominator of sex for money or for items of monetary value, there are different types of prostitutes and different types of prostitution in different environments.

Our experience has also shown that, on the whole, primary risk groups can be identified and targeted; are very receptive to targeted interventions; and can change high-risk behavior and sustain risk-reducing behavior. We also have found that the biggest obstacle to the development of interventions for high-risk groups are policy makers and health care providers. The problems we have encountered have included bureaucratic delays by Ministries of Health and National AIDS Committees; lack of interest and commitment by policy makers; and obstruction by religious groups.

With respect to interventions among prostitutes, we have learned that peer education is an acceptable and successful approach to reaching prostitutes; clients also need to be reached for a program to be successful; prostitutes may not regard sex with their regular partners (especially boyfriends) as high risk and will often not use condoms with them; social support organizations and groups exist that are willing to be involved with the intervention; and the availability of, and accessibility to, condoms is often a major problem.

Based on AIDTECH's experience, four major areas of research need have been identified: evaluation; basic behavioral research; operations research; and legal, ethical, and religious issues.

Evaluation of the efficacy of intervention activities, whether process or impact, must be carried out. Various intervention approaches need to be evaluated adequately, including peer education, STD clinic-based services, community-based activities, and social marketing efforts.

Basic behavioral research is needed to better understand high-risk behaviors in various subpopulations. This should include research on previously unresearched groups, including the general population and hard-to-reach and hard-to-change groups. It should also include research on secondary risk groups and studies to determine how to reduce their risk of acquiring HIV infection. There should also be research into normative behavior, which is a key component of behavior change at the community level. This research should address the question, "How does the normative behavior affect the ability of an individual who practices high-risk activity to initiate and sustain risk reduction behavior?"

In the area of operations research, experimental or quasi-experimental designs are needed to test various intervention models that allow the identification and manipulation of key variables. Results of such studies will lead to better design of intervention activities. Research in this area should include a study of the sustainability of risk reduction as well as the predictors and correlates of failure to reduce risk. An understanding of sustainability and risk reduction failure is necessary in order to identify the conditions under which individuals fail to respond to interventions. Operations research should also look at alternate strategies to behavior change, such as effective community-based control and prevention of STDs.

Research into legal, ethical, and religious issues is needed to determine how these impede public intervention activities and risk reduction. As long as legal, ethical, or religious obstacles exist, we will have great difficulty in affecting public perceptions of AIDS and risk-reduction interventions.

It is important for intervention programs targeting prostitutes to be sensitive and helpful regarding non-health-related needs of the prostitutes. This might involve helping out in cases of police harassment, problems with hotel proprietors, or even the loss of a family member. It must be remembered that prostitutes often have even fewer social and legal avenues open to them than do other underprivileged communities members.

Targeted interventions to prostitutes and clients are feasible and may be one of the most important approaches to reducing the spread of HIV infection. Knowledge of high-risk groups and high-risk behavior remains rudimentary. In order to improve AIDS intervention programs in high-risk groups, research must be carried out to address relevant behavioral questions. Furthermore, if these programs are to have any impact, they will need to reach the vast majority of high-risk groups. There is an urgent need to expand and replicate targeted AIDS intervention programs.

REFERENCES

1. Piot P, Laga M, Ryder R et al. The global epidemiology of HIV infection: continuity, heterogeneity, and change. *J AIDS* 1990; 3:403-412.
2. Piot P, Plumer F, Mhaki FS et al. AIDS: an international perspective. *Science* 1980; 29:573-79.
3. Pepin J, Plummer FA, Brunham RC et al. The interaction of HIV and other sexually transmitted diseases: an opportunity for intervention. *AIDS* 1989; 3:3-9.
4. Lamptey P. Intervention among high-risk commercial sex workers and their clients. The international Workshop on AIDS and Reproductive Health. Bellagio, Italy, November 1990.
5. CAREC (PAHO/WHO) in collaboration with AIDSTECH and USAID. AIDS, HIV, and STD surveillance in the Caribbean. Kingston, Jamaica, November 1989.
6. Quinn TC, Narain JP, Zacarias F. AIDS in the Americas: a public health priority region. *AIDS* 1990; 4:709-24.
7. Rwandian seroprevalence study group. Nationwide community-based serological survey of HIV-1 and other known human retrovirus infection in a central African country. *Lancet* 1989; 1:947-53.
8. Piot P. Control and prevention of STDs. In: The handbook for AIDS prevention in Africa. Lamptey P and Piot P, eds. Durham NC: 1990.

INTERVENTION RESEARCH NEEDS FOR AIDS PREVENTION AMONG COMMERCIAL SEX WORKERS AND THEIR CLIENTS

Barbara O. de Zalduondo

Johns Hopkins University

Mauricio Hernandez Avila

Instituto Nacional de Salud Publica, Mexico

Patricia Uribe Zuñiga

CONASIDA

INTRODUCTION

Given the absence of an effective vaccine against HIV infection, and the lack of effective and affordable therapies to mitigate disease progression in most high-prevalence countries, preventing further escalation of HIV/AIDS morbidity and mortality must focus primarily on educational interventions to reduce transmission of HIV. Responding to this challenge has created a wider awareness in public health circles that educational interventions are just as technically and operationally challenging to conceive, execute, and evaluate as are biomedical or environmental interventions to control disease.

Education is not merely the presentation of new facts or ideas. Individuals of all ages and cultures have beliefs and experiences that they use to "filter" (selectively acquire) new information, even about topics of interest to them. When learning occurs, it is not always stable; people reconfigure information over time in keeping with their actual experiences and/or their prior beliefs. Furthermore, for reasons that are rather well understood, learning does not lead to behavior change in anything like the direct and irreversible manner for which health educators strive (1).

In no domain of AIDS intervention research has this become more clear than in worldwide efforts to promote behavioral risk reduction among women in prostitution. Among the problems that challenge intervention development in this area is the diversity of sexual-economic exchange patterns that have been labeled "prostitution." In this chapter, we present a conceptual framework developed to assist in the design and implementation of population-based plans for AIDS education among the persons involved as sellers, buyers, or administrators/managers of commercial sexual services in diverse socio-cultural and economic settings. Although the strategy applies equally to male and female prostitution, our focus here is on female prostitution.

AIDS and Women's Reproductive Health
Edited by L.C. Chen *et al.*, Plenum Press, New York, 1991

REGIONAL EPIDEMIOLOGIC DIFFERENCES

Worldwide, the most prevalent mode of HIV transmission is through sexual intercourse. Whereas in the Western industrial countries (ICs) of Europe, North America, and Australia/New Zealand the HIV/AIDS epidemic was first identified among men who have sex with men, in many parts of the world the virus is most often sexually transmitted from men to women and from women to men. This pattern of HIV transmission, which, by extension, leads to relatively high rates of perinatal transmission, has come to be called "Pattern II" (2). It is found primarily in the developing countries (DCs) of Africa and the Caribbean, where heterosexual transmission is estimated to account for 80% of all HIV infections (2).

All unprotected sexual relations convey a serious health risk in the age of AIDS. There are, however, especially strong epidemiological and social reasons for directing a portion of AIDS prevention resources towards both female commercial sex workers (women in prostitution) and their customers (3,4,5,6,7,8). The women who "sell" sexual services and the men who "buy" them are at high risk of acquiring and transmitting HIV and other STDs (e.g., 3-6,9,10,11,12). Since both female commercial sex workers (FCSWs) and their clients have non-commercial sexual partners as well, people involved in commercial sex are implicated in the dissemination of infection in the heterosexual population at large (e.g., 4,5,6,13,14).

It is important to note that in Pattern I countries, rates of HIV infection among sex workers who do not inject drugs have been low, as have risks of transmission or acquisition of HIV through commercial sex (7,13). Until recently, attention has focused on prostitution and AIDS in Pattern II countries, where research has documented rapid increases in HIV prevalence among both FCSWs and heterosexuals in the population at large (e.g., 3,4,10,12,16-18). In countries such as Mexico, where the prevalence of HIV in the general population is still low at present (19), prompt interventions among FCSWs and clients may avert the tragic experience of some cities in central and East Africa, where HIV prevalence now exceeds 80% in selected samples of commercial sex workers, and exceeds 20% in the most sexually active age group (age 20-39) in the general population in locales hardest hit by the HIV/AIDS epidemic (e.g., 15,20,21).

PROGRESS TO DATE IN INTERVENTIONS

The first wave of AIDS interventions concerned with prostitution has had encouraging results, but leaves no room for complacency. In a number of socio-economic and cultural settings, women engaged in prostitution have proved eager to learn about AIDS and how to avoid it (e.g., 7,8,14,22-34). It is now rare to find reports of a sex worker population that is not well apprised of the risks of AIDS and of the protective value of condom use. By conventional measures of health program impact, several interventions have been extremely successful, achieving increases of 50% or more of the principal target behavior: condom use (e.g., 24,30,32). Although few programs have reported formal evaluation results, it is clear that many have been successful in the use of group discussions, one-on-one counseling, and peer education to increase motivation and impart skills for condom use, and reduce misconceptions about HIV transmission that persist despite high levels of knowledge about the existence of AIDS (22,24,25,28,30,34).

On the down side, starting rates of condom use in most studies have been so low (usually fewer than 10% of women report frequent client acceptance or use) that even after doubling or tripling the target behavior, rates still reflect partial, part-time, and/or inconsistent protection. While such results do impact the aggregate probability of HIV transmission and/or acquisition, they still leave individual FCSWs and clients at a grossly elevated risk. Projects producing much higher and more consistent rates of condom use are needed to stem the spread of the virus in these and other populations.

The persistence of risk-reducing behavior change is also not a foregone conclusion. Some investigators have observed a decline over time in the effectiveness of interventions. Brooke

Schoepf and colleagues (34) reported a precipitous fall-off of condom use among sex workers in Kinshasa, when news of the book *The Myth of Heterosexual Transmission* (35) reached their university student clientele. Decay in intervention effect is certainly not unique to FCSWs or to the AIDS prevention (1), but more longitudinal research to investigate causes of relapse or continuation of safer sex practices among sex workers is badly needed.

Several studies have indicated that FCSWs are less likely to use condoms with regular customers than with strangers (8,14,29,36,37,38). It is important to note that, in many settings, regular customers comprise a substantial proportion of FCSWs' clientele (e.g., 37,39,40). In addition, many studies have found that even FCSWs who use condoms consistently with their paying customers often do not do so with their lovers, husbands, or other non-commercial sexual partners (26,27,36,38,40,41,42). In regions where HIV prevalence is high among intravenous drug users (IVDUs) and where sex workers may use IV drugs or have steady (non-paying) partners who do so, FCSWs may be achieving little personal protection through condom use only in professional contexts. In commercial and personal sexual relations, women frequently report male resistance as the key reason for lack of condom use in sexual relations (8,14,23-25,29,33,36,41,42,43). Yet research by family planning programs has shown that women, too, have fears and concerns (e.g., that condoms will "get stuck" in the vagina) that dampen their commitment to condom use (e.g.,44).

To the concern of some advocates from both liberal and conservative ends of the political spectrum, few AIDS interventions among FCSWs have tried risk reduction strategies other than the promotion of condom use. In stark contrast to public health and social welfare campaigns of the past (e.g., 45,46), efforts to force or help women to find safer work, and other tactics that would reduce FCSWs' potential exposure to persons with HIV/STDs, have been scarce (e.g., 47,48). (Programs to "reform" or "redeem" sex workers through religious conversion, or by providing them with alternative employment, residences, and other resources, have, of course, existed for centuries [45,46,49].)

Perhaps interventions to mitigate economic pressures toward sex work are deemed too expensive to attempt; or perhaps it is politically difficult to justify education or employment services for FCSWs during an era when entire populations are in need of these oppportunities. Still, a variety of alternative intervention targets and tactics are conceivable, including many that have been ignored or passed over in programs that focus on condom promotion. Table 1 lists a range of such intervention targets and strategies, and Table 2 lists a range of different formats in which various combinations of targets have been or could be addressed. The cost estimates in Table 2 are hypothetical, for few studies have attempted to measure cost effectiveness empirically (but e.g., 24). Even fewer projects have made serious attempts to reach the clients of FCSWs (14), although there are notable examples demonstrating that it is possible to do so (30,50,51,52). The paucity of intervention efforts directed toward clients is striking because FCSWs so frequently report that client resistance is the biggest deterrent to condom use in the commercial setting. Furthermore, qualitative studies have encountered numerous reports of the weak negotiating position of most FCSWs, which makes it difficult or impossible for them to refuse a client who refuses to accept condom use (8,14,36,43,53).

SOCIAL VERSUS BEHAVIORAL DEFINITIONS OF PROSTITUTION

Efforts to estimate the prevalence of HIV among FCSWs and promote protective behaviors, such as condom use, among FCSWs and their clients have been complicated by numerous factors. Not the least of these is the fact that commercial sex is covert, if not illegal, in most countries, making both FCSWs and their clients reluctant to talk freely about their trade — especially to outsiders identified with public institutions. Also important is the geographical mobility of FCSWs, which imposes difficulties for studies involving follow-up of individuals. Furthermore, in urban areas of any size, the settings and practices of commercial sex work are rarely homoge-

Table 1. Six types of objectives for AIDS interventions for commercial sex workers.

   I.   Provide Information*
           re. HIV/AIDS
           re. STDs, consequences, and proper treatment
           re. Safer sex
           re. Strategies for reducing no. of clients

  II. Change Attitudes and Motivate Behavior Change*, e.g., by stressing such goals as:
           Protect fertility
           Protect child welfare
           Protect family
           Protect non-commercial partners
           Avoid costs of STDs or AIDS

 III. Build Skills*
           Effective safer sex skills (e.g., correct use of condoms)
           Negotiation with clients, other partners, and/or managers
           Recognition of STDs (high-risk clients)
           Protection against injury
           Erotization of condom use

 IV.   Reduce Economic Pressure towards Commercial Sex
           Provide income-generating alternatives for FCSW
           Improve money management and savings*
           Raise price charged per client
           Increase "class" of clients served
           Decrease proportion of earnings paid to managers and others
           Increase use of contraception (avoid additional dependents)
           Assist with housing and education
           Provide vocational training
           Assist in finding employment

  V. Improve Condom Supply
           Increase reliability and amount of supply
           Decrease costs
           Facilitate access (supply in FCSW meeting places)
           Improve quality and/or packaging

 VI. Treat STDs
           Diagnose and refer sex workers and/or clients to existing clinics for Rx
           Diagnose and treat sex workers and/or clients
           Establish routine, voluntary, anonymous, free STD screening and treatment

    *Likely focus of ARHN intervention trial

---

neous (8,14,29,36,42,54). Beyond these obvious problems in describing and reaching a marginalized population, there are serious questions about the conceptual definition of prostitution as an epidemiologically, as well as socially, significant category (54,55).

    The spectrum of sexual-economic exchange ranges from conventional marriage, in which long-term economic obligations and social relationships among kin groups accompany the sexual contract, to impersonal, brief sexual contracts between strangers, paid for in advance at an agreed unit price. Boundaries on this spectrum — from relations that are valued and deemed moral to those that are not —are not objective or self-evident, and vary by culture and class (e.g., 14,34,36,43,54,55,56). Empirical evidence complicates definitions and counters stereotypes of participants in commercial sex; both "buyers" and "sellers" of sex have proved difficult to characterize. Participants in commercial sex tend to span the cultural and socio- economic spectrum characteristic of the locale in question. In their review of literature concerning sexual relations in sub-Saharan Africa, for example, Caldwell, Caldwell and Quiggen observed:

Table 2. Possible types and cost-intensiveness of intervention formats.

Relative Cost per Person	Intervention Format	Intervention Goals Compatible With Format
$	Distribution of tailored print materials (e.g., pamphlets, photo novelas)	a)Promote awareness b)Provide information (limited) c)Modify attitudes
$$	Group education sessions (questions and answers with or without materials)	a, b, c, plus d)Correct misconceptions e)Suggest individualized strategies to meet goals, handle problems, etc. f)Promote inter-FCSW/client communication, mutual support and self-help
$$*	Tailored video	a, b, c, plus partial d, e, and f
$$$	Small-group work-shops (e.g., 4 to 8 hours)	a, b, c, d, e, and f plus g)Teach new skills h)Provide role-playing practice i)Train trainers
$$$$	Repeat individual counselling and/or social work	a, b, c, d, g, e, and j)Provide emotional support k)Provide assistance with continued problem solving l)Provide job placement and follow-up

*The cost of such videos will be modest only if a single video is appropriate and effective for a large audience. If class, age, ethnic, regional, and other differences require production of many videos for finely segmented audiences, the cost effectiveness of video strategies will be greatly reduced.

If a prostitute is a female who sells sex commercially, charging standard rates on the spot on each occasion, dealing for the most part with strangers and making no emotional commitment, and often operating from group commercial premises or a brothel that is primarily used for this purpose, then many of the women tested at clinics treating sexually transmitted diseases and described as "prostitutes" in reports are probably not being accurately named (55).

In recent studies, the definition of a prostitute as "someone who provides sexual services in exchange for money or goods" is widely used. This definition hinges on a criterion that is of no direct epidemiological importance: whether or not valuables change hands. Furthermore, it omits the social and behavioral criteria that differentiate prostitution from sexual-economic relations such as concubinage, and multiply risk of exposure to HIV: frequency of partner change; frequency of sexual intercourse; protective and/or harmful sexual practices; and exposure to or infection with other sexually transmitted diseases (54).

In this chapter, our focus is specifically on commercial sex work. The key criterion here is selection or acceptance of partners according to their ability to pay, without reference to rules governing normative social relations, and without explicit or implicit commitment for continued sexual or social relations. (The high frequency of partner change among FCSWs is directly related to this psycho-social aspect of sex work [54]). Thus, in this chapter we will not address the various informal multiple-partner sexual relations that may arise in the context of normative sexual relationships and that also imply risk of HIV acquisition or transmission.

DIVERSITY IN SEX WORK

Since norms of propriety and male and female sexual behavior are culturally constructed, major differences are observed in the values attached to the multiple-partner sexual relations that convey health risk. An international perspective has thrown some of these differences into high relief (see 36 for a condensed review). Consider, for example, the large urban centers of New York, Connecticut, or New Jersey, USA, where prostitution systems extend from the unorganized exchange of sex for crack cocaine in abandoned buildings (e.g., 29,43); to "street work," in which meetings and negotiations over services and cost takes place on public streets (37,50); to escort services, to which affluent clients may pay several hundred dollars for an evening of companionship in which sexual services may or may not be implicit in the contract (57). Consider, then, the range of commercial sexual exchanges — from "substitute wives" to bar girls, to street workers — that has been described by Louise White (58) and Nici Nelson (56) in Nairobi, Kenya. Although all of these types of people, places, and practices may be classified as pertaining to commercial sex, this common denominator is of little practical use. For purposes of intervention design, efforts to extract or identify objective, overt hallmarks, or the "essence," of prostitution miss the point (54). The real challenge is to understand and represent the diversity of situations and actors involved in commercial sex practices, and to develop a typology that disaggregates sites or populations with internally homogeneous and external distinct intervention needs.

Available typologies of female commercial sex work have called attention to regional differences (14,36) and to diversity in the types of work settings and services provided, and in the price or "class" of FCSWs and services (e.g., 29,42,58,59). Work settings, or "workplaces," refer principally to differences in the manner or place in which sellers and buyers find one another and conduct their sexual transactions. Some FCSWs work in or on the street (i.e., meet clients in designated public locations); others work at home, soliciting clients from their windows, or through advertising of various sorts. Still others find their customers in bars or nightclubs; others work in saunas, massage parlors, brothels, hotels, or other settings. Each national and regional location can be expected to have a unique configuration of types of commercial sex workplaces. The social and economic dynamics governing commercial sexual transactions may well vary across workplaces with superficially similar characteristics. For example, in terms of sexual behavior, singles bars in American cities may resemble "bar prostitution" in other locales, yet the two have rather different social and economic meanings. In specific areas of Addis Ababa, Mexico City, Nairobi, and New York City, FCSWs and clients solicit one another on the street. In New York City and Mexico City, street work is tightly managed by third parties (pimps or representatives of the FCSWs). In Addis Ababa and Nairobi, this kind of exploitation and/or management is not typical (60).

This diversity suggests that classification of commercial sex in colloquial "workplace" terms does not provide an adequate basis for transnational intervention prescriptions for FCSWs and their clients. What is needed is a way to describe and evaluate the following factors that more proximally affect the types and roles of actors, and their abilities to alter risk behavior in the sex work context:

• variations in meeting place (e.g, public or private; distant from, near, or on the sex site)
• variations in the facilities in which sexual services are rendered (e.g., automobile, room with or without facilities for bathing; room with or without safety features, such as alarms to control risk of abuse)
• variations in the degree of control the FCSW has over her own work (e.g., work schedule, client acquisition rate, selection of clients) and over specific encounters
• variations in the price FCSWs charge for services, and in the proportion of that sum that FCSWs surrender to others
• variations in the type(s) of services provided (i.e., types of sexual practices and other services expected)
• variations in the sexual culture and social meanings of commercial sex

In addition to these "professional" factors, of course, the amount of economic pressure or need perceived by the FCSW has an overarching impact on the FCSW's motivation and options in sex work.

In summary, the label "prostitution" has obscured important variations among FCSWs and clients within, as well as across, countries. The veneer of the universal and the familiar has obscured the profound diversity in sexual-economic exchange relations and notions about the nature and meaning of prostitution. Interventions that hinge on these conditions and meanings can not be uncritically transported from one cultural context or country to another (36,54,61,62). Because the diversity in sex work has been glossed over, more work needs to be done to "segment the market" for AIDS and reproductive health interventions that aim to reach persons with high-risk sexual behavior. In the remainder of this chapter we present a framework that we have developed for organizing research around the types and extent of heterogeneity in commercial sex work and the significance of this heterogeneity for intervention programs.

MODELS FOR INTERVENTION DEVELOPMENT

Identifying Modifiable Determinants of Prostitution

Whether the objective is to reduce participation in sex work, or to make participation safer for FCSWs and their clients, decades of research in the health and social sciences make clear that interventions should be based on some understanding of why high-risk behaviors occur (e.g., 1,63,64). Identifying the range of modifiable determinants of health risks, a routine public health strategy, has received relatively little attention in the prostitution and AIDS field. One possible explanation for this gap is the widespread assumption that these determinants are already known, and are unmodifiable (6,27,36). Drives for sexual release or sexual variety have often been assumed to be essential and natural male characteristics, irreducible constants producing an inevitable market for commercial sex (for contrasting views, see 54,56,66,67).

Research and debate about the "supply side" of prostitution go back over a hundred years in the social scientific, medical, and criminological literature of the West, as scholars tried to discern why women — idealized in Western intellectual circles as being "above the passions" — would participate in meeting this demand (45,49,65,68,69). Many of these analyses stressed explanations such as deviant sexuality, psychiatric illness, or victimization by economic need. Such theories have often proved simplistic, for as noted previously, empirical studies tend to find a broad spectrum of individuals in, and diverse paths to, prostitution.

While examining paths to prostitution is of great importance, our interest here is in the motivations and constraints for continuing to engage in sex work, and for learning about, adopting, or ignoring safety measures. These determinants include personal and environmental factors. The

Table 3. Classes of determinants of sexual risk reduction behavior among FCSWs.

I. Personal Determinants

      Perceived economic needs
      Role expectations and obligations
      Emotional attachments
      Personal domestic history
      Family context
      Health beliefs and behaviors
      Age
      Education
      Appearance
      Skills
      Personality, personal style

II. Environmental Determinants

  A. Professional determinants

      Degree of public exposure (e.g., street work, vs. indoors)
      Client selection process
      Types of facilities used
      Degree of individual autonomy
      Price charged per service
      Power of managers or clients to enforce work levels or practices upon the FCSW
      Safety features (e.g., provision of STD services, protections against client abuse, against
        manager abuse)
      Camaraderie, learning, and social support among FCSW
      Relations with authorities
      Degree of competition among FCSW and/or across groups of female and/or male CSW in the setting

  B. Contextual determinants

      Sexual culture of FCSW and their clients
      Degree of stigma associated with commercial sex
      Norms for gender relations
      Criteria for prestige and power
      Housing and employment opportunities for women
      Availability of health services
      Health beliefs of FCSW and their clients
      Availability and price of condoms
      Legal and policy status of commercial sex

---

latter category can be further divided to distinguish professional (workplace) influences from broader contextual influences that transcend prostitution settings (Table 3). Personal determinants include perceived economic needs; role expectations and obligations; emotional attachments; personal domestic history and family context; health beliefs and behaviors; and the individual's age, education, appearance, and skills. Professional determinants deal with those constraints upon individual FCSWs and clients that are a function of the type of workplace, or setting in which they work. The price a woman can charge per service; the ability of managers or others to impose quotas or to require particular practices; the degree of safety from threats or abuse by clients and/or managers; and the degree of isolation or sociability permitted and/or customary among FCSWs in the same workplace vary according to the type of workplace and the norms for that type in the given locale. Contextual determinants refer to broader societal factors ranging from the sexual, cultural, and socio-cultural norms for gender relations; to housing and employment opportunities; availability of health services; and the legal and policy status of commercial sex.

These factors are important because they affect FCSWs' and clients' motivations to engage in commercial sex; their motivations to engage in AIDS-protective behaviors; their access to resources needed for health protection (e.g., condoms, STD treatment); and the power dynamics between FCSWs and clients when conflicts of interest arise. Development of interventions should take into account these differences in both the personal and the environmental determinants of risky or protective behavior. The challenge now is to assemble information on the multiple actors and determinants of commercial sexual exchange into program guidelines that provide sufficient diversity to respond to the needs of the diverse circumstances and actors in the system.

Assessing Intervention Needs

Intervention program effectiveness depends upon achieving the appropriate content, format, and delivery system over the appropriate period(s) of time. If programs can fail from provision of inappropriate messages or services, it follows that planning effective services requires substantial knowledge of the targeted population(s). Decades of health education and communications work (1,70) indicate that education about the benefits of health behavior changes will be ineffective if the target audience does not understand the educational materials and does not consider the problem personally significant. Even if appreciated and understood, recommendations for health behavior change will be ineffective if the targeted individuals lack the means to adopt the preventive action, or if those recommendations conflict with strong perceived needs and/or environmental pressures.

Experience in the AIDS education field is congruent with the Health Belief Model (70) or one of its several sequellae (e.g., the AIDS Risk Reduction Model [64]). The Health Belief Model states that information about a health threat and its prevention is usually a necessary but not sufficient precondition for behavior change. Members of the target audience must consider the information personally relevant to them; consider the condition under discussion serious enough to warrant action; believe the proposed remedy or action will provide benefits of significant value; and judge that the costs of the health improvement strategy are worth bearing in order to achieve the predicted result (70). This suggests that appropriate recommendations to reduce sexual risk behavior will be those based on an understanding of the perceptions and determinants of risky behaviors in selected setting, and on a realistic picture of the resources that FCSWs and their clients have to support lower-risk alternatives.

Sexual risk behavior differs from many other unhealthy behaviors (e.g., sedentarism) in that it is interpersonal (71).* Recommendations for change can not be undertaken by half the sexual dyad without affecting and being affected by the other half. Moreover, in most locales, systems of female prostitution involve women providing sexual and other services for a fee, men buying those services, and various additional mediators (e.g., pimps), beneficiaries (e.g., rooming-house owners), and authorities (e.g., police). Since at least five classes of actors are involved in commercial sex, each with a different power position and interests, we postulate that interventions focused only on FCSWs are more likely to fail than are interventions that address all the key actors in the exchange (8,14). In settings where sex work is largely conducted independent of managers or other intermediaries, reaching FCSWs and clients may suffice. In settings where client access and/or FCSW actions are monitored and controlled by others, these mediators, beneficiaries, and authorities may be key targets for intervention.

Serious ethical dilemmas are raised by the involvement in intervention programs of third parties who exploit FCSWs. The objective of HIV/STD interventions is to prevent HIV/STD acquisition and transmission, not to affect the business of third parties. Rather than seek a uniform rule for resolving the surrounding dilemmas, the specific nature of the FCSW-"manager" relationship must be considered. For example, some "managers" train, promote, and protect "their" FCSWs, while others manipulate, extort, and abuse the women whose work they control. It will be less ethically perilous, and easier, to work with the former type of "manager" than the latter.

---

*The individual focus of health behavior change has probably been overrated with respect to many health problems. Smoking affects the environment of others, and radical changes in diet are very difficult for one household member to make without affecting the food preparation and diet of others in the household.

Methods for Intervention Strategy Development

Along with others (8,14,36), we have argued that prostitution is a complex system involving multiple sub-populations, actors, and types of settings within each country and city. In large urban areas, there is heterogeneity in the supply, demand, and settings of prostitution. The multiple actors involved, and the stigmatized or illegal status of the trade, make it particularly difficult to target FCSWs for research and interventions. This is made clear by the experiences of intervention projects to date. What remains debatable is whether a variegated, population-based research and intervention strategy to define and respond to the heterogeneous commercial sex market is feasible and/or worth the time, cost and effort needed to develop it.

The extent to which intervention strategies and materials can be usefully transferred across sub-populations or settings is currently unknown. As illustrated in Tables 1 and 2, intervention strategies can differ in many ways, not only in the language and packaging of materials, but also in the fundamental objectives and format of intervention delivery. Experience in the health education field suggests that materials have rather low transferability. On the other hand, we should be able to derive analytically the determinants of success or failure of intervention objectives and strategies through application of existing social and behavioral science data and theory (such as the Health Belief Model and theories concerning gender relations, sexuality, self perception and motivation, and the political economy of health). The strategies that prove most cost-effective over time for mitigating the health risks of commercial sex will be contingent upon the socio-economic, cultural, and political context as much as they will reflect attention to the participants in, and organization of, particular sex work settings. Information on the personal characteristics of FCSWs (much less measurement of known risk factors) is unlikely to suffice to guide program development. Information is needed on the environmental (workplace and context) determinants of commercial sex work as well.

The development of such an analytic framework requires several steps: compiling existing knowledge about the range of actors and workplaces implicated in commercial sex work; segmenting the commercial sex work system in terms of the significant educational, cultural, and socio-economic differences among participants that affect their intervention needs; setting priorities for intervention resource allocation in terms of rates of disease acquisition and transmission and/or likelihood of successful intervention; and implementing and evaluating services with the help of target audiences.

The integration of qualitative and quantitative methods is essential in every phase of this endeavor. There is ample evidence for the importance of local, culturally constructed values and meanings in the shaping of sexual feelings and practices, in definitions of prostitution, and in the multiple needs and values that promote and discourage multiple sexual partner relations and commercial sexual-economic exchanges (e.g., 29,34,36,43,54,55,56,58,59,61,72). These can only be explored and explained through qualitative methods, such as participant observation, open-ended interviews, and focus groups. Harnessing this qualitative information and assessing its generality and importance requires systematic sampling and survey methodologies. Quantitative methods are also required to measure the prevalence of HIV/STD morbidity and mortality and provide representative measures of program impact.

To our knowledge, while heterogeneity in commercial sex work is now widely recognized, programs to date have not attempted a population-based approach to interventions for FCSWs, or planned a range of treatment choices for diverse actors in the FCSW system. Shortfalls in program impact up to now may have been due to ineffective models, or to effective models applied to the wrong population(s).

CONCLUSION

Encouraging results are currently emerging from pilot HIV/STD interventions with FCSWs in every corner of the globe. These can only be extended and fortified by systematically matching interventions to FCSW and client needs and to the perceptions and roles of other actors who play parts in the particular prostitution system. Preliminary findings from Aids and Reproductive Health Network (ARHN) research on FCSWs in Mexico City confirm that no single intervention model, no matter how carefully or elaborately designed, can efficiently meet the education and support needs of such a diverse population (see chapter 15 in this volume).

As service providers in other locations plan to expand successful intervention programs and launch new ones with broader coverage, they will confront the diversity in sex work in their locales, and will need to reach for different models. For example, a successfull pilot program for street workers in Bangkok might be scaled up to reach all FCSWs in the region who work in comparable street settings, but entirely different models may be needed to reach FCSWs and their clients in the city's saunas, massage parlors, and tourist hotels. Whether or not the same mix of models will work in Chiang Rai or another urban Thai area will, we predict, depend on the degree to which the items listed in Table 3 are similar or different in specific sex workplaces in the two locales.

As the next generation of intervention projects increasingly attends to features listed in Tables 1, 2, and 3, health educators will be able to draw more easily and systematically on the experiences of colleagues in other locales. This implies preceding intervention development within an analysis of the range of actors and sex workplaces observed in the target area and the operative personal, professional, and contextual determinants of intervention needs in each local sex work setting. With these specifics in mind, program planners will be able to select and adapt a set of intervention models that identify and respond to the diverse needs of their heterogeneous target population, addressing personal-level and professional-level determinants of risk behavior within the broader socio-cultural context. Such efforts to see beyond individual intervention projects and populations, and to interpret appropriately and build on the experiences of others working in AIDS education today, are key challenges for the 1990s in the AIDS and reproductive health fields.

Acknowledgments

The research for this paper was supported by grants from the Mexican Ministry of Health, the U.S. National Institutes of Health, and the American Foundation for AIDS Research through the AIDS and Reproductive Health Network. We gratefully acknowledge the technical contributions made by Martha Lamas, Victor Ortiz, and Laura Elena de Caso, and the expert assistance of Miriam Gomez and Gloria D. Williams in the preparation of the manuscript.

REFERENCES

1. Sisk JE, Hewitt M, Metcalf KL, Behney, CJ. *How effective is AIDS education?* Washington: Health Program Office of Technology Assessment, 1988.
2. Piot P, Plummer F, Mhalu FS, Lamboray JL, Chin J, Mann J. AIDS: An international perspective. *Science* 1988; 239:573-579.
3. Kreiss JK, Koech D, Plummer FA et al. AIDS virus infection in Nairobi prostitutes. *N Engl J Med* 1986; 314:414-418.
4. Piot P, Kreiss JK, Ndinya-Achola JO, Ngugi EN, Simonsen JN, Cameron DW, Trelnar H, Plummer, FA. Editorial Review: Heterosexual transmission of HIV. *AIDS* 1987; 1:199-206.
5. Carael M, Van de Perre P, Allen S, Clumeck N, Butzler, JP. Sexually active young adults in central Africa. In: *AIDS in children, adolescents, and heterosexual adults*, edited by Schinazi RF and Nahmias, AJ. New York: Elsevier, 1988, p. 346-349.
6. Shelton JD, Harris JR. Role of condoms in combatting global AIDS: The application of Suttons' law to public health. In: *Heterosexual transmission of AIDS*, edited by Alexander NJ, Gabelnick HL, Spieler JM. New York: Wiley-Liss, 1990, p. 327-337.

7. Rosenberg MJ, Weiner JM. Prostitutes and AIDS: A health department priority? *American Journal of Public Health* 1988; 78(4):418-423.

8. Biersteker S. Promoting safer sex in protitution: Impedents and opportunities. In: *Promoting safer sex*, edited by Paalman M. Amsterdam: Swets & Zeitlinger, 1990, p. 144-152.

9. Giordano M, Pape J, Blattner W, Johnson WD. The seroprevalence of HTLV-1 and HIV-1 co-infection in Haiti. V International Conference on AIDS, Montreal, Canada. Abstract M.G.P.3.

10. Piot P, Ngugi EN, Rouzioux C. Retrospective seroepidemiology of AIDS virus infection in Nairobi populations. *Journal of Infectious Disease* 1987; 155:1108-1112.

11. Piot P, Taelman H, Minlangu KB. Acquired immunodeficiency syndrome in a heterosexual population in Zaire. *Lancet* 1984; II:65-69.

12. Mann J, Neilambi N, Piot P, N'galy B, Mpunga K. HIV infection and associated risk factors in female prostitutes in Kinshasa, Zaire. *AIDS* 1988; 2:249-254.

13. Haverkos H, Edelman R. Heterosexuals. In: *The epidemiology of AIDS: Expressions, occurrence and control of human immunodeficiency virus type I infection*, edited by Kaslow R and Francis D. New York: Oxford Press, 1988, p. 136-152.

14. WHO, Consensus statement from the consultation on HIV epidemiology and prostitution.*Weekly Epidemiologic Record* 1989; 49(8):377-382.

15. Konde-Lule JI, Berkley SF, Downing R. Knowledge, attitudes and practices concerning AIDS in Ugandans. *AIDS* 1989; 3(8).

16. de Lalla F, Rizzardini G, Santoro D, Galli M. Rapid spread of HIV infection in a rural district in Central Africa. *AIDS* 1988; 2:317-321.

17. Chiphangwi J, Keller M, Wirama J. Prevalence of HIV-1 infection in pregnant women in Malawi. IV International Conference on AIDS, Stockholm, Sweden, 1988; Abstract 324.2.

18. Odehouri K, De Cock KM, Krebs JW, Moreau J et al. HIV-1 and HIV-2 infection associated with AIDS in Abidjan, Côte d'Ivoire. *AIDS* 1989; 3(8):509-12.

19. Sepulveda-Armor J, Valdespino JL, Garcia ML, Izazola JA, Rico B. Caracteristicas epidemiologicas y cognositivas de la transmission del VIH en Mexico.*Salud Publica de Mexico* 1988; 30:513-527.

20. Chiphangwi J, Dllabeta G, Saah A, Liomba G, Miotti P. Risk factors for HIV infection in pregnant women in Malawi. VI International Conference on AIDS, San Francisco, CA, 1990. (Abstract).

21. Killewo J, Nyamuryekunge K, Sandstrom A, Bredberg-Raden U, Wall S, Mhalu F, Biberfeld G. Prevalence of HIV-1 infection in the Kagera region of Tanzania: a population-based study. *AIDS* 1990; 4:1081-1085.

22. Stephens CP, Hayes BJ, Adams R, Gross M. Women working as prostitutes; anticipatory/concensus-based planning for provision of mobile prevention, risk reduction, and seroprevalence activities. V International Conference on AIDS, Montreal, Canada, 1989. (Abstract).

23. Wilson D, Chiroro P, Lavelle S, Mutero C. Sex worker client sex behavior and condom use in Harare. *AIDS Care* 1989; 1(3):269-280.

24. Ngugi EN, Plummer FA, Simonsen JN, Cameron DW, Bosire M, Waiyaki P, Ronald AR, Ndinya-Achola JO. Prevention of transmission of human immunodeficiency virus in Africa: Effectiveness of condom promotion and health education among prostitutes. *Lancet* 1988; 15:887-890.

25. Monny-Lobe M, Nichols D, Zekeng L, Salla R , Kaptue L. Prostitutes as health educators for their peers in Yaounde: Changes in knowledge, attitudes and practices. V International Conference on AIDS, Montreal, Canada, 1989. (Abstract).

26. Aim G, de Vincenzi I, Ancelle-Park R, Brunet Jean-B, Catalan F. HIV infection in French prostitutes. *AIDS* 1989; 3(11):767-768.

27. Wofsy CR AIDS and prostitution. In: *AIDS in children, adolescents and heterosexual adults*, edited by Schinazi RF and Nahmias AJ. New York: Eslevier, 1988, p. 168-169.

28. Lamptey P, Neequays A, Weir S, Potts M. A model program to reduce HIV infection among prostitutes in Africa. IV International Conference on AIDS, Stockholm, Sweden, 1988. (Abstract).

29. Shedlin M G. An ethnographic approach to understanding high-risk behaviors: Prostitution and drug abuse. In: *AIDS and intravenous drug use: Future directions for community-based prevention research*, edited by Leukefeld CG, Battjes RJ, Amsel Z. Washington: Government Printing Office, 1990, p. 134-149.

30. Williams E, Efem S, Weir S, Lanson N, Lamptey P. Implementation of an AIDS intervention program in the Cross River state of Nigeria. Paper presented at the USAID AIDS mini-conference, Rosslyn, Virginia, USA, February 5-6, 1990.

31. Suarez E, De la Rosa G, Welsh M, Ponce de Leon R. Community-based AIDS prevention in Cuidad Juarez. VI International Conference on AIDS, San Francisco, CA, 1990 (Abstract).

32. Sakondhavat C, Werawatakul Y, Bennet A. Promoting condom-only brothels through solidarity and support for brothel managers. VI International Conference on AIDS, San Francisco, California, 1991. Abstract W.D.53.

33. Herasme L, Pareja R, Bello A. Convincing clients to use condoms. AIDSCOM, Washington D.C., 1990.

34. Schoepf B, Rukarangira N, Walu E, Payanzo N. Action research on AIDS with women in central Africa. *Social Science and Medicine* (in press).

35. Fumento M. *Myth of Heterosexual transmission*. Basic Books: New York, 1990, pp. 404.

36. Day S. Prostitute women and AIDS: anthropology. *AIDS* 1988; 2:421-428.

37. Freund M, Leonard TL, Lee N. Sexual behavior of resident street prostitutes with their clients in Camden, New Jersey.*The Journal of Sex Research* 1989; 26(4):460-478.

38. Ortiz V, de Caso LE. Personal communication, Mexico City, November 1990.

39. McLeod E.*Women working: Prostitution now*. London: Croom Helm Ltd, 1982. pp. 1-177.

40. Sittitrai W. Personal communication, Bankok, Thailand, 1990.

41. Padian NS. Prostitute women and AIDS: Epidemiology. *AIDS* 1988; 2:413-419.

42. Hernandez Avila M, Zuñiga PU, de Zalduondo BO. Diversity in Commercial Sex Work Systems: Preliminary Findings from Mexico City and their Implications for for AIDS Interventions. Chapter 15 in this volume.

43. Worth D. Sexual decision-making and AIDS: why condom promotion among vulnerable women is likely to fail. *Studies in Family Planning* 1989; 20(6):297-307.

44. Allman J, Desse G, Rival A. Condom use in Haiti. Working paper for Center for Population and Family Health, Columbia University, New York, 1985.

45. Connelly MT *The response to prostitution in the progressive era*. Chapel Hill: University of North Carolina Press, 1980.

46. Walkowitz JR. Male vice and female virtue: Feminism and the politics of prostitution in nineteenth century Britain. In: *Powers of Desire. The Politics of Sexuality*. Snitow A, Stansell C, Thompson S, eds. New York: Monthly Review Press, 1991, pp. 419-438.

47. Abenia MC, Guerrero E, De Moya EA. The development of micro-enterprises as work alternatives for female sex workers in Dominican Republic. V International Conference on AIDS, Montreal, Canada, 1989. (Abstract).

48. Society for Women and AIDS in Africa (SWAA). Women and AIDS in Africa. Workshop report of the First Workshop on Women and Aids in Africa, Society for Women and AIDS in Africa (SWAA), Harare, Zimbabwe, 1989.

49. Bullough V, Bullough B.*Women and prostitution: A social history*. Buffalo, NY: Prometheus Books, 1987.

50. Leonard TL. Male clients of female street prostitutes: Unseen partners in sexual disease transmission. *Medical Anthropology Quarterly* 1990; 4(11):41-55.

51. Williams EE, Hearst N, Udofia O. Sexual practices and HIV infection of female prosti-

tutes in Nigeria. V International Conference on AIDS, Montreal, Canada, 1989. (Abstract).

52. Wallace J, Mann J, Beatrice S. HIV-1 exposure among clients of prostitutes. IV International Conference on AIDS, Stockholm, Sweden, 1988 (Abstract).

53. Sittitrai W, Brown T. Female commercial sex workers in Thailand, a preliminary report. VI International Conference on AIDS, San Francisco, CA, June 1990. (Abstract).

54. de Zalduondo, BO. Prostitution viewed cross-culturally: Toward recontextualizing sex work in AIDS intervention research.*The Journal of Sex Research* 1991; 28(2):223-248.

55. Caldwell JC, Caldwell P, Quiggin P. The social context of AIDS in sub-Saharan Africa. *Population and Development Review* 1989; 15(2):185-234.

56. Nelson N. Selling her kiosk: Kikuyu notions of sexuality and sex for sale in Mathare Valley, Kenya. In: *The cultural construction of sexuality*, edited by Caplan P. London: Tavistock Publications, 1987, p. 217-237.

57. Barrows SB *Mayflower madame*. New York: Arbor House, 1986.

58. White L. Prostitution, identity and class consciousness in Nairobi during World War II. *Signs* 1986; 11(21):255-273.

59. Sittitrai W. Commercial sex work in Thailand. Paper presented at the AIDS in Asia and Pacific Conference, Canberra, Australia, 1990.

60. Bishaw M. Commercial sex work in Ethiopia: History and current situation. Paper presented at the meeting of the AIDS and Reproductive Health Network, Bangkok, Thailand, January, 1990.

61. de Zalduondo BO, Msamanga GI, Chen LC. AIDS in Africa: Diversity in the global pandemic. *Daedalus* 1989; 118(3):165-204.

62. Parker R. Acquired immunodeficiency syndrome in urban Brazil. *Medical Anthropology Quarterly* 1987; 1(2):155-175.

63. O'Reilly K. Risk behaviors and their determinants. Paper delivered at the Annual Meeting of the American Academy for the Advancement of science, Boston, Massachusetts, 1988.

64. Catania JA, Kegeles SM, Coates TJ. Towards an understanding of risk behavior: an AIDS risk reduction model (ARRM). *Health Education Quarterly* Spring 1990; 17(1):53-72.

65. Caplan P. Introduction: Sex, sexuality, and gender. In: *The cultural construction of sexuality*, edited by Caplan P. London: Tavistock Publications, 1987, p. 1-30.

66. Symons D.*The evolution of human sexuality*, New York: Oxford University Press, 1979.

67. Potts M, Feldblum PJ.Changing behavior: Barrier methods in high-risk populations. In: *Heterosexual transmission of AIDS. Proceedings of the 2nd contraceptive research and development (CONRAD) program*, edited by Alexander NJ, Gabelnick HL and Spieler JM. New York: Wiley-Liss, 1989, p. 69-79.

68. Pomeroy WB. Some aspects of prostitution. *Journal of Sex Research* 1965; 1:177-187.

69. Hobson BM. *Uneasy virtue: The politics of prostitution and the American reform tradition*, New York: Basic Books, 1987.

70. Janz NK, Becker MH. The health belief model: A decade later. *Health Education Quarterly* 1984; 11(1):1-47.

71. Nathanson CA. Private behavior and personal control: Contraceptive management strategies of adolescent women. In: *Dangerous Passage. The social control of sexuality in women's adolescence*. Nathanson CA. Philadelphia: Temple University Press, 1991, pp. 178-204.

72. Schoepf BG, Nkera R w, Schoepf C, Engundu W, Ntsomo P. AIDS and society in Central Africa: A view from Zaire. In: *AIDS in Africa: The social and policy impact*, edited by Miller, N. and Rockwell, R.C. Mellon Press, 1988, p. 211-235.

DIVERSITY IN COMMERCIAL SEX WORK SYSTEMS: PRELIMINARY FINDINGS FROM MEXICO CITY AND THEIR IMPLICATIONS FOR AIDS INTERVENTIONS

Mauricio Hernandez Avila

Instituto Nacional de Salud Publica, Mexico

Patricia Uribe Zuniga

CONASIDA, Mexico

Barbara O. de Zalduondo

Johns Hopkins University

The Federal District (DF) of Mexico City is one of the largest cities in the world (area: 1,320 square kilometers; 1990 population: 15 million). As the national capital, it is a cosmopolitan commercial, cultural, and administrative center of national as well as international significance. Although spared by high altitude from a variety of tropical disease threats (such as dengue and malaria) that affect other regions of Mexico, the infant mortality rate for Mexico City is high: 37 per 1000 (1). The leading causes of death in the city are chronic diseases, injury, and infectious diseases (2). The city is a mosaic of residential, commercial, and industrial districts (it generates 27.4% of Mexico's GNP) (3) and of affluent and poor neighborhoods (*colonias*). Indeed, it presents in microcosm much of the national spectrum of educational, economic, and ethnic diversity.

The scale and diversity of Mexico City present unique challenges for health promotion and disease prevention. They highlight the urgent need for a diversified AIDS education strategy, not only in the capital, but throughout the country.

Female and male prostitution is well known to occur in diverse forms in Mexico City. Thus, the city provides a good testing ground for the conceptual framework and intervention strategy described by de Zalduondo and Hernandez in chapter 14 of this volume (4). Implementation of the intervention research has been expedited and strengthened by building upon the epidemiological surveillance and counseling service infrastructure of CONASIDA, Mexico's national AIDS prevention and control program, and upon the previous work of the General Directorate of Epidemiology (GDE).

The Mexico research team, comprised in large part of CONASIDA and GDE professional staff, is now in the first phase of implementing a multi-disciplinary, multi-site project, developed through the AIDS and Reproductive Health Network, to identify, assess and respond with appropriately tailored interventions to the AIDS and STD education and prevention needs of female commercial sex workers (FCSWs) and their clients in this diverse "market". Underway since 1990, phase I of the project comprises an integrated program of descriptive baseline research using ethnographic, focus group, and structured interview techniques. Analysis of these data and comparison across three sites (the other two are in Ethiopia and Thailand), will support development, pilot implementation, and evaluation of a varigated set of intervention approaches for FCSWs and other actors in the local commercial sex system.

BACKGROUND

The cultural history of commercial sex in Mexico is beyond the scope of this chapter. However, it is important to note that, in Mexico as in many other countries, ambivalence toward FCSWs has a long history (5). Records from Spanish missionaries, upon their arrival in ancient Mexico, described the presence of prostitutes in Nahua (indigenous Mexican) religious ceremonies, as well as in houses where high officials and warriors were frequent customers. While their roles were deemed important, most FCSWs were viewed as slaves, and/or were women who had been presented to the Nahua in tribute by other tribes (6). We can speculate that this history of marginal but legitimate commercial sex work was not entirely wiped out by the adoption of the Christian doctrine that strongly opposes extramarital sexual behavior. Rather, it is possible that this history may have contributed to the tolerance and elaboration of the prostitution system in Mexico over the subsequent four centuries.

In 1926, the Mexican Congress issued legislation governing the practice and control of commercial sex. This legislation required prostitutes to register and be licensed by the public health authorities, restricted their activities to certain areas and types of organizations, and required them to be inspected periodically by qualified physicians (7). In 1940, this body of legislation was overruled when Mexico City joined the international abolitionist movement that aimed to wipe out prostitution altogether, as opposed to regulating it. The abolitionist strategy was to eliminate prostitution by eliminating its economic attractions. Thus, in 1940, the practice of commercial sex was banned in Mexico City (8). Any individual who practiced commercial sex, according to law, was to be fined the equivalent of 15 to 30 days minimum wage or held in detention for 24 to 36 hours. This form of regulation was intended to make prostitution unprofitable so as to prevent the persecution and exploitation of women, who were assumed to be selling sex under duress. It also aimed to minimize the visibility of sex work, which, while considered unavoidable, was deemed offensive and immoral by the privileged classes (9).

Today, under this legislation, police continue to organize "round-ups" of women in the street in notorious areas from time to time. Arrests are allegedly made, not because of the suspicion of prostitution, but because the women's personal appearance is considered offensive to "modesty and good customs." In Mexico, as in other countries, men who solicit or purchase the services of sex workers are rarely arrested or prosecuted (9-11). In 1985, the Mexico City Household Survey on young adult reproductive health found that 6% of males aged 15-24 reported having their first sexual intercourse with a FCSW (n=1539) (12). The proportion of adults who are at least occasional clients of FCSWs is undoubtedly higher.

Other states in Mexico did not join the international abolitionist movement. In some states, the regulations of, or laws against, commercial sex work are more severe; in other states less so. Throughout Mexico, and from the earliest recorded times, most women in prostitution have had a marginal socio-cultural status. In Mexico City today, prostitution is tolerated and excused, but is neither legal nor condoned. This type of marginal status has often served to deprive FCSWs and clients of health information, health services, and legal protection of their constitutional rights. At the same time, it has done little or nothing to prevent entry into sex work or use of the services offered (13).

EPIDEMIOLOGY

Since 1983, the Mexican Ministry of Health has been conducting surveillance of HIV status among FCSWs through provision of free, voluntary, anonymous HIV testing and supportive counseling services at CONASIDA centers, and through sero-surveys at sites where commercial

Table 1. Demographic and other characteristics of 395 female commercial sex workers attending HIV-1 screening in Mexico City.*

Characteristic	No.	(%)
Married	20	(5.1)
Single	266	(68.4)
Divorced	34	(8.7)
Other	69	(17.8)
Currently living with father of her children	37	(12.8)
Housing (Proxy for income)		
rented	238	(64.5)
owned	92	(24.0)
other	41	(11.05)
Frequency of prostitution		
every day	193	(58.5)
3-4 times per week	105	(31.8)
1-2 times per week	25	(7.5)
less than 1 per week	7	(2.1)
Claims knowledge about AIDS		
yes	175	(49.3)
no	180	(50.7)
Now Using Family Planning Method:	202	(66.4)
Oral contraceptives 38A	80	
IUD 38B	43	(21.0)
Hormonal IM 38E	62	(32.0)
Spermicides 38C	1	(0.4)
Transfusion ever	33	(8.5)
Reported Hx of STD	No.	(%)
Gonorrhea 49-EV	42	(11.2)
Syphilis 50-1	3	(0.8)
Condiloma 50-2	21	(5.7)
HIV	4	(1.0)

* The total sample size differs between variables because of missing information.

sex takes place. In contrast to the rates among self-selected gay or bisexual men*, prevalence rates of HIV among self-identified FCSWs** who present themselves for testing have been remarkably low. All surveys have also reported a prevalence of HIV below 3% (14–17). Between 1984 and 1990, the CONASIDA staff has screened more than 2,000 FCSWs in the metropolitan area of Mexico City. Among these women, the reported prevalence of HIV has been 2%. Dr. Valdespino and co-workers from the GDE (15,17) have conducted several sero-surveys at work sites of FCSWs. They observed a prevalence of 0.3% HIV-positive among 613 women tested in 1987 and 1,384 women tested in 1988. These figures are comparable to the rates observed among FCSWs in other parts of the country (14,18,19). From the serum bank comprised of blood samples from the aforementioned 2,000 FCSWs, we screened a random sample of 678 for syphilis, where twelve percent (n=83) were positive by Veneral Disease Research Laboratories (VDRL) and confirmed by Fluorescent Treponemal Antibody Absorption (FTA-ABS) test.

The low prevalence of HIV among FCSWs is partly explained by its low prevalence in the background population (6 per 10,000), and the rarity of intravenous drug use in this population. The persistence of this low rate since 1984 contrasts with other settings where a precipitous increase among FCSWs has been observed since 1987. In Ethiopia and Thailand, for example, prevalence of HIV, while still low in the general population, has risen to over 30% in some FCSW samples in Ethiopia, and over 70% in some FCSW samples in northern Thailand. This has occurred during the same period in which the rate remained quite stable in Mexico (22,23).

More detailed data collected by CONASIDA in an expanded pre-test interview suggested that the results from Mexico do not reflect misclassification of low-risk women (Table 1). 58% of the 395 women who reported prostitution as their occupation reported selling sex on a daily basis, and another 30% work 3-4 days per week, serving an average 13.5 clients per week. In basic socio-demographic characteristics, the populations of self-referred women match closely those encountered in "on the job" worksite screening (17). The mean age of the women who sought testing was 26 years. Less than half completed elementary school (six years schooling), and while over half the women have children, only 12% are living with the father of their children. It is likely that these women do not represent the full spectrum of sex workers in Mexico City (see below). We believe that very low income FCSWs — perhaps the majority — are underrepresented in this self-selected population.

Relative to reports from U.S. and European samples (24–26), these Mexican FCSWs report a limited range of services (Table 2). Nearly all report that vaginal coitus is "always" performed; 89% "never" perform oral sex with clients. The low reported rates of anal intercourse (97% "never" engage in anal intercourse with clients) are not surprising in light of findings elsewhere (30). 72% of the FCSWs report having changed their behavior since learning of AIDS; among those, 87% report an increase in condom use. Low rates of reported STD history suggest that these women's relative freedom from STDs predates their awareness of AIDS. Especially striking is the fact that 83% of these women report "always" using condoms in coitus with clients.

In contrast to their behavior in "professional" contacts, 85% of the women report "never" using condoms in sex with their lovers or husbands. Thus, in Mexico, as in many other sites where FCSWs have been studied, the contrast between personal and professional sexual relations is pronounced in behavior and in meaning. It is important to note that most of these Mexican FCSWs report a lifetime number of personal sexual partners that is well within the range of the general population (28), for which abstinence from pre-marital sex and lifelong female monogamy are cultural ideals. In contrast to the inferences of the psychological theories about FCSWs that were popular in the 1950s (5,10,29), focus group data from comparable Mexican FCSWs suggest that here, as elsewhere (e.g., 26,30), women in prostitution emotionally com-

---

* GDE studies have encountered rates from 0-30% HIV-seropositive in urban samples of self-referred gay and bisexual men, and from 9-16% among male CSWs (21).

**All testing center clients are asked their occupation as well as their sexual histories. Women who report prostitution as their occupation are categorized as an FCSW.

Table 2. Sexual behavior and other characteristics of 395 female commercial sex workers in Mexico City.*

Practice/Behavior	With Clients No. (%)	With Non-Clients No. (%)
Vaginal sex		
always	313 (98.6)	355 (98.0)
never uses condom	51 (16.5)	312 (86.7)
always uses condom	196 (63.2)	17 (4.7)
Anal intercourse		
never	283 (97.0)	288 (86.0)
Oral sex		
never	284 (89.0)	287 (80.6)

	No. (%)	
Who taught to use condom		
the leader	11 (4.5)	(not applicable)
co-worker	86 (34.0)	
the client	61 (24.0)	
self-taught	68 (27.5)	
Use of lubricant		
yes	28 (11.0)	
Change of behavior after AIDS		
yes	246 (72.0)	
Increase in condom use	214 (87.0)	
Decreased # of partners	46 (19.0)	

*The total sample size differs between variables because of missing information.

partmentalize their professional versus private sexual behavior, the former involving little or no affective involvement or erotic pleasure (62). For the women discussed here, interventions should support and encourage condom use in professional encounters, and should focus on strategies to promote reduction of HIV exposure through commercial sex (e.g., client screening or reduction of number of clients). At the same time, they should stress the need for protection in personal sexual relationships.

The high rates of condom use with clients, as reported to CONASIDA interviewers, is surprising in light of the common perception of male resistance to condom use in Mexico. Perhaps the national CONASIDA campaign has had such success that FCSWs insist on condom use and come supplied, and male clients no longer refuse to wear condoms and no longer offer extra money for sex without them. It is much more likely, however, that these FCSWs over-report condom use to CONASIDA personnel, as CONASIDA's emphasis on condom promotion is well-known. Certainly, selection bias and information bias must be considered. These women may only represent "the converted" among Mexico City FCSWs, those who have learned about AIDS/STDs and have taken the dangers so to heart that they accept the risked loss of business from rejecting prospective clients who refuse condoms. Indeed, many of these women have quarterly encounters with a public health institution (CONASIDA) to obtain anonymous screening for HIV.

Table 3. Prevalence of self-reported STDs and HIV infection in different groups of female commercial sex workers in Mexico City.*

STD	Street Low n=155 %	Street High n=35 %	Bar n=159 %
Gonorrhea	30(19)	1(2.8)	8(5.0)
Syphilis	3(2)	0	0
Condiloma	16(10)	1(2.8)	0
HIV	3(2)	0	1(0.06)
Change of behavior after AIDS?			
Yes	139(90)	21(65)	69(54)
If Yes, type of change:			
Increase in condom use			
	139(100)	18(85)	37(53)
Decrease in # of partner			
	4(2.8)	3(14)	32(46)

*The total sample size differs between variables because of missing information,

Given the low prevalence of HIV and reported STDs (Table 3), demostrating a protective effect of condom use will be difficult. These observations illustrate the problems faced when data are not available on "both halves" of the sex work dyad (seller and buyer). Even "hard" output measures, such as HIV or STD rates, are inconclusive indicators of behavior change if one cannot assess the prevalence of HIV/STDs among FCSW clients and other sexual contacts. Our observations also make clear the risks of basing policy or interventions upon clinic samples unless the representativeness and generalizability of those samples is precisely known and one can be sure the clinic setting is not causing bias in crucial responses. Selection and setting effects can only be determined by empirical work in a range of natural (non-clinic) settings.

HETEROGENEITY OF SEX WORK IN MEXICO CITY

Field research by staff from CONASIDA and the Center for Public Health Research was launched in 1990 in order to develop a population-based estimate of the variability of commercial sex in Mexico City, and better understand its characteristics and social dynamics. The initial phase has clarified the different types of commercial sex, and has enabled us to identify key informants and opinion-shapers to serve as liaisons with the numerous communities involved.

Overt prostitution in different forms is found to occur in clearly bounded, geographically defined zones in Mexico City. Approximately 10-15 areas are known sites for FCSWs; 4 areas are known sites for male CSWs; and 2 areas for male transvestite CSWs. The socio-economic and occupational diversity of men who frequent these areas suggests that the location and gross characteristics of these sites are common knowledge throughout the city. Within each of these three main categories of sex work zones, commercial sexual services are diverse and hierarchically structured by a competitive market.

Key informants report that women who meet clients on the street have the lowest status; next are those who contact clients in bars or nightclubs (this occurs in specific zones); next are women who work in massage parlors (*esteticas*) and those who work as call girls. These establishments usually operate during business hours. They are usually controlled by experienced FCSWs who employ 15-20 women as masseuses or stylists. Each woman performs the services the client requests and pays a percentage to the owner of the shop. At the top of the status and price hierarchy are women who work in a few very expensive bars, call girls, and women who work in brothels or houses of prostitution (*casa de citas*). The latter tend to consist of luxurious apartments in the residential areas of Mexico City, in which women attend to customers and waiters may serve beverages at extremely inflated prices.

Our observations indicate that the price/class hierarchy is not clearly defined by workplace, as some street work locations serve middle-class clients and charge fees similar to those charged by FCSWs at massage parlors. Another important factor to consider is that, while participants in street and bar work are publicly on display, most *esteticas* and *casas de citas* locations, personnel, and clients are secret. This makes them far less accessible to health service delivery and to intervention research.

CONTRASTS IN WORKPLACE TYPES

The diversity in workplace type can be illustrated by contrasting street work with work in bars or nightclubs. Tables 4-6 list key socio-demographic and behavioral characteristics of the women in the CONASIDA sample who reported working on the street in low- and high-priced areas and those working in bars or nightclubs. Bars and nightclubs are ranked higher than street work in status, and so it could be expected that they would attract (and be open to) women with fewer domestic responsibilities who can spend more on their clothing and appearance. However, the differences in socio-demographic features, other than those indexing socio-economic status (home ownership and education) are unremarkable. (We have not tested the differences for statistical significance because these preliminary data require further cleaning and standardization.) The sexual risk behaviors reported by these women are also not very different, except with regard to two crucial variables. Bar workers report an average of 3.2 clients per week, whereas street workers report 16.2 per week on average, and bar workers report far less consistent condom use with clients (Table 5). These differences cannot be understood without reference to the behavioral, social, and political context of these types of sex work.

The basic structure of street work is that FCSWs put themselves on display on the street; prospective clients "shop," walking or cruising by one or more women; men make the initial selection (by stopping to talk); FCSWs and prospective clients negotiate terms face to face; if they reach agreement, they go off to an agreed location for the service (e.g., a room in a hotel). As elsewhere in the world, women who work on the street in Mexico City require liaison/negotiation with, and protection from, the authorities (26,31). For this main reason (according to key informants), street women are organized in groups controlled by pimps (*lenones, representantes, padrotes*), or by other representatives (see below), to whom they pay a portion of their earnings. These agents negotiate for control of a specific site (*punto*) where "their girls" (*chavas*) are permitted to await and negotiate with potential clients with minimal police interference. The number of FCSWs at the *punto* at any time is tightly controlled, and women's names must be registered (by their pimp/leader) with the police. This keeps mobility to a minimum. The women may stand on the street or may circulate (on foot or in their own cars) around the block. The "success rate" of FCSW/client negotiations is low: approximately one out of 20 clients/cars who stop to negotiate in a moderately priced street zone actually go through with the transaction (32). Price is

Table 4. Demographic and other characteristics of different groups of female commercial sex workers in Mexico City.

Characteristic	Street Low (N=155) No. (%)	Street High (N=35) No. (%)	Bar (n=159) No. (%)
Married	18 (11.4)	6 (17.1)	28 (17.5)
Single	119 (75.8)	22 (62.8)	98 (61.6)
Divorced	14 (8.8)	7 (19.9)	29 (18.2)
Other	6 (3.1)	0	4 (2.9)
Currently living w/ father of children	12 (11.2)	2 (8.3)	18 (14.0)
Housing			
rented	118 (79.2)	21 (70.0)	81 (52.6)
owned	10 (6.71)	4 (13.3)	62 (40.2)
Frequency of prostitution			
every day	92 (58.6)	22 (81.4)	49 (44.1)
3-4 times per wk	56 (35.6)	5 (18.5)	39 (11.8)
1-2 times per wk	9 (5.73)	0	16 (14.4)
1 per wk	0	0	7 (6.3)
Have knowledge about AIDS?			
yes	57 (38)	17 (51)	86 (60)
no	90 (62)	16 (48)	55 (39)
Contraceptive use	100 (68)	13 (59)	135 (70)
oral contraceptives	5 (57)	4 (30)	11 (8)
IUD	9 (9)	1 (7)	17 (12)
hormonal IM	34 (34)	(46)	44 (32)
spermicide	1 (1)	1 (7)	1 (0.007)
Transfusion ever	9 (5.8)	4 (11.7)	20 (8.7)

strictly dependent on the zone of the city and on the duration and type of service provided. The more affluent the zone, the higher the price. However, many other things are negotiated in these discussions, including duration of the encounter, kinds of practices, how much clothing the FCSW will remove, and where the contact will take place. Some, but not all, FCSWs also discuss condom use in these early negotiations. (We do not have data on the effect of such discussions on pick-up rate.) Preliminary arrangements commonly take 15 minutes, so most women spend the bulk of their working time on the street.

FCSWs who work in bars or nightclubs in Mexico City have fewer clients than do street workers and receive most of their income in salary from the bar or club owner who employs them to encourage customers to buy drinks. In some nightclubs, FCSWs supplement their salary with money that they collect from dancing with customers. After the night club closes, an FCSW may reach an agreement about sex with a client, who must pay in advance for the services desired, to be provided in a nearby hotel. Bar girls in Mexico City can usually provide sexual services to only one client per night. By contrast, in the provinces of Mexico, where laws to abolish commercial sex work never existed, certain bars have adjacent rooms where women can take their

Table 5. Characteristics of different groups of female commercial sex workers in Mexico City.

	Street (n=230)			Bar (n=159)		
	mean	std	range	mean	std	range
Age (yrs)	25.3	5.8	18-46	28.0	6.5	8-59
No. of children	1.8	1.1	0-8	2.5	1.4	0-9
Yrs of education	5.2	3.4	0-16	7.2	3.0	0-14
Age 1st intercrse	16.7	2.3	9-26	16.6	3.7	9-48
Age first charged	22.2	4.8	13-43	23.8	4.7	14-37
Clients per week	16.2	10.2	1-60	3.2	6.4	0-40
Lifetime Non-Clients	2.1	1.9	1-15	3.6	3.5	1-20

Variable	Street Low (n=155)			Street High (n=35)		
	mean	std	range	mean	std	range
Age (yrs)	24.7	5.6	18-46	24.6	4.2	18-31
No. of children	1.7	1.1	0-8	1.8	1.0	0-4
Yrs of education	4.6	3.1	0-16	7.54	2.9	0-12
Age 1st intercrse	16.6	2.4	10-26	16.8	2.8	9-23
Age first charged	21.5	4.3	13-43	22.7	3.9	15-30
Clients per week	17.1	10.2	1-60	16.0	12.5	1-60
Lifetime Non-Clients	1.7	1.2	1-10	3.6	2.3	1-10

clients for brief sexual encounters. These bar girls are, therefore, not limited to a single customer per night.

Since bars/nightclubs are private property, and since those in Mexico City do not have rooms for rent, this form of commercial sex is less often subjected to interference from the authorities. Perhaps this is why there appears to be fewer social networks among women who work in bars than among street workers. To illustrate this difference, about half the street workers in this study, but only one-fifth of bar/nightclub workers, report having learned how to apply condoms from their co-workers. Bar work also differs from street work in that clients who go to bars have a more diversified entertainment agenda, including drinks, music, and dancing, so the relation between client and FCSW is, overtly, more social and multidimensional. (See 26,30 on the range of tactics some clients use to avoid acknowledging that these encounters are, from the woman's point of view, impersonal business.) A woman who has invested an evening in enlisting a given man as a sex partner has a lot more to lose than does a street worker in rejecting this client, if upon reaching the room she discovers he has genital lesions and/or refuses to use condoms. We think this explains the comparatively low rate of condom use among bar workers (30% report

Table 6. Sexual behavior and other characteristics of different groups of female commercial sex workers in Mexico City.

Characteristic	Street Low n=155 no. (%)		Street High n=35 no. (%)		Bar n=159 no. (%)	
Vaginal sex with non-clients						
always	134	(98)	35	(100)	150	(97)
never uses condom	116	(84)	30	(85)	130	(84)
Vaginal sex with clients						
always	156	(99)	27	(100)	94	(93)
always uses condom	131	(83)	19	(70)	31	(30)
Anal intercourse with non clients						
never	119	(95)	30	(88)	111	(77)
Anal intercourse with clients						
never	137	(98)	25	(96)	92	(95)
Oral sex with non clients						
never	133	(99)	23	(67)	111	(72)
Oral sex with clients						
never	155	(99)	19	(70)	90	(90)
Who taught to use condom						
the leader	3	(2.1)	1	(4)	4	(7)
co-worker	59	(43)	14	(63)	10	(17)
client(s)	9	(.6)	0		19	(32)
self-taught	36	(26)	5	(23)	14	(24)
Use of lubricant						
yes	15	(10)	6	(26)	2	(3)
Change of behavior after AIDS?						
yes	139	(90)	21	(65)	69	(54)
If yes, type of change:						
Increase in condom use	139	(100)	18	(85)	37	(53)
Decrease in # of partner	4	(2.8)	3	(14.2)	32	(46)

"always" using condoms with clients, whereas between 70% and 83% of street workers report "always" doing so). If clients prefer imagining that the contact is personal, their resistance to condom use may be higher, just as women's negotiating position appears to be weaker, in bar/nightclub-based commercial sex. Clearly, this population needs a different format and content of intervention materials from those directed at street workers. In addition, given these behavioral differences, the prevalence of bar work versus street work should be expected to drastically affect the rate of HIV dissemination. A population-based assessment of FCSWs will be essential in order to project HIV trends in Mexico City as a whole.

VARIATION WITHIN WORKPLACE TYPES

Within particular types of workplaces of comparable economic status, virtual price lists are observed and defined in relation to the type of service rendered and the beauty, age, social class, ethnic group, and education of the FCSW involved. A key informant reported on the price range for services of known street work areas; the price ranged from about $5 U.S. in a low-priced area to $50 U.S. in a middle-class area. Within workplace types, socio-economic disparities are also observed, not only in the price lists and characteristics of the participants, but in the entire complex of participants, behaviors, and settings. Data gathered at CONASIDA centers in 1989-1990 on the sample of self-referred FCSWs discussed above serve to illustrate some of these differences (Table 6). Comparisons must be viewed with caution, however, since almost five times as many women working in a lower socio-economic status district came to CONASIDA for screening (n=155 from low-priced zones and n=35 from high-priced zones). We present the quantitative results in the context of our growing qualitative data base on heterogeneous contexts of sex work.

In addition to continued ethnographic work with key informants from different FCSW groups, psychologists on the team (Laura Elena de Caso and Victor Ortiz) conducted an initial round of nine focus group discussions (FGDs) with experienced and inexperienced FCSWs from these two zones. Street workers often move in groups for protection and support, and it was impossible to recruit women for FGDs who did not know each other. FGDs addressed the organization of, and participants and behaviors involved in, the FCSWs' work, as well as their life contexts and concerns. While we cannot rule out selection or setting biases in this initial round of FGDs, differences in the personnel and routines described by high-priced and low-priced zone FCSWs are worth noting.

FCSWs working in low-priced street zones (LPS) work during the day. This is largely because of safety concerns. FCSWs working in higher-priced *puntos* (HPS) work only after dark. Some LPS women stand in specific alleys outside compounds where small, stall-like rooms are available for short-term rent. Prospective clients line up and stare at the FCSWs, awaiting their turn to engage a chosen girl in negotiations. Other LPS women circulate singly around the block, weaving in and out of shops and market stalls on the lookout for customers (and for angry shopkeepers and police). Male pimps are known to manage and control the FCSWs working in the LPS areas, and to manage recruitment of new women into commercial sex work. Whether out of loyalty or fear, the LPS women would reveal nothing about the proportion of earnings taken by their pimp (*padrote*) or about the services he does or does not provide.

Informants report that a police crack-down several years ago has imposed this solitary work format on LPS women. The police action not only accentuated the women's need for protection (and, thus, dependence upon their *padrotes*) (9,13,29), it also indirectly prevented development of social or financial support and friendship among women working in this area. More of these women reportedly regret their current occupation, and endeavor to keep it secret from neighbors and family. LPS and HPS street workers have very similar numbers of clients per week, despite the fact that LPS women work fewer days per week, but the quality of LPS services is reportedly very basic. Normally, LPS FCSWs do not take off their clothes. Hygiene facilities in the LPS zone consist of a bucket of cold water, so the FCSWs often do not wash their own genitals until they go home in the evening. Anonymity, speed of the transaction, and personal safety appear to be their principal concerns. A degree of powerlessness and resignation was expressed by LPS FCSWs in focus group discussions. This may reflect the women's lower educational attainment and their more rural origins — both economic liabilities in the capital city. Observations by the field team suggest that the clients that "shop" in these areas appear to be relatively poor, uneducated, and unsophisticated as well. However, if the LPS women's reports are true (of which we are not convinced), the high rate of condom use in these dyads suggests these women are smarter than many of the women in the more "sophisticated" groups.

In contrast to LPS FCSWs, HPS FCSWs work in teams, and most of the groups' leaders are women, former FCSWs. While waiting for clients to cruise by and talk, they joke, laugh, and share experiences and information with one another. They support each other in negotiations with clients, and watch out for each others' safety. In negotiations with the police and other intermediaries, these women are represented by one prostitute, usually an experienced or semi-retired FCSW, who takes legal and political responsibility for the group. She negotiates with police and has the responsibility of recruiting new workers. Each of the prostitutes pays a fee to the representative in order to maintain her access to the *punto* and for protection arrangements. After arrangements are set with prospective clients, most HPS FCSWs take clients to a hotel, at which they have an arrangement with owners for use of a room several times during the night. Most of the rooms we visited had adequate hygiene facilities. To our knowledge, FCSWs do not pay hotel owners any proportion of their earnings (their client usually pays for the room), but there is an agreement that the hotel will provide some security for the sex worker. In some areas, HPS groups have organized elaborate safety precautions, including the provision of a driver to take the FCSW to the hotel and to wait to take her back to the *punto* after the job. HPS women were able to describe in detail STDs that they had identified in their clients (they described gonorrhea and condilomas). They also claimed to clean and inspect thoroughly clients' genital areas and to reject clients if a disease is detected. Most of HPS FCSWs expressed a clear understanding of how to use a condom and were able to describe good strategies (verbal and tactile) to increase condom acceptance by clients.

CONCLUSIONS

While we are still in the early stages of research and analysis in this study, the field research reported here has convinced us of the value of and need for this multi-method, population-based approach to women and men involved in prostitution. We see important differences in reported risk factors for HIV and conventional STDs among FCSWs, not only related to socio-economic status, but also to workplace type. Follow-up is needed, of course, to validate reported rates of condom use and other key behaviors, and reported rates of STDs should be confirmed by medical examinations (and treated), in at least a sub-set of the population. The variation in risk behaviors and health outcomes among FCSWs of different types supports our hypothesis that researchers should stratify their samples by type of sex work, and any quantitative projections or generalizations about disease transmission should involve a weighting procedure to account for the relative prevalence of types.

While clients of FCSWs in Mexico City span the socio-economic range of society, our research indicates considerable matching of clients and sex workers based on education, economics, and ethnicity, all of which can be expected to reflect individual preferences in keeping with their sexual culture. It will simplify intervention development within areas (reducing the range of materials needed per site) if clients and sex workers frequenting one area are indeed homogeneous in culture and class. Our findings make clear that the diffusion of interventions across workplaces may be low. In addition, the findings emphasize the importance of monitoring outcome variables (behavior and STD rates) among both clients and FCSWs. Studies of HIV prevalence among blood donors in Mexico City have demonstrated that poor individuals who sell blood have much higher prevalence of HIV and other infectious diseases than do more affluent individuals who give blood voluntarily (33). Since variance in the prevalence of HIV among clients of FCSWs is to be expected, we must measure HIV rates in both clients and FCSWs in order to interpret results of intervention campaigns.

We have seen how the different patterns of sex work call for considerably different intervention program delivery strategies. Different workplaces and work styles attract or admit women with different personal characteristics with respect to education/literacy and alternative resources, for example. Practically speaking, women who work at night are more likely to be available to attend skill building workshops during the day, as opposed to women who do street work all day and then escape back to their families and communities in the evening. Ways must be found to reach women controlled by pimps, and other exploitative agents. In Mexico, these women appear to be more frightened of health service contact, more isolated and anxious about their work, and more suspicious of outsiders, including outsiders "in the trade" than are the HPS and bar women reached by the project to date. In Mexico, reaching these women will require working face-to-face. Most of the LPS women cannot read, and radio messages targeted for street working women are politically unfeasible in Mexico City.

Table 7. Information needed for intervention design.

ABOUT THE WORKPLACE

- Independent or managed

- Degree of privacy (e.g., outdoor vs. indoor meeting points)

- Accessibility and cooperativeness of managers and beneficiaries

- Quality (e.g., competition) and frequency of interactions among networks or groups

ABOUT THE FCSW

- Education/Literacy

- Access to diverse media

- Amount and accuracy of knowledge about AIDS, STDs, and reproductive health

- Periodicity of work

- Degree of concern about secrecy/anonymity

- Degree of dependence on CSW

- Degree of concern and commitment to intervention

ABOUT THE CLIENTS

- Education/Literacy

- Access to diverse media

- Amount of knowledge and accuracy of understanding about AIDS, STDs, and reproductive health

- Degree of concern about anonymity/secrecy re. their purchase of sexual services

- Intensity and periodicity of motivation to purchase sexual services

- Selectivity and selection criteria

- Norms and ideals re. health, family, citizenship, with which to articulate intervention

Our informants report that women in groups controlled by other women, as opposed to those controlled by pimps, are more supportive and concerned about AIDS prevention, operating more like a family or community than a set of competing individuals. If it is true that in capital cities the supply of hapless girls from the provinces is unlimited, and if it is true that exploitative managers care little for the health or survival of "their girls," then it would be naïve to appeal to the humanism and public spirit of FCSW managers in Mexico City to encourage risk-reduction behaviors if these behaviors impair business. Other pressures, such as increasing client demand for safer commercial sex, may need to be applied to managers and profiteers. Alternatively, strategies are needed to identify and assist women who want to try alternate work or alternative sources of protection.

These preliminary findings illustrate important interactions between the legal/policy environment and the intervention process in the area of commercial sex work in Mexico City. The debate about the legal status of commercial sex work is not closed in Mexico, despite the conservative nature of public policy. Indeed, at an assembly in Mexico City in August 1990, representatives of the government, of health and social services, of male and female CSW organizations/groups, and of the communities where commercial sex work occurs, showed considerable interest in reviving legalization with regulation. This would change the negotiating position of FCSWs with their managers and clients, and could make it easier for individuals to accumulate cash so as to leave the business.

Yet, some of the most important consequences of the political and social marginalization of FCSWs occur at a level that is often ignored. Clearly, where commercial sex work is classified as dangerous deviance by mainstream society, all who practice or intervene in it are in social, perhaps legal, jeopardy. It is likely that FCSWs would come forward for education more readily if their occupation were legal. In addition, FCSWs' constant concerns about safety take shape at other levels. A client can beat a FCSW without fear of legal prosecution; a pimp or other profiteer can extort or steal an FCSW's hard-won earnings with the same impunity. At a more poignant and subtle level, shopkeepers in the LPS zone prevent FCSWs from standing in a group on the street (bad for business), condemning the women to work alone all day, without the camaraderie, information, or protection from fellow workers that HPS FCSWs enjoy. It is not surprising that the LPS FCSWs seemed depressed and ashamed in focus group discussions, whereas the tone among the HPS FCSWs was more open and cheerful.

This project has raised many questions, which we cannot yet answer, about the risk behavior, social context, and social epidemiology of sex work in Mexico City. When merged with the work by collaborators under way in Ethiopia (Debrework Zewdie, Mekonnen Bishaw) and Thailand (Werasit Sititrai, and colleagues), the data will provide guidance, not only to support intervention design *in situ* (Table 7), but to predict the intervention needs and strategies that can be expected to work in other zones, towns, cities, and countries where commercial sex takes place in unsafe environments.

Acknowledgments
We are pleased to acknowledge the susbstantive and technical contributions of Laura Elena de Caso, Marta Lamas, and Victor Ortiz. Interview material was collected as a routine component of CONASIDA services, funded by the Ministry of Health, Mexico. Ethnographic and focus group work were made possible by a grant from the American Foundation for AIDS Research and The Rockefeller Foundation.

REFERENCES

1. Soberon B, Frenk J, Sepulveda J. The health care reform in Mexico before and after the earthquakes. *Am J Pub Health* 1986; 76:673-80.
2. Informacion Prioritaria en Salud. Consejo Asesor en Epidemiología, Mexico 1990.
3. Atlas de la Ciudad de Mexico. Departamento del Distrito Federal, Colegio de Mexico, 1987.

4. de Zalduondo B, Hernandez-Avila M, Uribe P. Intervention research needs for AIDS prevention among commercial sex workers and their clients: Responding to diversity in actors and settings. Chapter 14 in this volume.

5. Bullough V and Bullough B. Women and Prostitution: A Social History. Buffalo, NY: Prometheus Books, 1987.

6. Zubieta-Mendez R. Prostitucion masculina y femenina: un estudio exploratorio de personalidad. Facultad de Psicologia Tesis, Universidad Nacional Autonoma de Mexico, 1984.

7. Franco Guzman R. *La Prostitucion*. Mexico: Editorial Diana, 1973.

8. Sinopsis del XXV Ciclo de conferencias en "Eugenecia" No 50, febrero 1944, Mexico.

9. Walkowitz JR. Male vice and female virtue: Feminism and the politics of prostitution in nineteenth century Britain. In: *Powers of Desire. The Politics of Sexuality*. Snitow A, Stansell C, Thomson S, eds. New York: Montly Review Press, 1983, 419-438.

10. Connelly MT. *The Response to Prostitution in the Progressive Era*. Chapel Hill: University of North Carolina Press, 1980.

11. Lara MA. Entrevista conducida por Garcia–Flores M. Entrevista del suplemento SIEMPRE 1978; 839.

12. Morris L, Nunez L, de Velasco A, Bailey P, Cardenas C, Whatley A. Sexual experience and contraceptive use among young adults in Mexico City. *International Family Planning Perspectives* 1988; 14(1):147-152.

13. Biersteker S. Promoting safer sex in prostitution: impediments and opportunities. In: *Promoting Safer Sex*. Paalman M, ed. Amsterdam: Swets & Zetlinger, 1990, pp. 144-152.

14. Vazquez Valls E, Torres-Mendoza MB, Ayala-Chavira MN, Ayala G. Prevalence d'anticorps contre le virus d'immunodeficience humaine (VIH) chez les prostitutees a Guadalajara (Mexique). *Contraception-fertilite-sexualite* 1989; 17:265-268.

15. Magis CL, Loo E, Garcia L, Valdespino JL. Caracteristicas sociodemograficas y practicas sexuales en mujeres que pratican la prostitucion. II Congreso Nacional de SIDA, Mexico, 1989.

16. Uribe P, Hernandez-Avila M, De Zalduondo B, Lamas M, Hernandez G, Chavez-Peon F, Sepulveda-Amor J. HIV spreading and prevention strategies among female prostitutes. VII International Conference on AIDS, Florence Italy, 1991; Abstract W.C.3135.

17. Informe Técnico Evaluación del Impacto de la Estrategia Educativa para la Prevención del SIDA en México 1987-1988: Poblacion dedicada a la prostitucion. Secretaria de Salud, México, 1991.

18. Guerena-Burgueno F, Benenson AS, Sepulveda-Amor J. HIV-1 prevalence in selected Tijuana sub–populations. *Am J Public Health* 1991; 81:623-625.

19. Mendoza G, Diaz A, Aleman ME, Suarez S, Gomez EA. Prevalencia de anticuerpos anti–HIV en grupos voluntarios de alto riesgo en el Puerto de Veracruz. II Congreso Nacional de SIDA, Mexico DF, 1989.

20. Hernandez-Avila M, Uribe P, Avila C, De Caso LE, Gortmaker S, MUeller N, Sepulveda–Amor J. Homosexual and bisexual males at a testing center in Mexico City. HIV-1 seropositivity, risk, sexual behavior and condom use. Submitted for publication.

21. Izazola-Licea JA, Valdespino-Gomez JL, Gortmaker SL, Townsend J, Becker J, Palacios-Martinez M, Mueller NE, Sepulveda-Amor J. HIV-1 seropositivity and behavioral and sociological risks among homosexual and bisexual men in six Mexican cities. *J Acq Immune Def Synd* 1991; 4:614-622.

22. Sawanpanyalert P, Ungchusak K, Thanprassertsuk S, Akarasewi P. Seroconversion rate and risk factors for HIV-1 infection among low–class female sex workers in Chiang Mai, Thailand: A multi- cross-sectional study. VII International conference on AIDS, Florence, Italy, June 1991; Abstract W.C.3097.

23. Bishaw M. Commercial sex work in Ethiopia: History and current situation. Interim report for the AIDS and Reproductive Health Network Multi-Site Intervention Research Project on Prostitution and AIDS, 1991.

24. Rosenberg MJ, Weiner JM. Prostitution and AIDS: A health department priority? *Am J Public Health* 1988; 78(4):418-423.

25. Freund M, Leonard T, Lee N. Sexual behavior of resident street prostitutes with their clients in Camden, New Jersey. *J Sex Research* 1989; 26:460-78

26. McLeod E. *Women Working: Prostitution Now.* Guildford and King's Lynn, Great Britain: Biddles LTD, 1982.

27. Padian NS. Prostitute women and AIDS: epidemiology. *AIDS* 1988; 2:413-419.

28. Informe Técnico Evaluación del Impacto de la Estrategia Educativa para la Prevención del SIDA en México 1987-1988: Poblacion General. Secretaria de Salud, México, 1991.

29. Hobson, BM. *Uneasy virtue: The politics of prostitution and the American reform tradition.* New York: Basic Books, Inc., 1987.

30. Shedlin, MG. An ethnographic approach to understanding high–risk behaviors: Prostitution and drug abuse. In: *AIDS and intravenous drug use: Future directions for community–based prevention research.* Leukefeld CG, Battjes RJ, Amsel Z, eds. Washington, DC.: Government Printing Office, 1990; pp. 134-149.

31. Gomez JF. *Sociologia de la prostitucion.* Mexico: Ed Nueva edicion, 1978.

32. Lamas M, Personal communication, Mexico City, January 1991.

33. Avila C, Stetler HC, Sepulveda J et al. The epidemiology of HIV transmission among paid plasma donors, Mexico City, Mexico. *J AIDS* 1989; 3:631-33.

CONCLUSION

AIDS AND REPRODUCTIVE HEALTH WORKSHOP
RECOMMENDATIONS: REPORTS FROM THE WORKING GROUPS

I. EPIDEMIOLOGY/TRANSMISSION

(Working group members: Seth Berkley, David Hunter, Phyllis Kanki, Souleymane M. Boup, Frank Plummer, Mary Wilson)

At the start of the second decade of HIV/AIDS research, it is important to reassess epidemiologic research priorities. Although much descriptive and risk factor information is still needed, greater emphasis now needs to be given to intervention studies.

Research priorities have been categorized according to the life cycle conceptual framework. Within each category, priorities are listed in approximate order of importance. However, the heterogeneity of the HIV/AIDS epidemic worldwide means that an urgent priority in one area may be of lesser importance elsewhere. Finally, research priorities listed apply both to HIV-1 and HIV-2.

Epidemiologic Research Priorities

1. Contraception
   a. Determine the effect of available contraceptive methods on susceptibility and infectiousness. Current studies of spermicides should be extended to include memphigol, quaternary ammonium compounds, and gossypol.
   b. Develop new contraceptive and virucidal agents that will prevent HIV transmission; evaluate these agents among persons with a high frequency of sexual intercourse. Development of female-controlled methods is urgent.
   Note: Greater involvement of the population research community will substantially enhance progress in this area.
2. Conception
   a. Assess impact of HIV infection on fertility.
   b. Evaluate menstrual cycle variations in susceptibility and infectiousness.
3. Pregnancy
   For HIV-negative women:

a. Evaluate susceptibility of pregnant women to HIV.

b. Assess men's behaviors that may increase risk of HIV infection to pregnant women (e.g., men seeking other sexual contacts during or after pregnancy).

For HIV-infected women:

c. Evaluate impact of HIV infection on maternal health during pregnancy and in the post-partum period.

d. Evaluate impact of pregnancy on disease progression.

e. Evaluate effect of pregnancy on infectiousness.

f. Determine co-factors for, and markers of, in utero transmission.

g. Determine HIV effect on pregnancy outcome.

h. Determine whether co-infection of the mother with syphilis predisposes to congenital syphilis.

i. Assess role of route of infection (iv drug use, sexual) on priorities d-f.

4. Birth and Infancy

a. Develop diagnostic tools for early detection of HIV infection in infants.

b. Assess relationship of method of delivery to probability of perinatal transmission; examine morbidity of obstetric interventions in HIV-infected women.

5. Breast-feeding

a. Determine role of breast-feeding in perinatal transmission; include studies of viral shedding and role of potential transmission through nipple lesions/cracks.

b. Assess risk of transmission from HIV-infected babies to wet nurses.

Note: the potential role of breast-feeding in perinatal HIV transmission may increase if successful interventions to prevent in utero or conatal transmission are developed.

6. Childhood

a. Determine natural history of HIV infection (and relevant clinical markers) in children.

b. Assess risk of and timing of routine immunization in HIV-infected children or in areas where HIV prevalence is high; consider supplemental immunizations or other preventive strategies for HIV-infected children.

c. Determine role of injections in HIV transmission to children.

d. Determine role of transfusions in HIV transmission to children.

e. Assess impact of HIV infection on infant mortality rates, including impact of maternal HIV infection on non-infected children.

f. Assess impact of HIV status on bonding, care and development.

g. Determine role of child sexual abuse in HIV transmission.

7. Adolescence

a. Identify cultural differences in early sexual experience and their potential role in sexual transmission of HIV.

b. Assess prevalence and identify determinants of male and female adolescent prostitution.

c. Assess role of social factors (economic, homelessness, broken families) in HIV-relevant risk behavior.

d. Determine whether immaturity of cervical epithelia predisposes to HIV.

Note: as every year a new uninfected cohort of adolescents commences sexual activity, interventions specifically designed for adolescents merit particular priority.

8. Adulthood

a. Assess natural history of HIV infection, taking into account geographic variation and differences in prevalence of opportunistic infections and treatment.

b. Determine efficacy of male-to-female, female-to-male, and same sex HIV transmission.

c. Determine efficacy of HIV transmission via different sexual practices.

d. Determine effect of personal "hygienic" factors in transmission (e.g., douching, astringents, etc.).

e. Assess role of individual sexually transmitted diseases (STDs), including nonclassical infections, on infectivity or susceptibility to HIV.

f. Determine prevalence and attributable risk of STDs in different settings.

g. Stimulate development of rapid and affordable STD diagnostics, particularly for STDs in women.

h. Assess role of HIV on transmission of other STDs, their natural history and response to therapy.

i. Assess role of circumcision (male and female) in infectiousness or susceptibility.

j. Develop descriptive epidemiology of prostitution for different areas/cultures.

k. Develop and evaluate therapies to decrease infectiousness of HIV-infected people.

l. Develop methods to reduce frequency of blood transfusion by early intervention in anemia and childbirth. Rapid and affordable diagnostic blood screening methods are needed.

m. Assess occupational risk to health workers and develop cost-effective risk reduction measures and protective equipment.

Note: Although data are not adequate to define all risk factors for HIV transmission, currently available information mandates immediate intervention to prevent HIV spread while simultaneously studying the risk factors. Evaluations of interventions are important in prioritizing limited resources.

9. Death

a. Promote autopsy studies to define spectrum of opportunistic infections in different settings.

b. Assess demographic impact of HIV in general and in focal settings.

c. Evaluate HIV transmission risk associated with cultural practices related to dying (e.g., sexual cleansing rituals, marriage to a surviving relative).

Advocacy

Increasing global interdependence has blurred the concept of geographic barriers to the spread of infectious diseases. Yet there is a risk that HIV will be seen as "just another tropical disease." Also, as pattern I and III countries increasingly develop features of pattern II transmission, the global relevance of knowledge about heterosexual transmission will increase. Nevertheless, currently more than 95 percent of AIDS-related resources are devoted to research, prevention, and care in industrialized countries. This situation must change.

Potential advocates for change include: UN agencies, governments, nongovernmental organizations (including women's groups), researchers, and the ARHN. Potential targets for advocacy include: UN agencies, industry, universities, governments, other funders, and research institutions.

Research on treatment must become a high priority given the projected future caseload from the millions of persons currently infected with HIV.

Limitations in trained manpower will become more acute as each area becomes increasingly involved in research, prevention and care. In responding to the epidemic, this will become the limiting factor in some areas. Therefore, part of all research efforts must involve developing local capacity for conducting research, including training, support, institution strengthening, and technical support. Local capability strengthening efforts should focus on in-country training and the building and reinforcement of equal partnerships or networks. Failure to address these critical needs may stifle the response to the epidemic.

Epidemiologists should consider the meaning of their study results for prevention and seek opportunities to help translate research into action. Communication between epidemiologists and AIDS program managers and policy makers is often inadequate. Opportunities should be sought to increase interactions between the providers and consumers of epidemiologic research.

II. SEXUAL BEHAVIOR

(Working group members: Richard Parker, Barbara de Zalduondo, Jonathan Mann, Mauricio Hernandez, Katherine LaGuardia)

Sexual behavior includes both sexual practices and meaning at the individual and social/cultural level. Sexual behavior is a fundamental concern for both AIDS and reproductive health. In the past, the STD community, family planning, and other related fields did not consider sexuality as broadly as needed to contribute effectively to understanding determinants and patterns of sexual risk behavior. Accordingly, there is an urgent need to break out of the current paradigms that have directed the bulk of research on sexual behavior and AIDS.

Sexual Behavior Research Priorities

Sexual behavior research has suffered from barriers between the relevant research communities. First, there is a lack of integration of existing, potentially useful knowledge (e.g., literature on sex, gender and sexuality; power; sexuality in the socio-economic context; and sexuality as part of a system of roles and symbols). Second, much available knowledge is not relevant, for it either derives from sexology (often Western, Christian, heterosexual and culture-based) or from psychiatry, where sexuality has been studied from the perspective of "deviance" and pathology. Finally, there are major gaps in substantive material and in methodology on female sexuality, bisexuality, and male sexuality.

These barriers and gaps reflect a consistent lack of institutional and funding support for sexual behavior research; lack of professional legitimization, associated with a social stigma; lack of a critical mass of specialists; and dissatisfaction with, or exhaustion of, current research methods. Thus, there is not a long-standing tradition of theory and method to support research on sexual behavior.

In developing strategies against HIV/AIDS, and for promoting reproductive health, there is a danger that research will be limited to a narrow, short-term focus. However, as sexual behavior is, and will always be, such a fundamental dimension of human life and public health, there is a critical need for both short-term, focused intervention research and an ongoing commitment to long-term, basic research.

This broad research agenda will be critical for public health efforts on AIDS, STDs, family planning, and other reproductive health concerns.

Two working groups are proposed to develop the research priorities and promote the agenda for sexual behavior research: the Working Group on Public Health and Social Science and the Working Group on Sexual Behavior Research.

The Working Group on Public Health and Social Science will identify means of increasing communication between these two domains. Specific activities would include:

1. Promoting the agenda of sexual behavior research, including interdisciplinary AIDS and social science research.
2. Promoting interdisciplinary editorial expertise in specific disciplinary journals.
3. Preparing and distributing bibliographies of key documents.
4. Promoting representation of sexual behavior research in AIDS and reproductive health conferences.
5. Reviewing the professional resources and training needs required to achieve and sustain this agenda.
6. Seeking resources for training of sexual behavior researchers from both developing and industrialized countries.

The Working Group on Sexual Behavior Research will contribute to developing theory and methodology. Specific activities would include:

1. Analyzing the concepts and methods that have guided past research.

2. Critically examining how epidemiological and sexual behavior research theory and method can have inadvertent side-effects and negative impact on public health (examples include: the use of "risk group" concepts and the disproportionate frequency of HIV studies among high prevalence populations, such as commercial sex workers).
3. Examining sexual behavior in a dynamic framework, seeking to take into account behavior changes over the life course or in response to other issues and developments.
4. Developing new interdisciplinary conceptual and methodological frameworks for future sexual behavior research, including theoretical models bridging the biological and social sciences, and methodological approaches merging quantitative and qualitative investigation.
5. Seeking to disseminate these deliberations as widely as possible in order to expand and deepen discourse concerning the scientific study of sexual behavior. Specific means to this end may include: articles on impasses in sexual behavior research and the theoretical and methodological paradigms; articles on specific studies among different populations; and articles reviewing long-term research programs.

These two working groups are complementary and their relationship will evolve over time. The first working group has a political/advocacy function, as well as practical tasks that could be advanced in a relatively short period. However, the second working group, with a more extensive theoretical and methodological agenda, will require a long-term commitment.

III. WOMEN'S EMPOWERMENT AND REPRODUCTIVE RIGHTS

(Working group members: Adrienne Germain, Jody Heymann, Debrework Zewdie, E. Maxine Ankrah, Lincoln Chen, Olav Meirik, Judith Wasserheit)

Heterosexual transmission of HIV is increasing, and three million or more women worldwide are already HIV-infected. Women's disadvantaged position in society both increases their risk for HIV infection and magnifies its consequences. The unequal status of women puts them at a severe disadvantage in negotiating sexual encounters and in seeking and utilizing educational and health services. In addition, HIV infection reinforces women's social disadvantage. Social norms may cause women to be subject to stigma, ostracism, violence, and discrimination when they are known to be HIV infected. Finally, women rarely hold decision-making positions in health policies, programs, and research.

The focus of HIV/AIDS research on groups of women who are not representative (e.g., prostitutes, pregnant women) has led to frequent characterization of women as transmitters of infection. Relatively less attention has been given to women's own health and rights. Therefore, knowledge is largely lacking about HIV/AIDS in women, their susceptibility to infection, and the means that would enable them to protect themselves. In addition, current interventions have been inadequate in reaching women in the general population. Thus, women's rights are being abridged or compromised in HIV/AIDS research, programs, and policies that fail to provide women equal access to health services and technologies, or fail to recognize women's right to make informed choices regarding their own health care, reproduction, and sexual relations.

At the same time, it is essential to recognize that AIDS is only one of multiple threats to women's health related to their sexual activity and their unique role in reproduction. Therefore, work on HIV/AIDS is likely to be most effective and responsive to women's overall health needs and rights if it is undertaken in a women's health and sexuality framework. This framework should take into account the complex factors that determine women's sexual and health behavior, and the range of information and services required to empower women to protect and maintain their health.

Finally, it is essential that men's roles be recognized and that they share equally the tasks of prevention in sexual relationships, in the community, and in society.

Research Priorities

Research must acknowledge and act upon three principles: 1) involve more women and men concerned and knowledgeable about women's rights, health, and empowerment; 2) add a gender perspective to ongoing research; and 3) allocate human and material resources to research specifically on areas currently neglected with regard to women.

Specific research priorities involve issues of sexual and reproductive health; personal and political power; and violations of rights and access to choices.

1. Sexual and reproductive health
   a. Determine the progression of HIV/AIDS in women in the general population and in specific subgroups.
   b. Develop means of detecting and treating STDs in women (priority on simple, rapid, inexpensive STD diagnostics for women).
   c. Develop female-controlled methods to prevent HIV infection.
   d. Determine the interactions between HIV/AIDS and pregnancy.
   e. Determine the impact of breast-feeding on HIV-infected women.
   f. Determine the extent to which healthy women are exposed to HIV by improperly performed OB/GYN procedures.
   g. Determine the impacts of female contraceptive methods on the acquisition and natural history of HIV/AIDS in women.
   h. Determine the patterns of girls' and women's sexuality and how these influence their risks of HIV infection.
2. Personal and political power
   a. Determine the general characteristics of gender-power relations that affect girls' and women's ability to negotiate sexual encounters and protect themselves in sexual relationships, in the family and community, and in the society.
   b. Determine how gender power relations operate at the micro level with regard to women's ability to insist on effective condom use; timing of sexual initiation; women's knowledge of their partners' HIV risk factors; women's ability to leave a sexual relationship, determine the conditions of sex, and manage sexual practices; and exposure of girls and women to unwanted, abusive, and unsafe sex.
3. Violations of rights and access to choices
   a. Assess the extent to which health services discriminate against HIV-infected women.
   b. Assess whether HIV/AIDS programs and services respect women's right to make fully informed choices about contraception, abortion and breast-feeding. Is support provided for these decisions?
   c. Assess whether women identified as HIV-infected face special consequences, such as divorce, desertion, violence, disinheritance, or public blame for the epidemic.
   d. Assess the extent to which incest or other forms of sexual abuse increase the risk of infection of girls and women.
   e. Assess the sensitivity of research and service protocols to the particular social vulnerabilities of women, in particular to their right to privacy.
   f. Determine the extent, costs, and other consequences of women's roles in HIV/AIDS caretaking in the family and community.
   g. Assess the relevance, appropriateness, and effectiveness of public education strategies and messages for girls and women.
   h. Assess the best ways to reach women with information and services.

Advocacy

Key target groups for advocacy include: national AIDS committees and other agencies of government (ministries of health, education, women's affairs); religious bodies; international agencies; pharmaceutical companies; women's organizations; educators; politicians; media; and the scientific community.

Key areas of advocacy include:

1. Strengthening women's participation through:
   a. Representation of women and of women's perspectives in international, national, and local positions and bodies that set policy, including resource allocation, research, and service priorities; training; and legislation.
   b. Strengthening appropriate women's organizations by involving them in design and implementation of research, design and monitoring of service programs, and formulation of policies and legislation.
   c. Strengthening these organizations' basic institutional capacity to act so they can inform women about HIV/AIDS, including both health and rights issues, and also support women to exercise choice in sexual relations and reproduction.

2. Increasing financial resources for:
   a. Research on HIV/AIDS and women's reproductive health and rights, including development of female-controlled technologies.
   b. Women's organizations that provide information, services, and support, and that work for equal consideration of women in policies and programs.
   c. Educational and employment opportunities for girls and women in poverty because of the link between poverty, lack of choice, and high-risk behavior.

3. Educating the public about women and HIV/AIDS, including risks of infection, women's role in transmission, social discrimination against women, myths, and misconceptions.

4. Legislating reform on basic and reproductive rights (abortion, sexual abuses, etc.)

5. Improving basic education, employment opportunities, political participation, and other aspects of women's status.

IV. POLICY AND PROGRAM INTERACTION

(Working group members: Harvey Fineberg, Myron Essex, Jaime Sepulveda, Mbowa Kalengayi, Debrework Zewdie, Peter Lamptey)

Policies on AIDS and reproductive health should be coordinated and mutually supportive, yet the extent to which this applies in practice is unclear. One important aspect of policy analysis relates to the study and understanding of the policy-making process itself. Related to this analysis, guidelines could be developed for successful promotion of policies. These would need to be made pertinent to the particular local/national situation.

Alternatively, policy analysis can be approached prescriptively, by defining the optimal content of policies to be adopted. Finally, of at least equal importance is the critical question of how to carry out these policies.

Establishing Policy Priorities

One approach is to identify criteria for choosing among the array of policy issues to consider. Based on these criteria, key policy issues can be selected that deserve consideration. The state of preparedness to make policy recommendations can be specified, noting where further analysis could help determine the preferred option. A framework for analysis could include:

1. Identification of policy questions to consider (topics and issues).
2. Identification of criteria for selection, based on the importance or value of pursuing each question.
   Criteria could include:

a. Existence and magnitude of the problem.

b. Existence and adequacy of current policy dealing with the issue.

c. Potential impact if a new policy were adopted and implemented. Feasibility of policy adoption.

e. Implementability of the policy.

f. Indirect effects, both positive (i.e., solving another problem) and negative (i.e., opportunity costs).

3. Identification of audiences, including the target populations and the decision makers.

4. Determination of the methods of analysis that apply to the topics, questions and audiences:

a. Analytic (empirical data) vs. synthetic (combine available information to reach a policy recommendation).

b. Ethical and human rights considerations.

c. Economic, political, cultural, social, and organizational dimensions (related to both adoption and implementation).

Policy Issues to Consider

The following is a list of priority policy issues for consideration in the context of AIDS and reproductive health:

1. Breast-feeding: Should an HIV-infected woman breast-feed her baby?

2. Abortion: Should abortion be permitted, recommended, or mandated for pregnant HIV-infected women?

3. Condoms: Should condoms be promoted widely in public? Should they be promoted, permitted or denied to adolescents? Should they be promoted in school; and if so, at what level (high school, university)? Should they be promoted in connection with prostitution? Should they be advocated in all family planning, STD, and HIV programs? Should they be advocated in connection with other forms of birth control?

4. HIV screening: Should pregnant women, newborns and infants, and/or individuals to be married be tested for HIV infection; if so, all or a subset according to risk? Should testing be available, permitted, recommended, and/or mandatory? Should testing of prostitutes and clients be recommended or enforced; does the answer depend on whether prostitution is tolerated and/or legal?

5. Counseling: How can we ensure that adequate, culturally and personally sensitive counseling is available?

6. Prostitution: What is the appropriate policy and social attitude towards prostitution (both prostitutes and clients)?

7. Migration: Should countries test immigrants for HIV infection? Should non-nationals be denied admission or deported based on HIV status? Does the answer depend on their trade (i.e., migrant sex workers)?

8. STDs: Should some resources intended for HIV programs be redirected to STD control? To what extent should HIV programs and STD services be integrated?

9. Maternal and child health: To what extent should HIV programs be integrated with MCH/family planning services?

10. AIDS orphans: What planning and services should be undertaken to meet the needs of dependent survivors of people with AIDS?

11. Schooling: Should HIV-infected children be excluded from conventional schooling?

CONTRIBUTORS

Seth Berkley, M.D., M.P.H., is Assistant Director of the Health Sciences Division of The Rockefeller Foundation.

Manuel Carballo, Ph.D., is Chief of Research and Development in the Programme on Substance Abuse at the World Health Organization.

Lincoln C. Chen, M.D., M.P.H., is the Taro Takemi Professor of International Health at the Harvard School of Public Health.

Barbara O. de Zalduondo, Ph.D., is Assistant Professor in the Department of International Health at the Johns Hopkins School of Hygiene and Public Health.

Harvey V. Fineberg, M.D., Ph.D., is Dean of the Harvard School of Public Health.

Mauricio Hernandez Avila, M.D., Sc.D., is Director, Centro de Investigaciones en Salud Publica, Instituto Nacional de Salud Publica, Cuernavaca, Mexico.

Sally Jody Heymann, M.D., M.P.P., is a MacArthur Fellow at the Center for Population and Development Studies, Harvard School of Public Health.

David J. Hunter, M.P.H., Sc.D., is Assistant Professor of Epidemiology in the Department of Epidemiology, Harvard School of Public Health.

Mbowa Kalengayi, M.D., is Professor and Head of the Department of Pathology, University of Kinshasa Medical School, Zaire.

Phyllis J. Kanki, D.V.M., S.D., is Assistant Professor of Pathobiology in the Department of Cancer Biology, Harvard School of Public Health.

Katherine LaGuardia, M.D., M.P.H., is a Research Scientist in the Population Sciences Division of The Rockefeller Foundation.

Peter Lamptey, M.D., Dr.P.H., is Director of the AIDSTECH Division of Family Health International.

Jonathan M. Mann, M.D., M.P.H., is Professor of Epidemiology and International Health in the Departments of Epidemiology and Population and International Health, Harvard School of Public Health.

Japheth K. Mati, M.D., F.R.C.O.G., is Senior Scientist in the Population Sciences Division of The Rockefeller Foundation and Professor in the Department of Obstetrics and Gynecology at the University of Nairobi in Nairobi, Kenya.

Souleymane MBoup, Ph.D., is Professor of Bacteriology and Virology in the Department of Bacteriology and Virology, University of Dakar, Senegal.

Olav Meirik, M.D., Ph.D., is Medical Officer of the Special Programme of Research, Development and Research Training in Human Reproduction, World Health Organization.

Stephen Moses, M.D., M.P.H., is Visiting Lecturer in the Departments of Medical Microbiology and Community Health, University of Nairobi, Kenya.

Jackoniah O. Ndinya-Achola, M.B.Ch.B., is Senior Lecturer in the Department of Medical Microbiology, University of Nairobi, Kenya.

Richard G. Parker, Ph.D., is a Professor in the Institute of Social Medicine at the State University of Rio de Janeiro, Brazil.

Francis A. Plummer, M.D., F.R.C.P.C., is Associate Professor in the Departments of Medicine, Medical Microbiology, and Community Health Sciences, University of Manitoba, Canada; Visiting Lecturer in the Department of Medical Microbiology, University of Nairobi, Kenya; and Honorary Researcher at the Kenya Medical Research Institute.

Jaime Sepulveda Amor, M.D., D.P.H., is Subsecretaria de Organizacion y Desarrollo in the Ministry of Public Health of the Government of Mexico.

Sheldon J. Segal, Ph.D., is Distinguished Scientist of The Population Council.

Nebiat Tafari, M.D., is Professor of Pediatrics in the Department of Pediatrics and Child Health, Addis Ababa University, Addis Ababa, Ethiopia.

Judith N. Wasserheit, M.D., M.P.H., is Chief of the STD Branch, NIAID, National Institutes of Health.

Debrework Zewdie, Ph.D., is Deputy Director of the National Research Institute of Health in Addis Ababa, Ethiopia.

Patricia Uribe Zuñiga, M.D., is Director of the Centro de Informacion sobre SIDA, Zona Central, at CONASIDA, Mexico City, Mexico.

INDEX